Nancy Clark's

SPORTS NUTRITION GUIDEBOOK

Second Edition

Nancy Clark, MS, RD
SportsMedicine Brookline
Brookline, MA

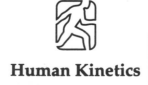

Human Kinetics

Library of Congress Cataloging-in-Publication Data

Clark, Nancy, 1951-
   Nancy Clark's sports nutrition guidebook / Nancy Clark. -- [2nd ed.]
      p. cm.
   Includes bibliographical references and index.
   ISBN 0-87322-730-1
   1. Athletes--Nutrition.   I. Title.   II. Title: Sports nutrition guidebook
   TX361.A8C54   1997
   613.2'024796--dc20   96-11313
   ISBN: 0-87322-730-1   CIP

Developmental Editor: Elaine Mustain; **Assistant Editors:** Susan Moore-Kruse, Jacqueline Eaton Blakley, and Sandra Merz Bott; **Editorial Assistants:** Amy Carnes and Coree Schutter; **Copyeditor:** Holly Gilly; **Proofreader:** Jim Burns; **Indexer:** Barbara E. Cohen; **Graphic Artist:** Ruby Zimmerman; **Graphic Designer:** Judy Henderson; **Cover Designer:** Jack Davis; **Illustrator:** Patrick Griffin; **Printer:** Versa Press

Human Kinetics books are available at special discounts for bulk purchase. Special editions or book excerpts can also be created to specification. For details, contact the Special Sales Manager at Human Kinetics.

Printed in the United States of America   10 9 8 7 6

Human Kinetics
Web site: http://www.humankinetics.com/

United States: Human Kinetics, P.O. Box 5076, Champaign, IL 61825-5076
1-800-747-4457
e-mail: humank@hkusa.com

Canada: Human Kinetics, 475 Devonshire Road, Unit 100, Windsor, ON N8Y 2L5
1-800-465-7301 (in Canada only)
e-mail: humank@hkcanada.com

Europe: Human Kinetics, P.O. Box IW14, Leeds LS16 6TR, United Kingdom
+44 (0)113-278 1708
e-mail: humank@hkeurope.com

Australia: Human Kinetics, 57A Price Avenue, Lower Mitcham, South Australia 5062
(08) 82771555
e-mail: humank@hkaustralia.com

New Zealand: Human Kinetics, P.O. Box 105-231, Auckland Central
09-523-3462
e-mail: humank@hknewz.com

Contents

DEDICATION

To my husband John McGrath,
son John Michael,
and daughter Mary.
Thank you for nourishing me with your love.

ACKNOWLEDGMENTS

With sincere thanks and appreciation to:

My clients, for teaching me about sports nutrition "in action." Their experiences allow me to better help others with nutrition concerns. I have changed their names in this book to protect their privacy.

Beth Goddard Parries, nutrition graduate student at Massachusetts General Hospital Institute of Health Professions, for being a dedicated research assistant.

Dr. William Southmayd, medical director of SportsMedicine Brookline, for his continual support.

Sue Luke, MS, RD, sports nutritionist in Charlotte, North Carolina, for her help and friendship.

Elaine Mustain, editor at Human Kinetics, for crafting the material into an easy-to-digest book.

Patrick Griffin, illustrator, for creatively capturing the messages in the text and translating them into tasteful art.

My family, for their patience, support, and love.

The recipe contributors, for sharing their culinary delights.

RECIPE CONTRIBUTORS

My special thanks go to the following food lovers who shared their special recipes. In some cases, I have adjusted their ingredients to meet my criteria for easier preparation and lower fat content.

Deb Allen, Weston, CT	Low-Fat Cheesecake Squares
Shawn Amirault, Nova Scotia	Zucchini Cake
Gabriella Andersen, Sun Valley, ID	Seedy Yeast Bread
Jane Balboni, N. Attleboro, MA	Maple Graham Shake
Donna Bambury, Middleton, MA	Chicken 'n Cheese
Annie and David Bastille, Holliston, MA	Pasta With Pesto Sauce
Mary Bernazanni, Boston, MA	Pizza Fondue
Joan Betterly, Sterling, MA	Cheesy Bean and Rice Casserole
Chris Brown, Concord, NH	Oatmeal-Orange Bread
Cynthia Carol, Concord, MA	Pasta Salad Parmesan
Caroline Clark, N. Dartmouth, MA	Apple Brown Betty
Janice Clark, Little Compton, RI	Goulash
Candace Crowell, Wakefield, MA	Blueberry Buckle
Molly Curran, Lynnfield, MA	Beans Baked With Apples
Karin Daisy, Taunton, MA	Low-Fat Oatmeal Cookies
Carol Davala, Port St. Lucie, FL	Sunshine Refresher
	Sweet Walnut Noodles
Patti Dillon, Boston, MA	Honey-Ginger Noodles*
Nancy Dowling, Milton, MA	Hot and Sour Soup
Pam Duckworth, Brookline, MA	Granola
Lorraine Evans, Orlando, FL	Pasta and Beans
Robyn Fass, Stockton, CA	Fruit Smoothie
Bill and Dottie Fine, Boston, MA	Lazy Lasagna
Linda Gould, Bedford, NH	No-Bake Peanut Butter Balls
Ellen Herbert, Newton, MA	Stir-Fry Pork With Fruit
Jane Houmes, Phoenix, AZ	Company Rice Salad
R. M. Lane, National Ski Patrol	Hot Spiced Tea Mix
Ann LeBarron, Waldorf, MD	Oven French Fries*
Patricia Lee, Mustang, OK	Creamy Pasta and Veggies
Sue Luke, Charlotte, NC	A to Z Cake
Sandy Miller, Watertown, MA	Hamburger-Noodle Feast
John McGrath, Waltham, MA	Chili
Emmy Norris, Cambridge, MA	Banana Frostie
Elaine Price, Boston, MA	Irish Tacos
Quaker Oats Company, Barrington, IL	Cinnamon Oat Bran Muffins
Fran Richman, Waltham, MA	Baked Chicken With Mustard
	Tofu Salad Dressing
Joan Riegel, Columbus, OH	Baked Chicken Chinese Style
Christine Ryan, Lynn, MA	Quick Potato Wedges
Dave Selsky, Boston, MA	Crunchy Fish Fillets
Jean Shanahan, Buffalo, NY	Irish Soda Bread
Diane Sinski, Belmont, MA	Chicken Stir-Fry With Apples and Curry
Jean Smith, Newton, MA	Potato Snacks
	Basic Oatmeal Yeast Bread
Evelyn Tribole, Irvine, CA	Easy Enchiladas
Susan Westin, Brockton, MA	Chocolate Lush

*Reprinted with permission from *The New York City Marathon Cookbook* by N. Clark, 830 Boylston Street, Brookline, MA 02167 ($23). Other recipes from *The New York City Marathon Cookbook* include Bran Muffins With Molasses and Dates, Oatmeal Pancakes, Cold Cereal Delight, Homemade Sports Drink, and Winter Squash Soup for One.

Preface

"I can't believe how much better I feel now that I've learned how to balance the right food into both my exercise program and my hectic lifestyle," commented Jim, a runner, dieter, and busy executive. "I have so much more energy and my workouts are stronger. What has helped me tremendously is your *Sports Nutrition Guidebook*. It's my nutrition bible!"

Jim is not the only one who has told me this story. So have many other health-conscious people from casual exercisers to high school athletes, Olympians, and senior citizens. The 150,000 people who have enjoyed my first *Sports Nutrition Guidebook* now have a surprise coming—a bigger and better book to enhance their health and performance both at work and at play.

If you are among the many readers who have called my first book "their nutrition bible," you'll like this book even more! It's filled with exciting nutrition news about

- how you can use food to help reduce your risk of heart disease, cancer, osteoporosis, and other diseases of aging;
- how you can lose weight successfully, keep it off, and be at peace with food;
- how you can healthfully feed an active family even when meals are replaced with snacks on-the-run; and
- how you can perform better by fueling optimally before, during, and after you exercise.

This expanded *Sports Nutrition Guidebook* is for anyone (athletes and non-athletes alike) who wants up-to-date food advice that is easy to understand and easy to use. In this latest edition of *Nancy Clark's Sports Nutrition Guidebook*, I've added more tips to help you win with good nutrition, whether you are a casual exerciser, an elite athlete, or simply a sedentary person thinking about buying some walking shoes and embarking on the road to good health.

This new edition is particularly valuable if you have concerns about your weight. Because so many of my readers ask for help with losing weight and learning how to be at peace with food and their bodies, I've enhanced the chapters on weight control and eating disorders. You'll learn how to reduce your body fat while maintaining energy to enjoy your exercise program. If you are among the many sports-active people who struggle with food, keep reading to find solutions to your weight and dieting concerns!

For those of you looking for the latest sports nutrition tips, you'll learn the latest on how to carbo-load properly, what to eat before competing, how to choose the best fluid replacers, how and what to eat for stamina, and how to bulk-up without getting fat.

For those of you who like to cook, the recipe section includes many new healthful recipes and menu ideas—quick, easy, and tasty! And for those of you who prefer to not cook, the simple "cook-free" food ideas can help you select a balanced diet even if you have limited kitchen skills. Because few athletes want to spend hours in the kitchen, most of my food suggestions are simple to fix. Enjoy them as they help you win with good nutrition!

Best wishes for good health, high energy, and success with food.

Nancy Clark, MS, RD
Director of Nutrition Services
SportsMedicine Brookline
830 Boylston Street
Brookline, MA 02167

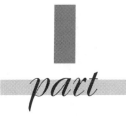

part

The Training Table

1
chapter

A Game Plan for Good Nutrition

Food is one of life's pleasures. Food is also important for fueling your body and investing in your overall health. As an active person, you may want to eat well but you struggle with juggling food and good nutrition with your busy schedule of work and workouts, family, and friends. Students, parents, businesspeople, and athletes alike repeatedly express their frustrations with trying to eat high quality diets. "I know what I should eat," they tell me. "I just don't do it." Although they take time to exercise, they don't always make time, or know how, to eat right.

One basic trick to winning with nutrition is to prevent yourself from getting too hungry. Hunger depletes the energy you need to choose the foods that both support your sports program and enhance your health. This book is dedicated to teaching you many tricks so you can easily enjoy an optimal sports diet. In this chapter, you'll learn how to design your personal good nutrition game plan, regardless of a busy lifestyle. Whether you are a fitness exerciser or an Olympic athlete, you can nourish yourself with wholesome foods, even if you are eating on the run. Keep reading!

SIX BASIC NUTRIENTS FOR HEALTH

Food is more than just fuel that stops your hunger. Food contains nutrients essential for maintaining optimal health and top performance. There are six types of nutrients.

3

Carbohydrates

Carbohydrates are a source of calories from sugars and starches that fuel your muscles and brain. Carbohydrates are the primary energy source when you're exercising hard. You should get about 60 percent of your calories from the carbohydrates found in fruits, vegetables, breads, and grains.

Fat

Fat is a source of stored energy (calories) that is burned mostly during low-level activity (e.g., reading and sleeping) and long-term activity (e.g., long training runs and gentle bike rides). Animal fats (butter, lard, fat in meat) tend to be saturated and contribute to heart disease and some cancers. Vegetable fats (e.g., olive oil, corn oil, canola oil) are generally unsaturated and less harmful. I recommend that my clients limit their fat intake to about 25 percent of their daily total calories.

Protein

Protein is essential for building and repairing muscles, red blood cells, hair, and other tissues, and for synthesizing hormones. Protein from food is digested into amino acids, which are then rebuilt into the protein in muscles and other tissues. Protein is a source of calories and can be used for energy if inadequate carbohydrates are available (e.g., during exhaustive exercise). About 15 percent of your calories should come from protein-rich foods such as fish, poultry, meats, tofu, and beans.

Vitamins

Vitamins are metabolic catalysts that regulate chemical reactions within the body. They include vitamins A, B complex, C, D, E, and K. Most vitamins are chemical substances that the body does not manufacture, so you must obtain them through your diet. Vitamins are *not* a source of energy.

Minerals

Minerals are elements obtained from foods that combine in many ways to form structures of the body (for example, calcium in bones) and regulate body processes (for example, iron in red blood cells transports oxygen). Other minerals are magnesium, phosphorous, sodium, potassium, chromium, and zinc. Minerals do not provide energy.

Water

Water is an essential substance that makes up about 60 to 75 percent of your weight. Water stabilizes body temperature, carries nutrients to and waste away from cells, and is needed for cells to function. Water does not provide energy.

THE REFERENCE DAILY INTAKES

To help you determine whether you are getting the right balance of these nutrients, the government has established the Reference Daily Intakes (RDIs) as a standard for nutrient intake. Their recommendations for protein, vitamins, and minerals exceed the average nutritional requirements to meet the needs of nearly all people, including athletes (see table 1.1).

In the following pages you will learn how to eat a high-energy, healthful combination of foods that provides the daily requirement of these important nutrients and promotes your health and fitness.

THREE BASIC KEYS TO HEALTHFUL EATING

When choosing your meals and snacks, try to base your nutrition game plan on these three important keys to healthful eating:

1. **Variety.** There is no one magic food. Each food offers special nutrients. For example, oranges provide vitamin C and carbohydrates but not iron or protein. Beef offers iron and protein but not vitamin C or carbohydrates. You'll thrive best by eating a variety of foods.

I often counsel athletes who severely restrict their diets. One runner, for example, limited herself to plain yogurt, rice cakes, and oranges. Besides lacking variety, her diet lacked iron, zinc, vitamins A, E, K, and much more.

2. **Moderation.** Even soda pop and chips, in moderation, can fit into a well-balanced diet. Simply balance out refined sugars and fats with nutrient-wise choices at your next meal. For example, compensate for a greasy sausage and biscuit at breakfast by selecting a low-fat turkey sandwich for lunch. Although no one food is a junk food, too many nutrient poor selections can accumulate into a junk food diet.

3. **Wholesomeness.** Choose natural or lightly processed foods as often as possible. For instance, choose whole wheat rather than white bread, apples rather than apple juice, baked potatoes rather than potato chips. Natural foods usually have more nutritional value and fewer questionable additives.

Table 1.1   Reference Daily Intake

The Reference Daily Intakes (RDIs) are not requirements but rather an estimate of safe and adequate nutrient intakes for proteins, vitamins, and minerals that will maintain good health for almost all people. The values are designed for the age group with the highest needs. For example, the RDI for iron is based on a woman's need and is a number overly generous for men. You should try to meet the RDIs on a daily basis. If your daily nutrient intake varies, but your average weekly intake meets the allowances, you are unlikely to suffer from nutritional deficiencies.

The Daily Values expressed in percentages of the RDIs on the nutrition facts on food labels are based on the following intakes:

Nutrient	Reference Daily Intake (RDI)
Protein	65 g
Vitamin A	5,000 IU
Thiamine (B-1)	1.5 mg
Riboflavin (B-2)	1.7 mg
Niacin	20 mg
B-6	2 mg
Folic acid	0.4 mg
Vitamin C	60 mg
Vitamin D	400 IU
Vitamin E	30 IU
Calcium	1,000 mg
Iron	18 mg
Zinc	15 mg
Vitamin K	80 μg
Chromium	120 μg
Selenium	70 μg
Manganese	2 mg

WHAT SHAPE IS YOUR DIET?

Whereas square meals and a well-rounded diet were once the shape of good nutrition, the food pyramid reflects nutrition for the 1990s. The U.S. Department of Agriculture has developed this new model that divides food into six groupings of varied sizes that stack into a pyramid. The pyramid supports the concept of a carbohydrate-based sports diet and offers the visual message that you should eat lots of breads, cereals, and grains for the foundation of your diet; generous amounts of fruits and vegetables; and lesser amounts of animal proteins and dairy foods. The tiny tip of the pyramid allows for just a sprinkling of sugars and fats.

DESIGNING A GOOD NUTRITION GAME PLAN WITH THE PYRAMID

When designing your good nutrition game plan, keep the Food Guide Pyramid in mind. Be sure to include a variety of foods, because each type of food provides different vitamins and minerals. You store these nutrients in your body. Some are stockpiled, such as the vitamin A made from the beta carotene in carrots, tomato sauce, and broccoli, and some are stored in smaller amounts, such as the vitamin C from orange juice, green peppers, and cantaloupe. These vitamins and minerals are the spark plugs your body's engine needs for top performance. After you've eaten your way to the top of the Pyramid, you can then enjoy a small amount of sweets and treats—the nutrient-poor sugars and fats that should take up only a little space in your food plan.

You can consume the reference daily intake (RDI) of the vitamins, minerals, and protein you need for good health within 1,200 to 1,500 calories if you wisely select from a variety of wholesome foods. Because many active people consume 2,000 to 5,000 calories (depending on their age, level of activity, body size, and gender), vitamin and nutrient excesses are more likely among hungry athletes than are deficiencies. For example, one of my clients, a football player, guzzled five times the RDI of vitamin C in his "snack" of a quart of orange juice. He also consumed excess protein and saturated fat, two problems that I'll discuss in chapters 2 and 8.

Unlike most hockey players, hikers, and cyclists (who are generally hearty eaters), weight-conscious athletes such as runners, wrestlers, and gymnasts often worry about fattening calories and they overlook the fact that food also provides essential nutrients. These athletes need to carefully select nutrient-dense foods—foods that offer the most nutritional value for the least amount of calories—to reduce the risk of a nutrient-deficient diet. By keeping in mind the recommendations the Pyramid makes for each of the food groups, and by always remembering the principle that fats and sugars should be limited, you can come up with a winning personalized nutrition game plan.

To help you select the nutrient-dense foods that fit your lifestyle, follow this good nutrition game plan.

Good Nutrition Game Plan: Grains and Starches

As illustrated by the Food Guide Pyramid, breads, grains, and cereals are the foundation of an optimal diet. They contribute to a sports diet

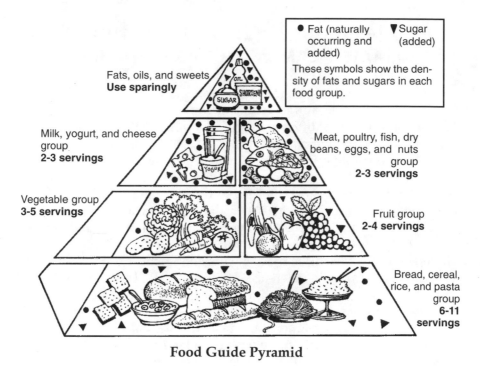

Food Guide Pyramid

by supplying 60 percent to 70 percent of the calories from carbohydrates. Grains and starches are excellent sources of carbohydrates, B vitamins, and fiber. They

- fuel your muscles,
- protect against needless muscular fatigue,
- reduce problems with constipation if they're fiber-rich, and
- enhance weight reduction programs if they're low in fat and calories.

Eating a sports diet based on wholesome starches and grains is akin to choosing high octane gasoline for your body's engine. The trick is to limit the fats that often accompany carbs: butter on bread, cream cheese on a bagel, or oil on fried rice. Low-fat carbohydrate cuisine requires careful selection, especially if you are eating fast foods.

How Much Is Enough?

About 60 percent of calories in a sports diet should come from carbohydrates. Starches and grains contribute much to that. You should strive to eat at least 6 to 11 servings of grains every day. Although this may sound like an overwhelming amount of food, it's not. You simply need to understand the definition of "serving." Serving sizes are shown here:

Grain food	Serving size	Athlete's portion	Number servings
Recommended intake: 6 to 11 servings per day			
cereal	1 ounce	2-4 ounces (1 big bowl)	2-4
bread	1 average slice	2 slices per sandwich	2
bagel	1/2 small	one big	3-4
pasta	1/2 cup cooked	2-3 cups	4-6
rice	1/2 cup cooked	1-2 cups	2-4

Six to 11 grain servings is only 2 to 4 servings per meal, or the equivalent of about 150 to 300 calories— not much for hungry exercisers who require about 600 to 900 calories per meal. Most active people commonly eat double or even triple the servings of grains per meal.

VARIETY IN THE DIET

Most people naturally vary and balance their food choices. They enjoy a variety of foods and consume a variety of nutrients. With little effort, their daily food choices stack into a pyramid.

But some active people are eating a linear diet: bagels, bagels, bagels; apples, apples, apples. One of my clients ate spaghetti for breakfast, lunch, and dinner day after day and month after month. This repetitive eating kept life simple, minimized decisions, and simplified shopping. But it also resulted in an inadequate diet and chronic fatigue.

A collegiate athlete ate the same foods every day because she disliked most of the school's food. She existed solely on corn flakes for breakfast, turkey sandwich on white bread for lunch, a colorless salad for dinner, and lots of cookies for snacks. I encouraged her to eat different brands of cereal topped with different fruits for breakfast, different types of sandwiches and breads for lunch, and to add dark, colorful vegetables to the salad.

If she preferred to limit her food choices, I suggested that she at least choose the best foods with the most nutrients: bran and other whole grain cereals, bananas, orange juice, dark sandwich breads, and colorful salad veggies. To optimize her diet, she just needed to choose more of the best foods and less of the rest!

Some Top Carbohydrate Choices

When selecting grains, try to choose the ones that have been only lightly processed, if processed at all. For example, brown rice, whole wheat bread, and stoned wheat crackers offer more B vitamins, potassium, and fiber than refined white rice, white bread, and white crackers (see table 1.2). Chapter 7 explains in greater detail the importance of wholesome starches and grains in a sports diet.

For premium nutrition, choose from among the following best bets.

Bran cereal.   Bran cereals are rich sources of fiber, B vitamins, and often iron (if they are enriched with this nutrient). Bran flakes with low-fat milk, a banana, and orange juice constitute a breakfast of champions. See chapter 3 for more information on cereals.

Oat bran.   When cooked into a tasty hot cereal, a bowl of oat bran makes a wonderful breakfast that helps lower elevated cholesterol and protects against heart disease. This microwaveable meal-in-a-minute is quick, enjoyable, and good for your health!

Bagels and muffins.   Bagels (pumpernickel, rye, whole wheat) and whole grain muffins (bran, corn, and oat bran) are more healthful than white flour-based muffins, doughnuts, buttered toast, croissants, or pastries. A bagel or muffin (preferably low in fat) along with yogurt and orange juice creates a well-balanced meal-on-the-run that's easily available from a convenience store or cafeteria, if not from home.

Whole grain and dark breads.   When it comes to choosing bread products, remember that whole grain breads tend to have more nutri-

---

Table 1.2   Refined Versus Whole Grain Breads

In general, breads made with whole grains tend to have more nutritional value than products made from refined flour. This chart compares the nutrients in breads made with dark versus light flours.

Bread (2 slices)	Fiber (g)	Potassium (mg)	B-6 (mg)	Magnesium (mg)
Whole wheat	3.2	90	0.10	45
Rye with seeds	2.6	100	0.04	10
Pumpernickel	2	280	0.10	45
French	trace	65	0.02	10
White, enriched	trace	55	0.02	10
Suggested intake:	*25-35*	*>3,500*	*2.0*	*400*

Nutrient data from food labels and J. Pennington, 1992, *Bowes & Church's Food Values of Portions Commonly Used*, 16th ed. (Philadelphia: Lippincott).

tional value than white breads. Look for whole grain (such as whole wheat) listed among the first ingredients. When at the sandwich shop, request the turkey with tomato on dark rye or whole wheat. At the supermarket, select the hearty brands that have whole wheat listed as the first ingredient. Keep fresh breads in the freezer so you'll have a supply on hand for toast, sandwiches, or a snack.

Stoned wheat and whole grain crackers.   These low fat munchies are a perfect high carbohydrate snack for your sports diet. Be sure to study nutrition labels so you can choose wholesome brands with low fat content, not the ones that leave you with greasy fingers!

Good Nutrition Game Plan: Fruits

As the Food Guide Pyramid shows, fruits help build a strong foundation for your sports diet. They are rich in carbohydrates, fiber, potassium, many vitamins (especially the antioxidant vitamin C), and health-protective phytochemicals (see table 2.6). The nutrients in fruits are important to

- improve healing;
- reduce risk of cancer, high blood pressure, and constipation; and
- aid recovery after exercise.

How Much Is Enough?

The recommended 2 to 4 fruit servings per day may seem like a lot, but it can be attained with only one or two *large* choices. If you rarely manage to eat fruit during the day, simply plan it into your breakfast routine. Bananas and orange juice are popular breakfast items, and they are among the most nutritious fruits so you'll be getting a good start to the day. A tall glass of orange juice and a large banana on your cereal will cover your minimum fruit requirement for the entire day.

Fruit	Pyramid serving size	Athlete's portion	Number servings
Recommended intake: 2 to 4 servings per day			
Orange juice	6 ounces	12 ounces	2
Apple	1 medium	1 large	2
Banana	1 small	one large	2-3
Canned fruit	1/2 cup	1 cup	2

Some Top Fruit Choices

If you have trouble including fruit in your diet because it is not readily available or because it spoils before it gets eaten, the following tips will help you balance your intake better and make these foods a top priority in your good nutrition game plan.

Citrus fruits and juices.   Whether whole, juice, fresh, frozen or canned, citrus fruits such as oranges, grapefruits, and tangerines surpass many other fruits or juices in vitamin C and potassium content.

If the hassle of peeling citrus fruit is a deterrent for you, just drink its juice. The whole fruit has slightly more nutritional value, but given the option of a quick glass of juice or nothing, juice does the job! Just six ounces of orange juice provides the daily requirement of 60 milligrams of vitamin C, all the potassium you might have lost in an hour's workout, plus folic acid, a B vitamin needed for building protein and red blood cells. Orange juice also has fewer calories and more nutrients than many other juices, such as cranberry, apple, and grape.

To boost your citrus juice intake, stock up on cans of the frozen orange juice concentrate, buy juice boxes for lunch or snacks, and look for cans of citrus juice in vending machines. Or better yet, stock whole oranges and grapefruits in your refrigerator.

Bananas.   This low-fat, high-fiber, and high-potassium fruit is perfect for busy athletes and nonathletes alike, and even comes prewrapped! Bananas are excellent for replacing potassium lost in sweat. The potassium also protects against high blood pressure. To boost your banana intake, include bananas on cereal, pack one in your lunch bag for a low-calorie dessert (a medium-sized banana contains only 100 calories), or keep them on hand for a quick and easy energy-boosting snack. My all-time favorite combination is banana with peanut butter, stoned wheat crackers, and a glass of milk—a well-balanced meal that includes a variety of foods (fruit, protein, grains, dairy).

To prevent bananas from overripening, store them in the refrigerator. The skin may turn black from the cold, but the fruit itself will be fine. Another trick is to keep banana chunks in the freezer. These frozen nuggets taste just like banana ice cream, but they have far fewer calories.

Without a doubt, bananas are among the most popular sports snacks. I have even seen a cyclist with two bananas safely taped to his helmet, ready to grab when he needed the energy boost!

Cantaloupe, kiwi, and strawberries.   These nutrient-dense fruits are also good sources of vitamin C and potassium.

Dried fruits.   Convenient and portable, these are rich in potassium and carbohydrates.

If you are eating too little fruit, be sure that the fruit you do eat is nutritionally the best. The information in table 1.3 can help guide your choices.

Table 1.3   Comparing Fruits

Fruit	Amount	Calories	A (IU)	C (mg)	Potassium (mg)
Apple	1 medium	80	75	10	160
Apple juice	1 cup	115	0	2	300
Apricots	10 halves dried	85	2,550	1	480
Banana	1 medium	105	90	10	450
Blueberries, raw	1/2 cup	40	70	10	65
Cantaloupe	1 cup pieces	55	5,150	70	495
Cherries	10 sweet	50	145	5	150
Cranberry juice	1 cup	150	—	110	60
Dates	5 dried	115	20	—	270
Figs	1 medium raw	35	70	1	115
Grapefruit	1/2 medium pink	35	320	45	160
Grapefruit juice	1 cup white	95	25	95	400
Grapes	1 cup	60	90	5	175
Honeydew melon	1 cup cubes	60	70	40	460
Kiwi	1 medium	45	135	75	250
Orange, navel	1 medium	65	255	80	250
Orange juice	1 cup fresh	110	50	125	500
Peach	1 medium	35	465	5	170
Pear	1 medium	100	35	5	210
Pineapple	1 cup raw	75	35	25	175
Pineapple juice	1 cup	140	1	25	335
Prunes	5 dried	100	830	2	310
Raisins	1/3 cup	150	4	2	375
Strawberries	1 cup raw	45	40	85	245
Watermelon	1 cup	50	585	15	185
Recommended intake:			>5,000	>60	>3,500

Nutrient data from J. Pennington, 1992, *Bowes & Church's Food Values of Portions Commonly Used*, 16th ed. (Philadelphia: Lippincott).

Good Nutrition Game Plan: Vegetables

Like fruits, vegetables are important for the foundation of your sports diet. Vegetables are what I call "nature's vitamin pills," because they are excellent sources of vitamin C and beta and other carotenes (see chapter 12, page 211), potassium, magnesium, and many other vitamins, minerals, and health-protective substances such as phytochemicals. In general, many vegetables have more nutritional value than do fruits. Hence, if you don't eat much fruit, you can simply eat more veggies and get the same vitamins and minerals, if not more.

How Much Is Enough?

The recommended intake is 3 to 5 servings per day. Many of my clients sheepishly confess they rarely eat that even in a week! Again, the trick is to eat large portions when you do eat vegetables—a big pile rather than a standard serving.

Vegetable	Pyramid serving size	Athlete's portion	Number servings
Recommended intake: 3 to 5 servings per day			
Broccoli	1 small stalk	2 big stalks	3-4
Spinach	1/2 cup	10-oz box frozen	3
Salad bar	small bowl	big bowl	3-4
Spaghetti sauce	1/2 cup	1 cup	2

Some Top Vegetable Choices

Dark, colorful vegetables usually have more nutritional value than paler ones. For example, the deeper green or deeper yellow a vegetable is, the more beta carotene it contains. If you are struggling to improve your diet, don't stuff yourself with pale lettuces, cucumbers, zucchini, mushrooms, and celery. Instead, feast on colorful broccoli, spinach, green peppers, tomatoes, and carrots, which offer far more nutrients.

Here's the scoop on the top vegetable choices.

Broccoli, spinach, and green peppers.   These low-fat, potassium-rich vegetables are loaded with vitamin C, health-protective phytochemicals, and carotenes that are the precursors of vitamin A. One stalk (1/2 cup) of steamed broccoli offers you the RDI for vitamin C, as does half a large green pepper or a spinach salad (4 ounces). I enjoy munching on a green pepper instead of an apple for an afternoon snack; it offers more vitamins and potassium and fewer calories. What a nutritional bargain!

Tomatoes and tomato sauce.   In salads or on pasta or pizza, tomato products are another easy way to boost your veggie intake. They are good sources of potassium, fiber, phytochemicals, and vitamins C (one medium-sized tomato provides half the RDI for vitamin C) and A. Tomato juice and vegetable juice are additional suggestions for fast-laners who lack the time or interest to cook. Those speedsters can simply drink their veggies! Commercial tomato products tend to be high in sodium, however, so people with high blood pressure should limit their intake or choose the low sodium brands.

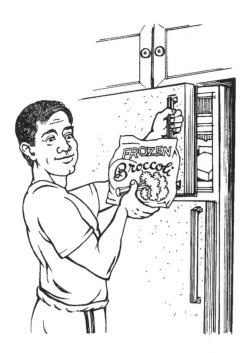

Cruciferous vegetables (members of the cabbage family).   Cabbage, broccoli, cauliflower, brussels sprouts, bok choy, collards, kale, kohlrabi, and mustard greens may protect against cancer, as may the carotene-rich choices such as carrots, winter squash, and greens. Surveys suggest that people who consume significant amounts of these vegetables have lower cancer rates. Do your health a favor by focusing on these choices! You can't go wrong eating piles of these.

Fresh, frozen and canned vegetables all have similar nutritional value. Of course, fresh from the garden is best, but that's often impossible to get. Frozen vegetables are a good second choice; freezing destroys very little nutritional value. Overcooking is a prime nutrient destroyer, so be sure to cook fresh or frozen vegetables only until they are tender-crisp, preferably in the microwave oven, steamer, or wok.

Because canned vegetables are processed quickly, they retain many of their nutrients. (One half-cup serving of canned peas, for example, has 8 milligrams of vitamin C, the same as frozen peas that have been cooked, and similar to the 11 milligrams in cooked fresh peas—but all of these cooked peas have much less C than the 29 milligrams in raw peas.) Using the water in canned vegetables for soups or stews minimizes the loss. The higher sodium level of canned vegetables can be reduced by rinsing them with plain water.

For more information on vegetables, see table 1.4 and read chapter 5, Super Bowls of Salads.

Table 1.4   Comparing Vegetables

Vegetable	Amount	Calories	A (IU)	C (mg)	Potassium (mg)
Asparagus	8 spears cooked	35	980	30	260
Beets	1/2 cup canned	45	5	5	170
Broccoli	1 cup cooked	50	2,500	80	340
Brussels sprouts	8 medium cooked	60	1,100	100	500
Cabbage, green	1 cup cooked	30	130	35	310
Carrot	1 medium raw	30	20,250	10	230
Cauliflower	1 cup cooked	30	20	70	400
Celery	1 7-inch stalk raw	5	55	5	115
Corn	1/2 cup frozen	70	200	5	115
Cucumber	1/3 medium	15	50	5	160
Green beans	1 cup cooked	30	800	15	370
Kale	1 cup cooked	40	9,600	55	290
Lettuce, iceberg	1 wedge	15	330	5	160
Lettuce, romaine	4 large leaves	20	2,800	35	400
Mushrooms	1 cup pieces	10	0	2	260
Onion	1/2 cup chopped	30	0	5	125
Peas, green	1/2 cup cooked	70	500	10	220
Pepper, green	1 cup diced	25	640	90	180
Potato	1 medium baked	110	Trace	15	420
Spinach	1 cup cooked	50	14,800	25	565
Squash, summer	1 cup cooked	35	250	10	345
Squash, winter	1 cup baked	80	7,200	20	890
Sweet potato	1 medium baked	120	25,000	30	400
Tomato	1 small raw	25	770	25	275
Tomato puree	1/2 cup canned	45	1,500	30	560
Recommended intake:			>5,000	>60	>3,500

Nutrient data from J. Pennington, 1992, *Bowes & Church's Food Values of Portions Commonly Used*, 16th ed. (Philadelphia: Lippincott).

Good Nutrition Game Plan: Meats and Protein-Rich Foods

Protein-rich animal foods (meats, seafoods, eggs,poultry) and plant foods (beans, nuts, tofu, legumes) are also important in your sports diet. They should be eaten daily along with breads, grains, fruits, and vegetables. Protein-rich foods provide the amino acids to build and repair muscles, assure proper muscle development, and reduce the risk of iron-deficiency anemia (if you eat darker meats with iron and zinc).

How Much Is Enough?

You should eat two to three servings of protein-rich foods every day. Athletes tend to either over or undereat protein, depending on their health consciousness or lifestyle. Whereas some athletes fill up on too much meat, others choose to bypass animal proteins and neglect to replace the beef with beans.

Slabs of steak and huge hamburgers have no place in a sports diet, or in any diet; excess protein isn't stored as bulging muscles or muscle fuel. However, smaller amounts of protein are important for building muscles and repairing tissues. The purpose of this section is to highlight quick and easy protein choices.

The protein rule of thumb is to include a total of 4 to 6 ounces of protein-rich food at lunch or dinner, or split them between each meal. Four ounces is tiny compared to the portions most Americans eat: 12-ounce steaks, 8-ounce chicken breasts, 6-ounce cans of tuna. Many athletes polish off their required protein by lunchtime and continue to eat one to two times more than they need.

Other people, however, miss out on adequate protein when they fuel up on only salads, plain pasta, or stir-fry veggies. Athletes who tend to choose exclusively low-fat carbohydrates commonly neglect their protein needs. See chapter 8 for more information on protein needs, vegetarian diets, and muscle-building foods.

Protein-rich food	Pyramid serving size	Athlete's portion	Number servings
Recommended intake: 2 to 3 servings per day			
Tuna	1/3 of 6-oz can	1 whole can	3
Chicken	2 oz drumstick	6 oz breast	3
Peanut butter	2 tablespoons	2-4 tablespoons	1-2
Lentil soup	1 cup	1 bowl	2
Kidney beans	1/2 cup	1 cup	2

Some Top Protein Choices

All types of protein-rich foods contain valuable amino acids, the building blocks of protein you need to make muscles (see chapter 8). The following popular choices can enhance your sports diet.

Lean beef. A lean roast beef sandwich made with two thick slices of bread for carbohydrates is an excellent choice for not only protein but also iron, which prevents anemia; for zinc, needed for muscle growth and repair; for B vitamins, which help produce energy; and for other nutrients that are important for the sports diet. In terms of heart health, a lean roast beef sandwich is preferable to a grilled cheese sandwich, tuna salad, or a hamburger because of these nutrients and the lower fat content. Top round, eye of round, round tip, and any cut with "round" in the name are among the leanest cuts of beef.

Chicken and turkey.   Poultry generally has less saturated fat than red meats, so it tends to be a more heart-healthful choice. Just be sure to buy skinless chicken, or discard the skin (which is high in fat) prior to cooking. Cooked until crispy, poultry skin can be a big temptation.

Fish.   Canned or fresh, fish not only is a great source of protein, but it also may protect your health. The recommended target is three fish meals (canned or fresh) per week, with the best choices being the oilier varieties such as salmon, albacore tuna, swordfish, sardines, and blue-fish. However, any fish is better than no fish.

Peanut butter.   What would we do without this "emergency food"? Although peanut butter by the jar full can be a dangerous diet breaker, a few tablespoons on whole grain bread, crackers, a bagel, or banana offers protein, vitamins, and fiber in a satisfying snack or a quick meal. Being a source of plant protein, peanut butter has no cholesterol. And if you buy the unprocessed, old-fashioned brands, you'll get more poly-unsaturated oils (as compared to saturated)—two pluses for people concerned about heart health.

Canned beans.   Vegetarian refried beans (tucked into a tortilla with salsa and grated low-fat cheese, then heated in the microwave oven), baked beans (on top of a baked potato), and canned garbanzo or kidney beans (added to a salad) are just three easy ways to boost your intake of these plant proteins that are also excellent sources of carbohydrates. If you tend to avoid beans because they make you flatulent, try eating them with Beano™, a product available at health food stores that takes the gas out of plant foods.

Tofu (soybean curd).   Tofu is a vegetable protein rich in phytochemicals that may reduce your risk of heart disease and cancer (Anderson et al. 1995; see chapter 8). It's an easy addition to a meatless diet because you don't have to cook it. Tofu has a mild flavor, so you can easily add it to salads, chili, spaghetti sauce, lasagna, and other mixed dishes. Look for it in the vegetable section of your grocery store. Buy "firm" tofu for slicing or cutting into cubes, and "soft" or "silken" tofu for blending into milkshakes or dips.

Even noncooks can easily incorporate adequate protein into a day's diet. Buy lean roast beef, roast chicken, or turkey breast at the deli counter; open a can of tuna or salmon; or resort to peanut butter, or nuts. Protein-rich canned beans, lentils, and legumes are quick and convenient during your busy week. For example, hummus (chick-pea spread, see recipe in part IV) is a tasty dip or easy pita filling. If you prefer to cook beans yourself rather than use the canned varieties, simply cook them in quantity on the weekend so you'll have enough to last through the week. Tofu is another healthful, versatile protein that you don't have to cook. Table 1.5 lists some popular protein-rich foods.

Good Nutrition Game Plan: Low-Fat Dairy Products

On the same level with protein-rich meats and dried beans in the Food Guide Pyramid, dairy products such as low-fat milk, yogurt, and cheese are also quick and easy sources of protein. And they are rich in calcium, a mineral that is particularly important for growing teens and women of all ages. A calcium-rich diet helps maintain strong bones, reduces

Table 1.5   Where's the Protein?

The following is a general summary of the amounts of protein in popular sports foods. For a more complete list, see table 8.1

Food	Serving size	Protein (g)
Meat, fish, and poultry	4 ounces cooked*	30
Egg	1 large	7
Tuna	1 6-ounce can	40
Beans, legumes, split peas	1/2 cup	7
Peanut butter	2 tablespoons	9
Tofu, firm	1/4 cake (4 ounces)	10
Milk or yogurt	8 ounces	8-10
American cheese	1 slice (0.75 ounces)	6
Hard cheese	1 ounce	7
Rice, noodles, pasta, potato	1/2 cup	2
Bread	1 slice	2
Cold cereal	1 cup	3
Peas, carrots, beets, corn	1/2 cup	2
Fruits	1 piece	<1

*Four ounces raw meat yields 3 ounces cooked meat; 3 ounces is about the size of a deck of cards.

Data from J. Pennington, 1992, *Bowes & Church's Food Values of Portions Commonly Used*, 16th ed. (Philadelphia: Lippincott).

the risk of osteoporosis, and protects against high blood pressure. Dairy foods are also rich in riboflavin, a B vitamin that helps convert food into energy.

Make no bones about it! Low-fat milk and other calcium-rich dairy products should be an important part of your diet throughout your lifetime. Because your bones are alive, they need calcium daily. The best choices include 1% or skim milk and yogurt and low-fat cheeses (part-skim mozzarella, string cheese, lite brands of cheddar). These sources of calcium are preferable to supplements because they include many other nutrients involved in bone health, such as vitamin D and phosphorous.

Children and teens need calcium for growing bones. Adults need calcium to maintain strong bones. Although you may stop growing by age 20, you don't reach peak bone density until age 30 to 35. The amount of calcium stored in your bones at that age is a critical factor that influences your susceptibility to fractures as you get older. After age 35, bones start to thin as a normal part of aging. A calcium-rich diet, in combination with exercise, can slow this process. In the next chapter, I will further discuss the serious health problem of osteoporosis.

Dairy products are not the only sources of calcium, but they tend to be the most concentrated, convenient, and accepted sources for eat-and-runners. Relatively few nondairy foods contain concentrated amounts of calcium, and what calcium they do contain may be poorly absorbed into your system. If you exclude or limit your consumption of dairy products, you'll be challenged to consume the recommended intake of calcium from natural foods. For example, to absorb the same amount of calcium that you would obtain from one glass of milk, you'd need to eat either 2-1/2 cups of broccoli, 8 cups of spinach, 2-1/2 cups of white beans, 6 cups of pinto beans, 6 cups of sesame seeds, or 30 cups of unfortified soy milk. The easier bet is to choose calcium-fortified foods, such as calcium-enriched orange juice or soy milk. Table 1.6 lists some nondairy calcium sources.

Dairy food	Pyramid serving size	Athlete's portion	Number servings
Recommended intake: 3 to 4 servings per day			
Milk, preferably low-fat	8 ounces	12 ounces	1.5
Yogurt	8 ounces	2 per day	2
Cheese on pizza	1.5 ounces	3 ounces (3 slices pizza)	2

Table 1.6   Nondairy Sources of Calcium

Although dairy products are among the richest dietary calcium sources, you can get significant amounts of calcium through other foods.

Animal food	Amount	Calcium (mg)
Sardines with bones*	3 ounces	370
Salmon with bones*	3 ounces	170
Shrimp, canned	3 ounces	100

Because plants contain oxalic acid and phytic acid, two compounds that inhibit calcium absorption, you have to eat big portions of some of the following foods to consider them a significant source of calcium. Note that the calcium in spinach is poorly absorbed; you're better off eating piles of broccoli for calcium.

Plant food	Amount	Calcium	Absorbable amount equal to 1 cup milk
Orange juice, calcium fortified	1 cup	300	1 cup
Tofu, processed with calcium sulfate**	4 ounces	150-250	5-8 ounces
Spinach, cooked	1/2 cup	120	8 cups
Turnip greens, cooked	1/2 cup	100	1 cup
Kale, cooked	1/2 cup	45	1.75 cups
Bok choy, cooked	1/2 cup	80	1.25 cups
Broccoli	1/2 cup	35	1.25 cups
Target intake	1,000-1,500 mg/day		

*You have to eat the bones to get the calcium!
**Read the ingredients on the label. If calcium sulfate is not listed, that brand of tofu is a poor source of calcium.

Data from C.M. Weaver and K.L. Plawecki, 1994, "Dietary calcium: Adequacy of a vegetarian diet," *Am J Clin Nutr* 59: 1238S-1241S.

How Much Is Enough?

For only 300 calories, even weight-conscious athletes can easily get the minimum 3 servings of low-fat dairy foods that are recommended per day (see page 20).

Here are the calcium intakes recommended in 1994 by the National Institutes of Health. (These recommended intakes are based on the latest research and are higher than the current RDI of 1,000 milligrams based on older data.) Be sure to get at least half, if not all, of your calcium requirements from food.

Age group	Optimal daily calcium (mg)	Number servings milk
Children		
1-5 years	800	3
6-10 years	800-1,200	3-4
Young adults		
11-24 years	1,200-1,500	4-5
Women		
25-50 years	1,000	3-4
>50 years, on estrogen	1,000	3-4
>50 years, not on estrogen	1,500	4-5
Amenorrheic athletes	1,200-1,500	4-5
Pregnant or breast feeding	1,200-1,500	4-5
Men		
25-65 years	1,000	3-4
>65 years	1,500	4-5

Some Top Calcium-Rich Choices

To consume the amount of calcium you need to build and maintain strong bones (1,000 to 1,500 milligrams per day), you should plan to include a calcium-rich food in each meal.

Low-fat and skim milk and yogurt.   These are among the richest sources of calcium. They are also among the healthiest because they have most of the fat removed, but retain all the calcium and protein. A glass of whole milk has the same amount of fat as two pats of butter, but skim milk has almost no fat.

Type of milk	Percent fat by weight	Percent fat by calories	Grams fat
Whole	3.5	50	8.5
2% lowfat	2	38	5.0
1% lowfat	1	28	2.5
Skim	trace	4	0

Plain yogurt is one of the richest food sources of calcium. Ice cream and frozen yogurt are only fair sources of calcium; I consider these foods treats that fit into the tip of the food pyramid, rather than basic sources of calcium. See table 1.7 for additional calcium-rich food suggestions.

Low-fat cheese.   Because many brands of fat-free cheese tend to be unpalatable, I suggest you first try the low-fat options. They are usually tasty and they add both calcium and protein to pasta, chili, and other vegetarian meals.

Dark green veggies.   Broccoli, bok choy (a vegetable common in Chinese cookery), and kale are among the best vegetable sources of calcium. Spinach also contains calcium, but your body can absorb very little of it.

Special Calcium Considerations

People who have trouble digesting milk because they lack an enzyme (lactase) that digests milk sugar (lactose) need to find alternate calcium sources. Some athletes who can't drink milk can tolerate yogurt, hard cheeses, or even small amounts of milk. Others enjoy Lactaid milk, a lactose free brand available at larger supermarkets. I also recommend a

FROZEN YOGURT

If you are a frozen yogurt fan, here is some information to help you put "fro-yo" into perspective.

• Frozen yogurt may be fat free, but it is not calorie free. A large serving (9 to 13 ounces) can easily contribute 225 to 400 calories to your diet. With the cone and a few mix-ins, you have the calorie equivalent of a small meal, but with far less nutritional value.

• Unlike regular yogurt that is a nutrient-dense food, frozen yogurt is a sugar-based food that has less calcium and protein than you might suspect. Frozen yogurt fits into the tip of the food pyramid; I consider it a sugar-based food that contains a little milk, not a milk-based food that contains a little added sugar. Yes, the sugar in frozen yogurt fuels your muscles, but it can fool your good nutrition intentions.

• Gourmet frozen yogurt tends to have the same fat content as reduced-fat ice cream. Be sure to read food labels so you don't get fooled!

Table 1.7   Calcium, Cholesterol, and Fat in Dairy Products

Dairy product	Amount	Calories	Fat (g)	Choles-terol (mg)	Calcium (mg)
Milk					
Whole	1 cup	150	8.5	35	290
2% low-fat	1 cup	120	5	20	300
1% low-fat	1 cup	100	2.5	10	300
Skim	1 cup	85	0	5	300
Skim, protein fortified	1 cup	100	0	5	350
Yogurt					
Dannon low-fat:					
Plain	1 cup	150	4	20	400
Vanilla	1 cup	210	3	15	400
Fruit	1 cup	240-260	3	15	350
Dannon fat free:					
Plain	1 cup	100	0	<5	400
Vanilla	1 cup	100	0	<5	350
Fruit	1 cup	100	0	<5	350
Cheese					
American	1 ounce	105	10	30	175
Cheddar	1 ounce	115	10	30	200
Cheddar, lite	1 ounce	70	4.5	15	200
Mozzarella, part skim	1 ounce	80	5	15	205
Ricotta, part skim	1/2 cup	170	10	40	340
Cottage, 1% fat	1/2 cup	90	1	5	70
Cottage, fat free	1/2 cup	80	0	10	100
Ice cream (vanilla)					
Regular	1 cup	260	15	60	190
Rich	1 cup	350	25	90	180
Light	1 cup	220	7	30	200
Soft serve	1 cup	220	5	20	275
Frozen yogurt					
Fat free	1 cup	220	0	0	100
Low-fat	1 cup	240	3	10	80
Shakes					
McDonald's vanilla	1 (15 oz)	340	5	25	320
Burger King	1 (10 oz)	310	7	20	240
Safe intake: Women		1,800-2,200+	45-60	<300	1,000
Men		2,200-3,500+	60-95	<300	1,000+

Nutrient data from food labels and J. Pennington, 1992, *Bowes & Church's Food Values of Portions Commonly Used*, 16th ed. (Philadelphia: Lippincott).

MILK MYTHS

Myths abound regarding milk for athletes.

• One high school swimmer who drank milk by the quart ("I can polish off four glasses at one dinner!") was concerned that this much milk would lead to calcium deposits. For most healthy people, this is unlikely. When you consume more calcium than your body needs, your body excretes the excess.

• One football player thought that milk causes cotton mouth. It doesn't. The dryness he experienced prior to competition was due to nervousness and anxiety, not to milk.

• A runner had heard that milk is hard to digest and causes stomach cramping. It doesn't unless you are lactose intolerant. Low-fat milk and dairy products are comfort foods that tend to digest easily.

• A skier hobbled into my office on crutches, wondering if his broken bone would benefit from his guzzling lots of milk. Drinking extra milk does *not* hasten the healing process! Six to eight weeks and a balanced diet are the two main keys to mending broken bones.

nutrition consultation with a registered dietitian to ensure appropriate calcium intake.

In most cases, calcium supplements are poor substitutes for calcium-rich dairy products. As I mentioned earlier, calcium pills supply far fewer nutrients than the power-packed dairy products that offer a full spectrum of important vitamins, minerals, and protein. For example, milk is rich in vitamin D, potassium, and phosphorous—nutrients that work in combination to help your body use calcium effectively. Milk is also one of the best sources of riboflavin, a vitamin that helps convert the food you eat into energy. Active people, who generate more energy than their sedentary counterparts, have higher needs for riboflavin. If you don't eat dairy products, your riboflavin intake is also likely to be poor.

Fats, Oils, and Sweets

The inclusion of fats and sugars in the tip of the Food Guide Pyramid suggests that you need not eat a "perfect" diet (that is, with no fat and no sugar) to have a good diet. Although fats and sugars are nutrient poor, they are an important part of a balanced diet because they add taste and flavor. Fats also help transport the fat-soluble vitamins (A, D, E, K) and provide essential fatty acids that the body can't make, such as the linoleic acid that is an essential part of cell membranes. Essential fatty acids help regulate cholesterol metabolism and are precursors for a group of hormone-like compounds (eicosonoids) that help regulate many physiological processes. They help the nutrient-dense foods taste better, add satiety (a pleasant feeling of fullness), and can appropriately be included with each meal. Few people will deny that a spoonful of brown sugar on oatmeal, a skimming of butter on a hot roll, or a little olive oil on a nice salad adds to the pleasure of a meal.

How Much Is Enough?

Some people eat too many fats, oils, and sweets from the tip of the food pyramid instead of eating a wholesome diet of grains, fruits, and vegetables from the base. If you have a junk food diet that topples the tip, you should correct this imbalance; you can easily do so by eating more wholesome foods from the base and body of the pyramid before you get too hungry. If you are like most active people, after you get too hungry, you'll tend to choose foods low in nutrients and high in fats and sugar. The simple solution to the "junk food diet" is to prevent hunger by first eating wholesome meals.

Some Top Choices for Fats and Sugars

Given that about 25 percent of your calories can come from fat, and about 10 percent can appropriately come from sugar, the following foods are some of the best ways to spend these calories.

Olive oil.   This monounsaturated fat is associated with low risk of heart disease and cancer. Use it for salads, sautéing, and cooking.

Walnuts.   Thought to be protective against heart disease, walnuts are a fine addition to salads, cooked vegetables, and even pasta meals. Try the recipe on page 344 for Sweet Walnut Noodles—yummy!

Molasses.   Confirming the rule "the darker the food is, the more nutrients it has," molasses is among the darkest of sugars, and it has the most nutrients. Molasses is a fair source of potassium, calcium, and iron—if you eat enough of it. Try adding a tablespoon to milk for "taffy milk," mix some in yogurt, or spread it on a peanut butter sandwich.

Berry jams.   Because of the seeds in raspberry, strawberry, and blackberry jams, these sweet spreads have a little fiber that somewhat boosts their healthfulness. Preferable to strained jellies, the jams offer slightly more fruit value, but you still have to count them as primarily sugar.

Your favorite sweet temptation.   Although rich desserts and gooey treats may not contribute vitamins, minerals or healthfulness to your diet, they do add pleasure. You can fit a small amount of any favorite food in your diet; there is no "bad" food.

In the next chapter, I will provide far more details about the best fats and in chapter 4 I'll discuss more about how to appropriately fit sweets into snacks and snack attacks.

Building Your Pyramid

Now that you have read this chapter, you know which foods are the best choices. The trick is to assemble the foods into wholesome meals and snacks. I recommend that you try to choose from at least three out of five food groups at each meal. Here's how this might work.

Foods made from a combination of ingredients can create a well-balanced meal in one dish. For example, vegetable pizza topped with peppers, onions, and mushrooms is far from a junk food. It offers calcium-rich dairy food (from the low-fat mozzarella); vegetables rich in potassium, beta carotene, and vitamin C (from the tomato sauce and vegetable toppings); and carbohydrate-rich grain foods in the crust. Choosing a dinner of thick crust pizza, with a foundation of carbohydrates, better fits the pyramid plan than does choosing a steak dinner that is mostly protein.

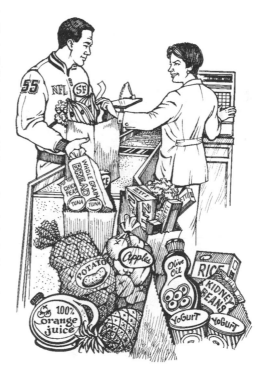

Shaping up your diet into a Food Guide Pyramid need not be a major task. It simply means knowing how to choose more of the best foods and less of the rest. The following chapters offer additional tips to help you fine-tune your choices so you can enjoy a tasty, pleasurable, nourishing, yet simple sports diet. Read on!

BOOSTING YOUR CALCIUM INTAKE

Here are some tips to help you boost your calcium intake to build and maintain strong bones:

• For breakfast, eat cereal with one cup low-fat or skim milk (300 mg). For crunchy cereal, use yogurt (400 mg/cup) in place of milk. For hot cereal, cook the cereal in milk or mix in 1/4 cup powdered milk (300 mg).

• When planning a quick meal, choose pizza with low-fat mozzarella cheese (200 mg/slice), or sandwiches with cheese, preferably low in fat (200 mg/oz).

• Make calcium-rich salads by adding grated cheese (200 mg/oz), lowfat cottage cheese (70 mg/1/2 cup), or tofu cubes (150 mg/4 oz calcium-processed tofu). Blend salad seasonings into soft tofu (150 mg/1/4 cake) or plain yogurt (400 mg/cup) for a calcium-rich dressing. Read the labels on the tofu containers, being sure to choose the brands processed with calcium sulfate; otherwise, the tofu will be calcium-poor.

• Drink low-fat or skim milk with lunch, snacks, or dinner (300 mg/cup).

• Add milk instead of cream to coffee (only 15 mg/1-ounce creamer). Take powdered milk to the office to replace coffee whiteners. Or, drink milk-based hot cocoa (300 mg/ 8 oz) in place of coffee.

• Snack on fruit-flavored yogurt rather than ice cream (350 vs. 180 mg/cup). Frozen yogurt, ice milk, and puddings are other tasty low-fat calcium treats (150-250 mg/half-cup).

• If you are a fish lover, canned salmon or sardines with bones (170 or 370 mg/3 ounces) are easy lunch options; serve with crackers.

• Add tofu (150 mg/1/4 cake) to oriental soups or stir-fry meals.

• Chow down on dark green, leafy vegetables such as broccoli, kale, and bok choy (about 200 mg/cup).

2
chapter

Good, and Good for You

Food is not only one of life's pleasures, it is also an important way to improve and maintain your health. Years ago, people were plagued by nutrition deficiencies. Today, nutrition excesses, in combination with a deficiency of exercise, are the biggest nutrition problems in America. A lifetime of nutrition excesses and inadequate exercise culminates in an aging process that is far more unhealthy than it should be. Excesses of saturated fat, cholesterol, refined foods, and gooey calories contribute to obesity, heart disease, cancer, hypertension, diabetes, kidney failure, and other diseases.

Fortunately, a proper diet in combination with a regular exercise program can help protect your health. And the same foods you eat to enhance your health also enhance your athletic performance. Everyone wins in the long run with a wholesome, high carbohydrate, moderate protein, and low-fat sports diet!

EAT TO YOUR HEART'S CONTENT

Being physically fit and eating wisely are two ways to reduce your risk of heart disease, which is the number one killer in America. Sports-active people often believe they are exempt from the low-fat rules about heart-healthy eating because they are athletic. They assume that being athletic will protect them from heart disease. Wrong! No one is exempt.

Even sports-active people can succumb to heart disease. Serious athletes and fitness exercisers alike should ration their intake of ice cream, cookies, cheese, and other foods bulging with saturated fat and cholesterol.

Some Important Questions

Unfortunately, most of us are confused by the constant updates and changes of heart-health information. This leaves us wondering what the real answers are to questions like the following.

Is Beef Good or Bad?

A few years ago, everyone shunned the stuff, believing it to be an artery clogger. Today, health experts tell us that small portions of lean beef aren't so bad after all, especially for athletes who need beef's iron, zinc, and other important nutrients. Despite popular belief, beef is not exceptionally high in cholesterol; it has a cholesterol value similar to chicken and fish. Beef tends to have more saturated fat than chicken or fish, so that's why it has a bad name among health watchers. This saturated fat is a bigger culprit than dietary cholesterol.

In the past decade, the healthfulness of beef and other meats has improved because farmers have learned how to raise animals that are leaner, and because butchers are trimming more of the fat from the meat at stores. Hence, you can easily fit beef (and pork and lamb) into a heart-healthy sports diet if you

- select lean cuts of beef, such as eye of round, rump roast, sirloin tip, flank steak, top round, and tenderloin; and
- eat smaller portions, limiting yourself to a piece of lean protein about the size of the palm of your hand.

Table 2.1 can help guide your choices, and the recipe section offers low-fat cooking suggestions.

Are Eggs Good or Bad?

Eggs have gotten a bad rap when it comes to healthy eating. Medical experts have told us that that eating eggs is bad because a single egg has 210 milligrams of cholesterol. This just about hits the American Heart Association's recommended limit of 300 milligrams per day. But recent studies suggest that egg cholesterol may have little effect upon the blood cholesterol level in many people, especially in combination with an overall low-fat diet (Ginsberg et al., 1995).

To date, it is unclear whether the cholesterol that you eat affects the cholesterol in your blood, because most of the blood's cholesterol is

Table 2.1   Fat and Calories in Red Meat

Although greasy red meat can be high in saturated fat and increase your risk for heart disease, moderate portions of the leaner cuts are a fine addition to your sports diet. The rule of thumb is when buying beef, look for the words *round* or *loin*; when buying pork, look for *leg* or *loin*.

Meat, 4 oz. cooked, trimmed	Percent calories from fat	Total calories	Total fat (g)	Saturated fat (g)
Beef				
Eye of round, roasted	25	185	5.5	2.5
Sirloin steak, broiled	35	225	8	3
Tenderloin, lean broiled	45	240	12	4
Rib roast, lean only	50	265	15	6
Hamburger, 10% fat	50	280	15	8
Lamb				
Roasted, shank half of leg	40	215	9	3
Shoulder chop, broiled	50	240	13	4
Pork				
Loin, tenderloin, roasted	25	190	5.5	2
Loin, top loin, roasted	30	230	8	3
Ham, canned, extra-lean	35	155	6	2
Ham, canned, regular	50	210	12	4
Spareribs, braised	70	450	35	14
Veal				
Cutlet, roasted	20	175	4	2
Sirloin, roasted	35	200	18	3

Data from J. Pennington, 1992, *Bowes & Church's Food Values of Portions Commonly Used*, 16th ed. (Philadelphia: Lippincott); and *Nutrifacts Update*, 1995, Food Marketing Institute, 800 Conn. Ave., NW, Washington, DC.

made in the liver. We do know that dietary fats affect the way the body disposes of cholesterol. In particular, saturated fats (such as butter and animal fats) appear to inhibit the body's ability to get rid of the bad form of cholesterol (low-density lipoprotein, or LDL) that clogs arteries. We also know that some people respond more readily than others to a low-cholesterol diet, and that dietary recommendations need to be individualized.

So, when it comes to eggs, you should limit your intake if you have a high blood cholesterol level and a family history of heart disease; the American Heart Association recommends a limit of four eggs per week, including those used in cooking. Otherwise, if you have low blood cholesterol and no family history of heart disease, this highly nutritious protein source may be eaten in moderation as a part of your balanced nutrition game plan. An estimated 85 percent of Americans can eat a high cholesterol diet with no elevation of blood cholesterol.

Is Cooking Oil Good or Bad?

Liquid oils are an acceptable type of fat to include in limited amounts in a heart-healthy diet. In particular, the monounsaturated fats in olive oil and canola oil seem to be health-protective heroes and are perhaps better choices than safflower, corn, sunflower, and other polyunsaturated vegetable oils. Use olive and canola oils with salads, pesto, and pasta and when sautéing. Just be sure to use only moderate amounts, so that most of your calories still come from carbohydrates.

When it comes to selecting heart-healthy cooking fats, the rule of thumb is "the softer the better." That is, soft (liquid) vegetable oils and tub margarines have a higher percentage of unsaturated fats compared to harder (solid) fats such as stick margarines and solid vegetable shortenings. Liquid oils are preferable to the animal fats that are solid at room temperature: butter, bacon grease, lard, and the fat on meats. Refer to table 2.2 for more information about comparing fats.

Ticker Tips

The following tips should help clear up any additional confusion about the best foods to eat to keep your heart ticking in good health.

Ticker Tip #1: Know Your Number

Know where you stand when it comes to heart disease. By knowing your cholesterol level, you can assess your risk of developing heart disease. Make an appointment with your doctor to get your blood tested for these health indicators:

• **Total cholesterol.** A waxy substance that contributes to hardening of the arteries, cholesterol accumulates in the walls of the blood vessels throughout the body, especially those in the heart. This buildup limits blood flow to the heart muscle and contributes to heart attacks.

• **HDL cholesterol.** High density lipoprotein cholesterol is the "good stuff" that carries the bad cholesterol out of the arteries.

• **LDL cholesterol.** Low density lipoprotein cholesterol is the "bad stuff" that clogs arteries.

• **Total cholesterol to HDL ratio.** At least 25 percent of your total blood cholesterol should be HDL. Because exercise tends to boost HDL,

Table 2.2   Good Fat, Bad Fat

Foods ladened with saturated fat can raise blood cholesterol level. Food with more monounsaturated or polyunsaturated fat is the better health bet. If you are watching your weight, note that all types of fats have about 120 calories per tablespoon.

Fat	Saturated (%)	Mono-unsaturated (%)	Poly-unsaturated (%)
Highly saturated vegetable fat			
Coconut oil	90	10	—
Palm oil	50	30	20
Animal fat			
Butter fat	65	30	5
Beef fat	50	45	5
Chicken fat	30	50	20
Monounsaturated oil			
Olive oil	15	75	10
Canola oil	5	60	35
Peanut oil	20	50	30
Polyunsaturated oil			
Safflower oil	10	15	75
Sunflower oil	10	20	70
Corn oil	15	25	60
Cottonseed oil	25	20	55

Data from J. Pennington, 1992, *Bowes & Church's Food Values of Portions Commonly Used*, 16th ed. (Philadelphia: Lippincott).

active people often have a high percent of this good cholesterol. Their total cholesterol may be higher than that of a sedentary person, but as long as 25 percent of it is HDL, these individuals have a lower risk of heart problems. The higher the HDL percent, the better.

If you're over 20, have your serum total cholesterol measured at least once every five years; this measurement should be made after a 12-hour fast. If your total cholesterol is high, you should have it remeasured, looking at both HDL and total cholesterol.

Genetics plays a large role in health, so you may have a blood cholesterol that puts you at a high risk for developing heart disease even if you eat a low-fat diet. One 28-year-old triathlete was shocked to discover his cholesterol was very high. He probably inherited this trait from his father and grandfather, both of whom had had heart attacks.

Is Your Blood Cholesterol Level on Target?

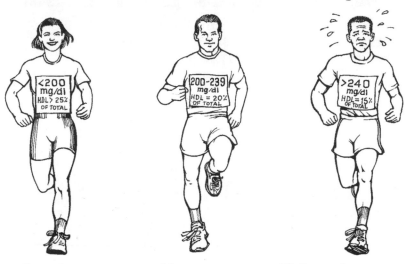

Good   Not so good   Talk with your doctor!

mg/dl = milligram of cholesterol per deciliters of blood
HDL = high-density lipoprotein cholesterol

After you know your blood cholesterol level, you'll be better able to determine how strict you need to be with your diet. For example, if your level is less than 180 milligrams and if your parents and 97-year-old grandparents are still alive and thriving, you can perhaps be a bit more lenient in your eating habits than your buddy whose cholesterol is a risky 250 milligrams and whose father and grandfather suddenly died of heart attacks in their 50s.

Ticker Tip #2: Cut the Fat.

Eat less fat, particularly saturated animal fat and tropical oils like coconut and palm. This means cutting down on fat-filled foods such as greasy hamburgers, pepperoni, fatty cheeses, and commercially prepared baked goods. Use small amounts of olive oil or canola oil for cooking, rather than butter, lard, or animal fat drippings. Both a sports diet and a heart-healthy diet limits fat to 25 to 30 percent of calorie intake, and to 20 percent if you have elevated blood cholesterol.

The American Heart Association advises a limit of 30 percent of daily calories to come from fat:

- At least 10 percent from olive or canola oil and other monounsaturated vegetable fats

- About 10 percent from corn or safflower oil and other polyunsaturated vegetable fats for essential fatty acids required for good health
- No more than 10 percent from butter or animal fats, or from coconut and palm oils, two highly saturated vegetable oils that are commonly used in processed foods

I advise athletes to aim for a 25 percent fat diet. The 5 percent fewer fat calories allows them to eat more carbohydrates to better fuel their muscles. Hence, if you are an active woman who eats about 2,000 calories per day, 500 of them could appropriately come from fat:

25% fat × 2,000 total calories = 500 calories from fat

By rationing your intake of foods obviously high in fat (butter, margarine, mayonnaise, salad dressing, ice cream, cookies, chips) you'll end up with a diet that's about 25 percent fat.

If you have a very high cholesterol level, your physician may recommend a diet that is 20 percent, or even 10 percent, fat. This restriction is for people clinically endangered by heart disease, not for healthy people who have low cholesterol levels. I talk often to food fanatics with low cholesterol who try to eliminate all fats from their diet. They have self-imposed a questionable dietary burden. As I've mentioned before, a low-fat diet need not be a no-fat diet. Some fat is appropriate for a well-balanced diet. (Refer to chapter 14 for more information on dietary fat.)

Your weight in kilograms (1 kilogram = 2.2 pounds) is a rough estimation of the number of grams of fat you can healthfully include in your diet. For a more precise calculation, follow these three steps:

1. Estimate how many calories you need per day. See "Thirteen Tips for Successful Weight Reduction" (pages 258-266) in chapter 14 for instructions.
2. Multiply your total daily calories by 25 percent (.25) to determine the number of fat calories you can appropriately eat. For example, .25 × 2,000 calories = 500 calories from fat.
3. Divide your allotted fat calories by 9 to determine the number of grams (g) of fat in your daily fat budget. (One gram of fat = 9 calories.)

   For example, if you are entitled to 500 fat calories, 500 fat calories ÷ 9 cal/g = 55 g fat.

Table 2.3 can help you determine your target fat intake. If you are underweight or very active, you may need more calories from fat to boost your total calorie intake. Plan to eat more of the heart-healthy fats, such as olive oil, old-fashioned peanut butter, and oily fish.

Table 2.3   Low Fat: What's That?

For a heart-healthy sports diet, you should limit your fat intake to about 20 to 30 percent of your total calories (20 percent if you have high cholesterol; 30 percent if you need more calories to prevent weight loss). In general, athletes can fuel their muscles better if they trade excess calories from fat for more calories from carbohydrates. Don't trade away too much fat, however, and be left with an unbalanced diet.

Calorie needs per day	Grams fat in diet		
	20% fat	25% fat	30% fat
1,500	30	40	50
1,800	40	50	60
2,000	45	55	65
2,400	55	65	80
2,600	60	70	85

Ticker Tip #3: Read Food Labels

The nutrition information on food labels can help you compare the types and amount of fat and cholesterol in specific foods. You can then use this information to wisely choose the foods that fit into your fat "budget" for the day. Here are the definitions for words used on the food labels:

- **Fat free.** Less than 0.5 grams of fat per serving.
- **Cholesterol free.** Less than 2 milligrams of cholesterol per serving.
- **Light or lite.** A food contains at least one-third fewer calories, or no more than half the fat as the original product.
- **Low fat.** Three grams or less of fat per serving.
- **Low saturated fat.** One gram or less of saturated fat per serving.
- **Low cholesterol.** Less than 20 milligrams of cholesterol per serving.
- **Lean.** Less than 10 grams of fat, 4 grams of saturated fat, and 95 milligrams of cholesterol per serving and per 3.5 ounces.
- **Extra lean.** Less than 5 grams of fat, 2 grams of saturated fat, and 95 milligrams of cholesterol per serving and per 3.5 ounces.
- **Reduced, less, or fewer.** The food contains 25 percent less fat than the standard product.

Table 2.4 offers additional information to help you count grams of fat and cholesterol.

Table 2.4   Fat and Cholesterol in Some Common Foods

Food Product	Amount	Fat (g)	Cholesterol (mg)
Milk			
Skim	1 cup	0	5
2% low-fat	1 cup	5	20
Whole	1 cup	8.5	35
Cheese			
Cheddar	1 ounce	10	30
Swiss	1 ounce	10	25
Mozzarella (part skim)	1 ounce	5	15
Ricotta (part skim)	1/2 cup	10	40
Cottage cheese, 1% fat	1/2 cup	1	5
Ice cream			
Expensive brands (16% fat)	1/2 cup	12-18	40-50
Less expensive brands (10% fat)	1/2 cup	5-10	30-35
Low-fat	1/2 cup	3-5	10-20
Lean meats and fish (cooked)			
Pork, roast loin	4 ounces	8	85
Beef, 10% fat hamburger	4 ounces	15	110
Lamb, roast leg	4 ounces	9	100
Ham, canned lean	4 ounces	6	50
Chicken, roast breast	4 ounces	2	95
Tuna, canned white	4 ounces	3	45
Shrimp, 16 large	4 ounces	2	175
Cereals			
Quaker 100% Natural	1/2 cup	7	0
Kellogg's Low-Fat granola	1/2 cup	3	0
Oatmeal, uncooked	1/2 cup	3	0
Oat bran, uncooked	1/2 cup	3	0
Post Grape-Nuts	1/2 cup	0	0
Snack and fast foods			
Potato chips	1 ounce	10	0
Potato chips (95% fat-free)	1 ounce	1.5	0
Pretzel twists	1 ounce	1	0
Tortilla chips, fried	1 ounce (6)	6	0
Tortilla chips, baked	1 ounce	1	0
Cheese curls	1 ounce (25)	8	2

(continued)

Table 2.4 *(continued)*			
Food Product	**Amount**	**Fat (g)**	**Cholesterol (mg)**
Popcorn, lite, popped	1 ounce (4 cups)	6	0
Popcorn, regular, popped	1 ounce	10	5
McDonald's Big Mac		28	80
McDonald's Filet-o-Fish	1	16	35

Nutrient data from food labels, McDonald's Corp.; *Nutrifacts*, 1995, Food Marketing Institute, 800 Conn. Ave., NW, Washington, DC; and J. Pennington, 1992, *Bowes & Church's Food Values of Portions Commonly Used*, 16th ed. (Philadelphia: Lippincott).

Ticker Tip #4: Eat More Foods Rich in Soluble Fiber, Such as Oats and Beans

The type of fiber found in oats (soluble fiber), and the soluble fiber in barley, lentils, split peas, and beans protect against heart disease. Find ways to include more of these foods in your diet! Bean and barley soups are easy to fit in, and so are oatmeal and oat bran. Research suggests that 2 ounces of oat bran each day can help people with high cholesterol attain lower cholesterol levels, especially when eaten as part of a low-fat diet (Van Horn et al., 1986, Jenkins et al., 1993).

Oat bran is available in the hot cereal section of supermarkets and health food stores. It is similar to cream of wheat but has a nutty flavor. Enjoy it either as a hot cereal (add chopped almonds and raisins for a nice texture contrast) or bake it into muffins. (See "Breads and Breakfasts," in part IV.)

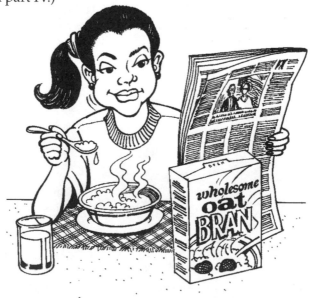

Foods high in soluble fiber are not only a heart-healthy choice, but are also excellent pre-exercise foods. They have what is called a *low glycemic index*. That is, they provide a sustained release of energy into the bloodstream, and they can enhance your endurance and stamina if you will be exercising longer than 60 to 90 minutes. (See chapter 7 for more information about the glycemic index.)

To easily include oatmeal—or better yet oat bran—in your daily sports diet, microwave it according to the directions on the package (but prepare it with low-fat milk instead of water) while you start to read the morning newspaper, cool it off with more milk to make it "soupy," drink it down, read the rest of the paper, and then, head out the door feeling comfortably fed and well-fueled.

I'll talk more about soluble fiber in the upcoming section on fiber.

Ticker Tip #5: Eat More Fish

Getting hooked on fish can boost the healthfulness of your diet. Although some recent research questions if a high intake of fish is associated with a lower risk of heart disease (Ascherio et al., 1995), fish meals that replace meat meals high in saturated fat continue to be a healthful choice. Eating at least two or three fish meals per week can replace meat meals filled with saturated fat, providing an excellent source of protein, and possibly helping reduce your risk of heart disease as well as hypertension, cancer, arthritis, and who knows what else! Some researchers believe that fish oils can help prevent heart disease from the beginning rather than merely having a beneficial effect after the disease has set in.

Table 2.5 can help guide your fish choices to help you include in your overall heart-healthy diet the fish highest in omega-3 fats—the oilier fish that live in cold ocean waters, such as salmon, mackerel, albacore tuna, sardines, and herring. These choices may or may not help enhance your health, but at least they will add variety to your diet. Just be sure that your fish is prepared in low-fat ways: not fried or broiled in butter. If you shy away from cooking fish, simply take advantage of canned fish, such as tuna (mixed with low-fat mayonnaise), salmon, and sardines.

If you are not a fish fan, you may be tempted to take the seemingly easier alternative, fish oil pills. Despite the fancy price tag, these supplements contain only a small amount of omega-3s compared to a fish dinner. For example, you might have to take 10 capsules of one popular brand to get the equivalent of one 4-ounce serving of salmon. Health professionals also question whether the supplements are as effective as the fish itself. To date, the consensus is to get hooked on fish, not on pills.

Table 2.5 Fish Highest in Omega-3 Fatty Acids	
Fish	Omega-3 fatty acids (g/7 oz raw or 5 oz cooked)
Atlantic mackerel	5
King mackerel	4.5
Pacific herring	4
Lake trout	4
Norwegian sardine	3
Bluefin tuna	3
Chinook salmon	3
Albacore tuna	3
Atlantic salmon	3
Sockeye salmon	2.5
Greenland halibut	2

F. Hepburn, J. Exler, and J. Weihrauch, 1986, Provisional tables on the context of omega-3 fatty acids and other fat components of selected foods. Copyright The American Dietetic Association. Reprinted by permission from *Journal of the American Dietetic Association*, Vol. 86: 788.

THE ANTICANCER CRUSADE

In the United States, cancer follows heart disease as the most frequent cause of death. Cancer deaths have risen 7 percent in the past 20 years. Cancer isn't one disease, it is many. Each has its own high-risk groups, its own attack and cure rates, and its own causes. Diet is a factor in an estimated 35 percent of cancer cases, and a healthier diet may cut your risk more than you may think.

Despite the gloomy news that two out of every five of us will get cancer, the encouraging news is that dietary changes can prevent perhaps one-third of cancer deaths. For example, people who eat at least 5 servings a day of fruits and vegetables have a 40 percent lower risk for certain cancers (lung, colon, stomach, esophagus, and mouth) compared to people who eat 2 or fewer servings of fruits and vegetables. A fruit-filled, low-fat, high-fiber, cancer protective diet is also a top performance sports diet. Indulge in good health for high energy!

Protective Nutrients

One key to the role of diet in preventing cancer may lie in an anti-oxidative capacity—that is, in a nutrient's ability to deactivate harmful chemicals in the body known as free radicals. Free radicals are formed daily through normal body processes. Environmental pollutants such as cigarette smoke, automobile exhaust, radiation, and herbicides also generate free radical precursors. These unstable compounds can attack, infiltrate, and injure vital cell structures. Fortunately, our bodies have natural control systems that deactivate and minimize free radical reactions within the cells. These natural control systems involve many vitamins and minerals, including these:

• **Carotenoids.** These precursors of vitamin A are found in plants and then converted into vitamin A in the body. Beta carotene, as well as the more than 40 other carotenoids found in orange and green fruits and vegetables, may help prevent the formation of free radicals. Some of the best sources include carrots, spinach, sweet potatoes, kale, apricots, and cantaloupe. (If you eat too many carotene-rich vegetables and fruits, your skin might turn yellow. If it does, cut back!) Although beta carotene supplements have been touted to protect health, the latest research shows no reduction in cancer or heart disease in supplement users (Hennekens et al., 1996). I recommend you invest in fruits and vegetables instead!

• **Vitamin C.** This vitamin guards against harmful reactions within the cells. The best sources include citrus fruits, broccoli, brussels sprouts, green and red peppers, and strawberries. A conservative recommendation for cancer protection is 1,000 milligrams per day; the RDI is 60 milligrams.

• **Vitamin E.** Vitamin E protects the cell walls from free radical damage. The best sources are vegetable oils (and foods made with them, such as salad dressings), almonds, peanuts, sunflower and sesame seeds, wheat germ, and whole grains. A conservative recommendation for cancer protection is 250 to 1,000 milligrams per day; the RDI is 8 milligrams for women and 10 milligrams for men.

• **Selenium.** Selenium protects the cell walls from free radical damage and enhances the immune system's response with increased resistance to cancer growth. The best sources of selenium include seafoods such as tuna fish, meats, eggs, milk, whole grains, and garlic. An adequate intake is between 50 to 200 micrograms. Supplements are not recommended due to the danger of toxicity with long-term supplementation over 200 micrograms.

Other cancer protectors include foods rich in fiber. Although population studies suggest that people who eat a lot of fiber from grains, fruits, and vegetables have a lower risk of cancer, scientists are unclear if the fiber is the protective nutrient. In addition to the known vitamins and minerals in grains, fresh fruits, and vegetables, these fiber-rich foods contain hundreds, perhaps thousands, of other lesser known substances called phytochemicals that may protect our health. (See table 2.6, and chapter 12.)

Although research suggests that high intakes of antioxidants and phytochemicals can reduce the incidence of some types of cancer, most health professionals emphasize the importance of obtaining these nutrients from food, not from supplements, because of unknown components in food that may prove beneficial and protective. Scientists have yet to pinpoint which of the thousands of substances in fruits and vegetables are protective. If you choose to take an antioxidant supplement, be sure to do so in addition to eating well. No amount of supplementation will compensate for a high-fat diet low in fruits and vegetables and a stress-filled, health-eroding lifestyle.

Table 2.6   Nutrition and Cancer Prevention

Why should you push yourself to eat 5 servings a day of fruits and vegetables, as well as 6 to 11 servings of whole grains? Because plant foods contain active compounds called phytochemicals (*phyto* is the Greek word for plant) that provide protection not only against cancer, but also against heart disease, hypertension, arthritis, and other degenerative diseases of aging. The following list contains some foods rich in phytochemicals that you should routinely incorporate into your food plan as you take steps to move toward the healthiest sports diet.

Food	Phytochemical	Action
Soy milk, tofu	Genistein	Inhibits the formation of blood vessels that assist in the growth of small tumors
Spinach, collard greens	Lutein	Reduces blindness in the elderly
Carrots, squash, apricots, peaches	Beta carotene	Protects the immune system
Fish oil	Omega-3 fatty acids	May decrease risk of heart disease
Rosemary	Quinines	Interfere with the action of cancer-causing substances
Chile peppers	Capsaicin	Prevents toxic molecules from invading and damaging cells, thereby discourages the growth of cancerous cells

Food	Phytochemical	Action
Beans, peas, peanuts	Isoflavones	Interfere with harmful estrogen action and may reduce the risk of breast and ovarian cancer
Cabbage, broccoli, cauliflower, kale	Isothyocynates, indoles	Block carcinogens from damaging a cell; interfere with the action of the harmful precancerous form of estrogen
Citrus fruits	Terpenes	Stimulate enzymes that block tumor growth
Strawberries, pineapple	Chlorogenic acid	Blocks the production of cancer-causing nitrosamines
Garlic, onions	Allylic sulfide	Intercepts and detoxifies carcinogens, slowing tumor growth
Flaxseed	Lignans	Interfere with estrogen action and may reduce breast and ovarian cancer
All fruits and vegetables	Flavenoids	Prevent carcinogenic hormones from attaching to cells

Cancer and Fat

Eating a low-fat diet may be a second dietary key to reducing cancer risk. Population studies suggest that people who eat low-fat diets have a lower incidence of cancer. The National Research Council recommends that we eat less than 30 percent of our total calories as fat, eat more fruits and vegetables rich in beta carotene and vitamin C (review the nutrients in fruits and vegetables in tables 1.3 and 1.4), and eat more whole grains. Voilà—a high-carbohydrate sports diet!

Cancer (and other health problems) can be affected by not only your diet, but also your lifestyle. According to wellness promoter Don Ardell

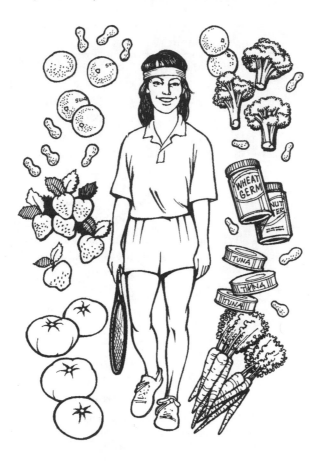

of Florida, relaxation, peace of mind, a positive outlook on life, a contented spirit, absence of envy, love of mankind, and faith are powerful, health-promoting factors without which optimal health cannot be achieved. This holistic approach to cancer prevention and health protection includes nourishing yourself with pleasant, well-balanced, low-fat meals; enjoying exercise as a part of your daily routine; and taking time to smell the roses.

SHAKE IT OR LEAVE IT: SALT AND HIGH BLOOD PRESSURE

High blood pressure, or hypertension, affects approximately 25 to 30 percent of Americans. By having your blood pressure measured, you can determine if it is in a healthy range. The normal pressure is 120 over 80, and a measure that exceeds 165 over 95 is considered high.

What Causes Hypertension?

Risk factors that can predispose people to hypertension include obesity, smoking, high stress, poor kidney function, and poor diet. Most health-conscious exercisers are not obese, do not smoke, and eat a healthier-than-average diet, thus eliminating several risk factors. Most active people, in fact, have low blood pressure. However, additional predisposing factors such as your genetics, age, and race cannot be changed, and they sometimes cause high blood pressure in spite of all your good health habits.

If you do have high blood pressure, you may believe the problem is caused by salt and that reducing salt intake will lower your high blood pressure, but that's not always true. Only 10 percent of American cases of high blood pressure have a known cause. In the remaining 90 percent, no one cause can be identified.

So Who Needs Salt?

Salt is a compound of 40 percent sodium and 60 percent chloride. The sodium helps maintain proper fluid balance between the water in and around your body's cells; thus, you do need some sodium—about 1,000 milligrams per day. Many Americans, however, routinely consume up to seven times that amount!

The suggested daily value is 2,400 milligrams, but that number seems questionably low for athletes with low blood pressure. Because you lose salt when you perspire heavily, a low-salt diet is a questionable restriction if you are very active and have normal or low blood pressure and no family history of hypertension. If you choose to restrict your sodium intake, your body will adjust by conserving more sodium and secreting less.

The best reason to limit salt intake may relate to bone health. The higher your sodium intake, the more calcium you excrete. This can contribute to reduced bone density. If you have a family history of osteoporosis, you should be aware of the sodium-calcium connection (Devine et al., 1995).

Salt for Athletes

Even sweaty athletes who prefer the natural taste of unsalted food can get adequate sodium from the sodium that naturally occurs in foods. For the most part, your body adapts to the heat by conserving salt and sweating proportionately more water. If you are unacclimatized to the heat, such as on that first warm spring day when you overexercise to clear out the winter cobwebs, you will notice that your sweat is far saltier than it is at the end of the summer when you've adapted to the heat. If you really need salt, you will crave it. Many ultramarathoners and long-distance cyclists seek salted crackers, chips, pretzels, and other salty snacks to satisfy their salt cravings.

Shaking the Salt Habit: Tips for People Who Want to Lower Their Sodium Intake

For some people, too much sodium, combined with any or all of the other risk factors, may raise blood pressure to an unhealthy level. For others, it may increase their risk for developing osteoporosis. Before you put yourself on a very-low-salt diet, you should first define your genetic predisposition for these conditions and then talk to your doctor and a registered dietitian about a sodium-restricted diet.

You can lower your intake by following these guidelines:

Foods to Limit

Table salt. Remove the salt shaker from the table. Train your taste buds to appreciate the flavor of unsalted foods. Because the preference for salt is an acquired taste, your taste buds can adjust to a lower salt intake within two months.

Obviously salty foods such as salted crackers, chips, pretzels, popcorn, salted nuts, olives, and pickles. Buy low-sodium versions, if they're available.

Smoked and cured meats and fish such as ham, bacon, sausage, corned beef, hot dogs, bologna, salami, pepperoni, lox, and pickled herring. Choose low-sodium versions, if you like these foods.

Cheeses, in particular processed and low-fat cheeses, some of which may be higher in sodium than the regular form.

Seasonings and condiments such as catsup, mustard, relish, Worcestershire sauce, soy sauce, steak sauce, MSG, and garlic salt.

Commercially prepared foods such as frozen dinners, canned soups, and instant meals unless they are labeled "low sodium."

Baking soda, seltzers, and antacids. Some laxatives may be high in sodium.

Foods to Select

The following general overview of the sodium in commonly eaten foods can help you keep track of your sodium intake. Food labels provide additional information. Your best bet is to buy foods in their natural state, such as raw unsalted peanuts, fresh (not canned) vegetables, and so on.

Food type	Average sodium content	Comments
Milk, yogurt (preferably low-fat)	125 mg/8 ounces	
Cheese (preferably low-fat)	200 mg/ounce	Moderate amounts; 1-2 ounces/day
Meat, fish, poultry	80 mg/4 ounces	
Eggs	60 mg/egg	
Fruit, juice	5 mg/serving	
Vegetables	10 mg per serving	Fresh and frozen. If canned, rinse well.
Breads	150 mg/slice	
Cereal (cold)	250 mg/ounce	Read food label
Butter, margarine	50 mg/pat	
Baked goods	250 mg/serving	

Cooking Tips

Omit or reduce salt from cooking and baking. You can leave it out without affecting the outcome. Substitute wines and vinegars for salt.

Experiment with herbs and spices. When you try a new seasoning, cautiously add a small amount. Some tried-and-true combinations are listed here:

- Beef—dry mustard, pepper, marjoram, red wine, or sherry
- Chicken—parsley, thyme, sage, tarragon, curry, white wine, or vermouth
- Fish—bay leaf, cayenne pepper, dill, curry, onions, garlic
- Eggs—oregano, curry, chives, pepper, tomatoes, pinch of sugar

Be Positive

Rather than focusing exclusively on reducing sodium to alleviate high blood pressure, you should also boost your intake of potassium and calcium, two protective minerals. Eating a potassium-rich diet seems to guard against hypertension and may control blood pressure more effectively than a low-sodium diet does. Potassium helps to make arteries stronger and better able to withstand the blood vessel damage that can occur with aging. A high-calcium diet is associated with low blood pressure. Calcium may offset the effect of too much sodium in the diet. See tables 1.3 and 1.4 for the potassium content of some popular fruits and vegetables and tables 1.6 and 1.7 for a list of calcium-rich foods.

For more information on potassium and sodium for athletes, see chapter 11.

INCREASING YOUR POTASSIUM INTAKE

Potassium is found in most wholesome foods—fruits, vegetables, whole grain breads and cereals, lentils, beans, nuts, and protein foods. Refined or highly processed foods, sweets, and oil foods (salad dressing, butter, etc.) are poor sources of potassium. You can increase your potassium intake by eating the following kinds of foods:

- Whole wheat, oatmeal, and dark breads instead of white bread and flour products
- More salads and raw or steamed veggies cooked in only a small amount of water, because the potassium leaches into the water. Steaming removes only 3 to 6 percent of the potassium, as compared to 10 to 15 percent with boiling. Microwaving is best for optimal potassium retention.
- Potatoes more often than rice, noodles, or pasta
- Natural fruit juices instead of fruit-flavored beverages or soft drinks

The suggested daily intake for potassium is 3,500 milligrams for the average person and 6,000 for the athlete not acclimated to the heat. The typical American diet contains 4,000 to 7,000 milligrams of potassium. One pound of sweat loss may contain 85 to 105 milligrams.

FIBER: JUMPING ON THE BRAN WAGON

Fiber is the part of plant cells that humans can't digest. Having heard claims that fiber promotes regular bowel movements, lowers blood cholesterol, improves blood sugar control, and protects against colon cancer, sports-active Americans are seeking out high-fiber, carbohydrate-rich foods—the fruits, vegetables, beans, legumes, and whole grains that easily fit into a sports diet.

Types of Fiber

Certain types of fiber have specific health benefits. For example, the insoluble fiber in wheat bran relieves constipation and may help prevent cancer. Wheat bran absorbs water, increases fecal bulk, and makes the stool easier to pass. By tripling stool volume, fiber dilutes the concentration of bile acids, substances that digest fat and are suspected cancer instigators. Some researchers believe bile acids irritate

Table 2.7   Fiber in Foods

Fiber is lost through food processing, such as milling whole wheat into white flour, peeling skins, pureeing vegetables, and juicing fruits. To reach the target intake of 25 to 35 grams of fiber per day, you should try to eat foods that have not been processed. You should also try to eat a *variety* of fiber-rich foods, because different types of fibers have different positive health effects.

Cereal (1 oz)	Fiber (g)	Grain (1 oz)	Fiber (g)
All-Bran with		Bulgur, 3/4 cup	6
Extra Fiber	15	Barley, 1 cup	6
All-Bran	10	Brown rice, 1 cup	4
Bran flakes	5	Branola bread, 1 slice	3
Corn bran	5	Spaghetti, cooked, 1 cup	2
Fruit & Fibre	6	White rice, 1 cup	1
Cheerios	3	Pita bread, 1 slice	1

Legumes (1/2 cup)	Fiber (g)	Fruits	Fiber (g)
Kidney beans	5	Prunes, 5 dried	3
Lentils	4	Apple/skin, medium	3
Chick-peas	3	Orange, medium	3
		Banana, medium	2
Vegetables	Fiber (g)	Kiwi, medium	3
		Raisins, 1/4 cup	2
Peas, 1/2 cup	3	Pear, 1 medium	4
Brussels sprouts, 8	4		
Corn, 1/2 cup	4		
Spinach, 1 cup	4		
Potato, 1 medium/skin	3		
Lettuce	trace		

Data from food labels and J. Pennington, 1992, *Bowes & Church's Food Values of Portions Commonly Used*, 16th ed. (Philadelphia: Lippincott).

the intestinal lining, leaving it open to attack from the carcinogens. A high-fiber, low-fat diet may reduce by 30 percent your risk of developing colon cancer, and with a fiber-rich diet that promotes regular bowel movements, you'll feel more comfortable during training and competitions. The information in table 2.7 on page 49 can help you choose the foods richest in fiber.

The soluble fiber in beans, legumes, oat bran, psyllium, and pectin and guar gums (two fibers often added to foods and listed among the ingredients) lowers blood cholesterol, particularly if you start off with elevated cholesterol. The soluble fibers transport bile acids (needed to make cholesterol) out of the body, which results in lower blood cholesterol. In one study (Van Horn et al., 1986) about 2 ounces of oat bran were added to a low-fat, low-cholesterol diet, and the subjects' serum cholesterol dropped 5 percent. Keeping in mind that a 1-percent drop in serum cholesterol reduces by 2 percent your risk of heart disease, the subjects lowered their risk by 10 percent.

You can try to do the same by eating more oat bran, oatmeal, and oatmeal breads, cookies, and muffins. Eating more beans and legumes will also help, and these are also excellent sources of carbohydrates and protein. Corn bran, barley, and rice bran are other rich sources that are becoming more readily available.

A Fiber Myth

Despite popular belief, fiber does not hasten the time it takes for food to pass through your system. It may increase fecal weight and the number of trips to the bathroom, but it usually does not increase transit time. Transit time varies for each person, but it normally averages between two and four days. This varies according to stress, exercise, and diet. Your best bet as an active person is to determine the right combination of fiber-rich foods that promotes regular bowel movements for your body. You may need to restrict your fiber intake if exercise itself becomes a powerful bowel stimulant.

BUILDING STRONG BONES FOR LIFE: CALCIUM AND OSTEOPOROSIS

Osteoporosis, or thinning of the bones with aging, results in hunched backs and brittle bones that break easily. It is a serious health problem primarily among older postmenopausal women; a woman at age 50 today has about one chance in two of developing osteoporosis in her remaining years. Osteoporosis is also a major concern for younger female athletes who have stopped having regular menstrual periods. Both amenorrheic and postmenopausal women lack adequate estrogen, a hormone that contributes to menstruation and helps to maintain bone density. The low bone density of a 29-year-old woman, a former amenorrheic runner, has left her living in pain from osteoporosis and doubting if her bones will be able to withstand the weight of a pregnancy.

You can reduce your risk of developing osteoporosis with these good-health habits:

- A lifelong calcium-rich diet
- A regular exercise program that includes both aerobic and strength-building exercises
- Adequate estrogen maintenance through a healthy diet. If you are entering menopause, you should discuss with your health care provider the option of estrogen replacement therapy.
- A low sodium intake. Because too much salt interferes with the retention of calcium (Matkovic et al., 1995), your best bet is to moderate your salt intake, especially if you have a genetic predisposition to osteoporosis.

Unfortunately, too many women follow too few of these guidelines.

In Chapter 1, I talked about how to include in your daily diet the calcium necessary for lifelong fitness. Unfortunately, the typical 25- to 40-year-old woman consumes only 600 milligrams of calcium daily, less than the current RDI of 1,000 milligrams and the suggested optimal intake of 1,000 to 1,500 milligrams. This may be one reason why an estimated 25 percent of women over 65 years are afflicted by osteoporosis (of whom 12 percent may die from medical complications). These women might have reduced their risk by consuming more calcium-rich foods throughout their lifetimes.

Elderly men also may lose enough bone calcium to suffer from osteoporosis. Regardless of gender, those who want to live a long and healthy life should make sure that they promote their future well-being by eating a calcium-rich diet today!

COFFEE: GROUNDS FOR CONTROVERSY

Some folks never touch coffee: "It makes me hyper and jittery." Others thrive on the stuff: "I'm useless without my morning brew."

Coffee, like tea and cola, contains the stimulant caffeine. Many research studies have tried to link coffee or caffeine to increased risks of cancer, high blood pressure, heart disease, and fibrocystic breast disease. The only confirmed correlation, to date, is that coffee drinkers who smoke cigarettes do have a significantly higher incidence of heart disease.

At-Risk Coffee Drinkers

There are others, in addition to smokers, who should abstain from caffeine:

• **Ulcer patients and others prone to stomach distress.** Caffeine stimulates gastric secretions and may cause "coffee stomach."

• **Pregnant and nursing women.** Caffeine readily crosses the placenta and, in excess, may be associated with premature birth. Caffeine also crosses into breast milk and can make babies agitated and poor sleepers.

• **Anemic athletes.** Substances in coffee and tea can interfere with the absorption of iron. Athletes are at higher risk for iron deficiency than most people, because heavy sweating results in significant loss of this nutrient. A cup of coffee consumed with a hamburger can reduce by about 40 percent the absorption of the hamburger's iron. If you suffer from anemia and routinely drink coffee or tea with meals or within one hour after a meal, you might be cheating yourself nutritionally. However, drinking caffeinated beverages within an hour before eating seems to have no negative effect on iron absorption.

How Are Your Coffee Habits?

If you are healthy, a moderate amount of coffee (1 or 2 cups per day) is unlikely to harm your health. If you are feeling guilty about your traditional morning mug, relax and enjoy it. The biggest health worries about coffee have to do with the following habits surrounding that beverage:

• **Adding cream or coffee whiteners containing coconut oil.** These add saturated fat that contributes to heart disease. At least switch to milk for whitening your coffee.

• **Drinking coffee instead of eating a wholesome breakfast.** A large coffee with two creamers and two sugars contains 80 nutritionally empty calories. Multiply that by three mugs, and you could have had a nourishing bowl of cereal for the same number of calories. Many people who say they "live on coffee" could easily drink much less if they would eat a satisfying breakfast and lunch. Food is better fuel than caffeine!

• **Drinking coffee to stay alert.** A good night's sleep might be a better investment. You could also try drinking a tall glass of ice water to perk yourself up. Sometimes dehydration contributes to fatigue, and you'd be better off drinking water than pumping caffeine.

These bad habits are more likely to harm your health than the caffeine itself.

Cutting the Caffeine

If you drink too much coffee, sleep poorly, and are chronically nervous, jittery, and irritable, then you should slowly cut back. Don't try to abstain cold turkey, because you're likely to suffer a withdrawal headache. Try reducing your caffeine intake by drinking more of the following caffeine-free hot beverages:

- Decaffeinated coffee
- Decaffeinated tea
- Herbal tea
- Hot water with a lemon wedge
- Postum, Pero, and other cereal-based coffee alternatives
- Broth, bouillon (low-sodium or regular)
- Alba, Ovaltine, and other hot milk-based drinks
- Mulled cider
- Hot cranberry or apple juice

Without a doubt, the best caffeine-free alternative to a coffee break is an exercise break. A quick walk and some fresh air may be far more effective than another cup of brew. The next time you start to feel drowsy, try waking yourself up with exercise rather than caffeine.

For more information about caffeine and performance, see chapter 12.

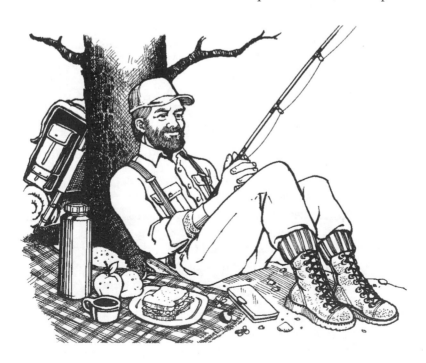

NUTRITION FOR THE PREGNANT ATHLETE

Each woman experiences a pregnancy unique to her. Some feel fine, eat well, exercise regularly, and breeze through the nine months of pregnancy. Others suffer from fatigue, nausea, low-back pain, and other discomforts and count every day of the nine months.

Regardless of your personal experience, your job during pregnancy is to eat as healthfully as you can and to focus on foods rich in calcium, protein, iron, and folic acid. Eat according to your appetite and drink plenty of wholesome fluids.

Your best bet for nutrition during pregnancy is to follow the good nutrition guidelines in the first two chapters of this book, as well as to read some of the pregnancy books suggested in the reading list. Your diet should focus primarily on calcium-rich foods, dark green or colorful vegetables, fresh fruits such as oranges and other citrus fruits, whole grains, and protein-rich foods.

For about two-thirds of women, tastes change during pregnancy. You may develop strong aversions to meat, vegetables, or coffee. If you can hold down nothing but a few crackers, rest assured that your baby will still manage to grow on the nutrients you've stored up from your prepregnancy diet. Experiment with eating a variety of wholesome foods until you (I hope!) find some that are palatable. If you eat a very limited intake due to nausea that lasts for more than three months, you might want to consult with a registered dietitian who can suggest ways to balance your diet.

If you experience unusual cravings, such as for salt, fat, or red meat, it's possible that nature is telling you that those foods have nutrients you're needing. Food cravings tend to be harmless and probably won't lead to a nutrient deficiency, so listen to your body and respond appropriately.

Try to resolve your cravings for sweets with the most healthful choices, such as frozen yogurt instead of ice cream or raisins and dried fruits instead of candy. The reality of the situation may be that there's only one food that will do the trick: the food you crave, no substitutions allowed! You want to eat a healthful, prepregnancy diet to be sure you start off well-nourished so your body can survive the strange cravings and morning sickness.

Trust that regularly scheduled meals and snacks will contribute to the weight gain appropriate for your body, the enjoyment of a comfortable exercise program, and to building a blue-ribbon baby.

Some women gain more weight than anticipated. Others gain according to the standard guidelines shown in this table.

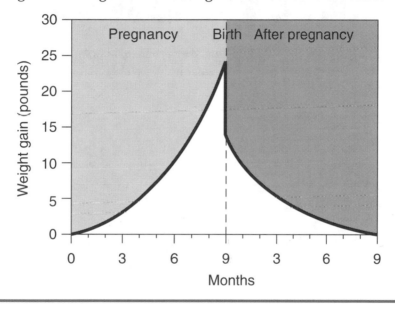

To Your Good Health

By combining the best food choices from the Food Guide Pyramid with a regular exercise program, you can invest in your future well-being. Although genetics does play a strong role with heart disease, cancer, hypertension, and osteoporosis, you can help put the odds in your favor by eating wisely. As Hippocrates once said, "Let food be thy medicine."

chapter

Breakfast *Is* for Champions

When it comes to eating a high-energy sports diet, I firmly believe that breakfast is the most important meal of the day. You've heard that from your mother, teachers, health professionals, coaches, the media, ad infinitum. And now you'll hear it from me!

DON'T SKIP BREAKFAST

Of all the nutritional mistakes that you might make, skipping breakfast is the biggest.

> Ginny, a collegiate rower, learned this the hard way: She fainted from low blood sugar after one of her morning workouts. After rowing for an hour, she felt very tired and hungry because she had no breakfast. When she got out of the boat, she fainted and ended up flat on the dock surrounded by her frightened teammates. She had blacked out because she had run out of fuel.

Ginny's story is a dramatic example of how skipping breakfast can sabotage your sports performance. A high-energy breakfast sets the stage for a high-energy day. Nevertheless, many sports-active people come up with familiar excuses for skipping the morning meal:

- "I don't have time."
- "I'm not hungry in the morning."
- "I don't like breakfast foods."
- "I'm on a diet."
- "If I eat breakfast, I feel hungrier all day."

Excuses, excuses. If you skip breakfast, you're likely to concentrate less effectively in the late morning, work or study less efficiently (Pollitt 1995), feel irritable and short tempered, or fall short of energy for your afternoon workout. For every flimsy excuse to skip breakfast, there's an even better reason to eat it. Keep reading!

YOU *DO* HAVE TIME FOR BREAKFAST

"I just don't have time to eat breakfast. I get up at 5:30, go to the swimming pool, train for an hour, then dash to school by 7:45," insisted Kayla, a high school competitive swimmer.

Obviously, Kayla's morning schedule didn't allow her to relax and enjoy a leisurely meal. However, she still needed the energy to tackle her high school classes. I reminded Kayla that breakfast doesn't have to be a sit-down, cooked meal. It can be a substantial snack after swim practice

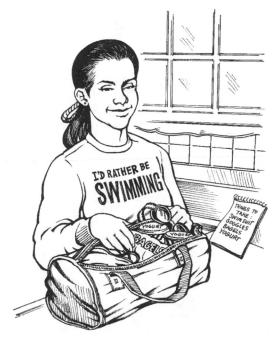

while riding to school. I advised her to plan and prepare a breakfast-to-go the night before. If she could make time to swim, she could make time to eat right for swimming.

Kayla discovered that her "duffel bag breakfast" was indeed worth the effort. Two peanut butter and banana sandwiches and two juice boxes satisfied her ravenous appetite and improved her ability to concentrate at school. No longer did she sit in class counting the minutes until lunch and listening to her stomach grumble. Rather, she was able to concentrate on her classwork and even improve her grades.

Jane, a runner and nurse, had the same excuse of no time for breakfast. She'd rise at 6:00 and be at the hospital by 6:45; she didn't want to eat breakfast at that early hour. However, by 10:00 she'd be ravenously devouring doughnuts—grease bombs that she didn't particularly like but that she ate anyway because they were in the nurses' station begging to be eaten!

I recommended that Jane eat some nutritious food between 8:00 and 9:00 to prevent the overwhelming hunger that contributed to her overeating and subsequent weight gain. Jane made the effort to do one of the following every day:

- Bring a sandwich to work to eat within four hours of waking.
- Buy a bagel, yogurt, and orange juice at the coffee shop.
- Take an early break and enjoy a hot breakfast at the cafeteria.
- Keep emergency food in her locker: crackers, peanuts, and dried fruits.

She soon became a breakfast advocate, feeling so much better when well-fueled rather than half starved.

No Morning Appetite?

If you are not hungry for breakfast, you probably ate too many calories the night before. I often counsel athletes who routinely devour a whole bag of chips while watching TV or raid the cookie jar at 2 A.M. These snacks can certainly curb a morning appetite, contribute to weight gain, and even result in inadequate diets if too many munchies replace wholesome meals.

Mark, a 35-year-old runner and computer programmer, wasn't hungry for breakfast for another reason: His morning workout killed his appetite. However, he did get hungry by 10:00 when his appetite came to life again. He'd try to hold off until lunchtime but he raided the candy machine three out of five workdays.

CREATIVE, QUICK-FIX BREAKFASTS

If you lack creative quick-fix breakfast ideas, these suggestions can help you make a fast break to becoming a regular breakfast eater.

- **Yogurt.** Keep your refrigerator well stocked; add cereal for crunch.
- **Banana.** Eat an extra-large one, and wash it down with a large glass of milk.
- **Blender drink.** Whip together juice, fruit, and yogurt or dried milk.
- **Raisins and peanuts.** Prepacked in small plastic bags, these are ready to get tucked in your pocket.
- **Bran muffin.** Add jam for more carbohydrates.
- **Bagel.** Spread it with low-fat cream cheese and drink a can of V-8 juice.
- **Graham crackers.** These are a refreshing favorite with low-fat milk, and a skimming of peanut butter.
- **Pita bread.** Stuff it with low-fat cheese, cottage cheese, sliced turkey, hummus, or other handy fillings.

I recommended that Mark take a bagel, yogurt, and banana to work. These portable foods are much more nutritious than candy, especially for breakfast! For morning exercisers like Mark, a wholesome breakfast of cereal, fruit, whole grain toast, bagels, or low-fat muffins promptly replaces the depleted glycogen stores and helps refuel the muscles for the next training session. Exercised muscles are hungriest for carbohydrates within the first two hours after a hard workout. The sooner you eat, the quicker you'll refuel. For more information on recovery foods, see chapter 11.

A recovery breakfast is particularly important if you do two workouts per day. Unfortunately, too many athletes who do double workouts say they're not hungry for breakfast after the first workout. They also skimp at lunchtime, afraid that a substantial meal might interfere with the afternoon session. They end up dragging themselves through a poor workout.

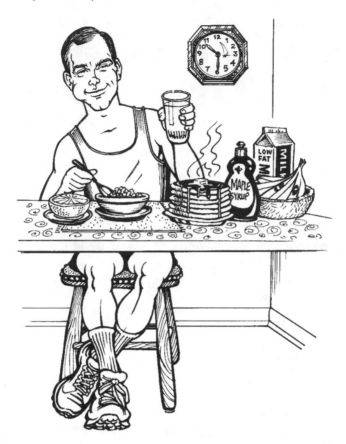

In this situation, I recommend having brunch or a substantial snack around 10:00 or 11:00. The food will be adequately digested in time to fuel the muscles that afternoon. Refreshing liquids, such as juices and smoothies, also can help refuel you as well as quench your thirst. You'll discover that you have more energy for the second workout.

BREAKFAST FOR DIETERS

Skipping breakfast to save calories is an unsuccessful approach to weight loss. Breakfast skippers commonly struggle more with body fatness than do breakfast eaters. If you are tempted to save calories by skimping on breakfast, remember that you don't get fat eating this meal. You are more likely to get fat if you skip breakfast, get too hungry, and then overindulge at night. If you are going to skip any meal, skip dinner but not breakfast.

By eating during the day, you'll have more energy to be more active and burn off the calories. In one study with subjects who needed about

2,000 calories per day to maintain their weight, the subjects all lost weight when they ate all 2,000 calories at one morning meal (Halberg 1983). When they moved these calories to an identical meal in the evening, four of the six gained weight; the other two lost less than they had when they ate breakfast only. The weight loss difference averaged about two and a half pounds. Breakfast is a dieter's aid.

Time and again I advise dieters to eat during the day and to diet at night. Time and again they look at me with fear in their eyes.

As Pat, a weight-conscious dancer explained, "If I eat breakfast, I get hungrier and seem to eat more the whole day." Her breakfast was only a slice of 50-calorie diet toast, enough to "prime the pump" and get the digestive juices flowing, but not enough to satisfy her appetite. When she ate a substantial 500-calorie breakfast, she felt fine and didn't blow it later in the afternoon. Although she initially couldn't believe that the following 500-calorie breakfasts would help her lose weight, she discovered they did.

Sample 500-Calorie Breakfasts (Appropriate for a 1,500-Calorie–Reducing Diet)

Breakfast type	Approximate calories
Breakfast at home	
1 cup orange juice	100
2 ounces cereal	220
1 cup low-fat milk	100
1 small banana	80
Total:	500
Breakfast on the run	
Bagel, large	300
Vanilla yogurt	200
Total:	500
Non-traditional breakfast	
2 slices pizza (leftover from dinner)	500
Total:	500
Splurge-on-a-diet breakfast	
(To be balanced with low-fat, wholesome meals for the rest of the day)	
Chocolate glazed donut	320
Coffee with cream and sugar	80
2 Powdered Sugar Munchkins	100
Total:	500

> Pam, a 28-year-old mother, tennis lover, and lifelong dieter, insisted that eating breakfast triggered her to overeat the whole day. I requested she experiment for just three days to determine if a substantial 500-calorie breakfast really did make her hungrier and fatter.

Pam quickly discovered that she no longer craved cookies at lunch and that she snacked less in the afternoon, played better tennis after work, and was able to enjoy a relaxed dinner rather than ravenously wolfing down whatever food was in sight the minute she walked in the door. She felt less hungry and snacked less throughout the night. By trading in the evening's 600 to 800 snack calories for 500 breakfast calories, she discovered that breakfast for her could become the most important meal of the day!

If you are watching your weight and for some reason overeat at breakfast, don't continue to overeat the rest of the day. Simply acknowledge that you ate part or all of your lunch calories early, and then eat less at lunch. You won't be hungry! Listen to your body instead of your mind, which probably is whining, "Keep eating because this is your last chance before The Diet starts again."

NONTRADITIONAL BREAKFASTS

If you skip breakfast because you don't like breakfast foods, just eat something else. Who said you have to eat cereal or toast? Any food you eat at other times of the day can be eaten at breakfast. I happen to love leftover pizza or Chinese food for a morning change of pace!

Your goal is to eat about one-third of your daily calories in the morning, so you might want to eat a dinner or lunch at breakfast. Try "planned-overs," a baked potato, a peanut butter and honey sandwich, a cottage cheese "sundae" with sliced fruit and sunflower seeds, tomato soup with crackers, or even special holiday foods. Save some of those high-calorie treats that may be left over from a special event and enjoy them for breakfast. You're better off eating them during the day and burning off their calories than holding off until evening, when you may succumb to overconsumption in a moment of weakness.

THE #1 BREAKFAST FOR CHAMPIONS

My sports-active clients commonly ask what I recommend for breakfast. My #1 choice is cereal.

What's So Great About Cereal?

I'm big on cereals because they are all these positive things:

• **Quick and easy.** Athletes of all ages and cooking abilities can easily pour a bowl with no cooking or messy cleanup.

• **Convenient.** By simply stocking the cupboard, gym bag, or desk drawer, breakfast will be ready for the morning rush. A handful of dry cereal is better than nothing.

• **Carbohydrate-rich.** Your muscles need carbohydrates for energy. Cereal, milk, a banana, and juice create a super carbohydrate-rich meal.

• **Fiber-rich.** When you select bran cereals, you reduce your risk of becoming constipated, an inconvenience that can certainly interfere with optimal sports performance, and you also consume a health-protective, anticancer food.

• **Iron-rich.** By selecting fortified or enriched brands, you can easily boost your iron intake and reduce your risk of becoming anemic. Drinking orange juice or another source of vitamin C with the cereal may enhance the iron absorption from the cereal.

• **Calcium-rich.** Cereal is rich in calcium when it's eaten with milk or yogurt. Women and girls, in particular, benefit from this calcium-booster that helps maintain strong bones and protects against osteoporosis.

• **Low in fat and cholesterol.** Cereals are a heart-healthier choice than the standard breakfast alternatives of buttered toast, a bagel slathered with cream cheese, or bacon and eggs.

• **Versatile.** Rather than getting bored by always eating the same brand, try mixing cereals to concoct endless flavors. I typically have 10 to 18 varieties in my cupboard. My friends laugh when they discover this impressive stockpile! I further vary the flavors by adding different mix-ins, such as banana, raisins, applesauce, cinnamon, maple syrup, or vanilla extract.

The Scoop on Cereals

Cereals, in general, are a breakfast for champions. However, some brands offer far more nutritional value than others. Here are a five tips to help you make wise choices.

1. **Choose Iron-Enriched Cereals.** Iron is particularly important for active people, because it is the part of the red blood cell that carries oxygen from your lungs to your muscles. If you are anemic (have iron-poor blood), you will feel tired and fatigue easily during exercise. Iron-rich breakfast cereal is a handy way to boost your iron intake, particularly if you eat little or no red meat (the best source of dietary iron). See table 3.1 for the brands enriched

What to Look for In a Cereal ...

If your favorite cereal doesn't meet these criteria, combine it with others to achieve a healthy mix.

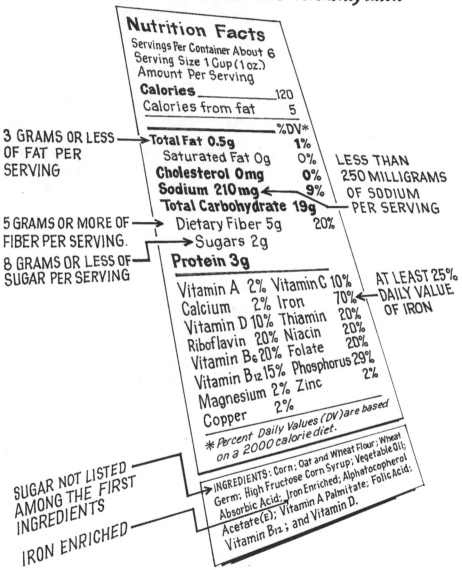

3 GRAMS OR LESS OF FAT PER SERVING

5 GRAMS OR MORE OF FIBER PER SERVING.

8 GRAMS OR LESS OF SUGAR PER SERVING

LESS THAN 250 MILLIGRAMS OF SODIUM PER SERVING

AT LEAST 25% DAILY VALUE OF IRON

SUGAR NOT LISTED AMONG THE FIRST INGREDIENTS

IRON ENRICHED

Nutrition Facts

Servings Per Container About 6
Serving Size 1 Cup (1 oz.)
Amount Per Serving

Calories	120
Calories from fat	5

	%DV*
Total Fat 0.5g	1%
Saturated Fat 0g	0%
Cholesterol 0mg	0%
Sodium 210mg	9%
Total Carbohydrate 19g	
Dietary Fiber 5g	20%
Sugars 2g	
Protein 3g	

Vitamin A 2% Vitamin C 10%
Calcium 2% Iron 70%
Vitamin D 10% Thiamin 20%
Riboflavin 20% Niacin 20%
Vitamin B6 20% Folate 20%
Vitamin B12 15% Phosphorus 2%
Magnesium 2% Zinc 2%
Copper 2%

* Percent Daily Values (DV) are based on a 2000 calorie diet.

INGREDIENTS: Corn; Oat and Wheat Flour; Wheat Germ; High Fructose Corn Syrup; Vegetable Oil; Absorbic Acid; Iron Enriched; Alphatocopherol Acetate (E); Vitamin A Palmitate; Folic Acid; Vitamin B12; and Vitamin D.

with iron to supplement the small amount naturally occurring in grains.

Because the iron in cereal is often poorly absorbed, you may enhance your body's ability to absorb iron by drinking orange juice or eating fruit rich in vitamin C along with the cereal (try oranges, grapefruit, cantaloupe, and strawberries). For more information on iron, see chapters 8 and 12.

2. **Choose High-Fiber Bran Cereals.** Bran cereals can provide far more fiber than most fruits and vegetables. High-fiber cereals include All-Bran, bran flakes, Fruit & Fibre, corn bran, raisin bran, oat bran, and any of the multitude of cereals with bran in the name (see table 3.1). You can also boost the fiber content of any cereal by simply sprinkling raw bran on it.

3. **Choose Wholesome Cereals.** By "wholesome cereals," I mean those not loaded with sugar. Some kids' cereals are 45 percent sugar. They fit better as a snack or dessert rather than as breakfast. Although sugar does fuel the muscles and is not the poison it is reputed to be, sugary cereals tend to pamper your sweet tooth rather than promote your health. To determine the calories of sugar per serving in a cereal, multiply grams of sugar (listed under Total Carbohydrate) by four calories per gram. For example, one cup of Cinnamon Life contains 14 grams of sugar (14 g sugar $\times$ 4 calories per g = 56 calories). That means 30 percent of the 190 calories per serving are from sugar.

Charlene, a 32-year-old rollerblade enthusiast and accountant, avoided all cereals with sugar listed among the ingredients, even the lightly sweetened ones such as Total, Wheaties, or bran flakes. She restricted herself to sugar-free Puffed Wheat, corn flakes, and shredded wheat, cheating herself of both iron and fiber. She failed to recognize that sugar is a carbohydrate that fuels, not poisons, the muscles.

The small amount of sugar in cereal is relatively insignificant in comparison to the sugar Charlene ate in frozen yogurt, fat-free cookies, and jelly beans. The overall healthfulness of the cereal breakfast far outweighed those few nutritionally empty sugar calories. Given this perspective, she decided to relax her sugar rules to include more variety, especially brands with health-protective fiber and iron.

4. **Choose Low-Fat Cereals.** Fat is a bigger health threat than sugar because it's linked with weight gain, heart disease, and cancer. If you like the higher-fat cereals, such as granola or Cracklin' Oat

Table 3.1   Nutritional Value of Some Commonly Eaten Cereals

Cereal	Amount	Calories	% Calories from sugar	% Calories from fat (g)	Fiber (g)	Iron (%DV)
All-Bran Extra Fiber	1/2 cup	50	0	11 (1)	15	25
Bran Flakes, Kellogg's	1 cup	100	22	trace	5	45
Cap'n Crunch	3/4 cup	120	44	12 (1.5)	—	25
Cheerios	1 cup	110	4	16 (2)	3	45
Corn bran	3/4 cup	90	27	7 (1)	5	45
Corn flakes	1 cup	110	7	trace	1	10
Cracklin' Oat Bran	3/4 cup	230	31	31 (8)	6	10
Crispy Wheats & Raisins	1 cup	190	42 *	5 (1)	4	25
Frosted flakes	3/4 cup	120	43	trace	—	25
Fruit & Fibre	1 cup	210	34 *	13 (3)	6	35
Grape-Nuts	1/2 cup	200	11	trace	5	45
Honey Nut Cheerios	1 cup	120	37	11 (1.5)	2	25
Life	3/4 cup	120	20	15 (1.5)	2	45
Muselix, Kellogg's	2/3 cup	200	32	14 (3)	4	25
Nutri-Grain Wheat	3/4 cup	100	24	trace (.5)	4	6
Product 19	1 cup	110	11	trace	1	100
Puffed wheat	1 cup	50	0	trace	trace	2
Quaker 100% Natural	1/2 cup	220	27	33.8	4	6
Quaker Lowfat Granola	1/2 cup	210	31	16 (3)	3	10
Raisin Bran, Kellogg's	1 cup	170	40 *	5 (1)	7	45
Rice Krispies	1-1/4 cup	110	11	trace	1	10
Shredded wheat	2 biscuits	160	trace	trace	5	8
Special K	1 cup	110	11	trace	1	45
Total	3/4 cup	100	20	trace	3	100
Wheat Chex	3/4 cup	190	10	9 (1)	5	70
Wheaties	1 cup	110	11	8 (1)	3	45

*Includes raisins

Compiled from information provided on the cereal box, 1995.

Bran, use them for a topping sprinkled on a foundation of a lower-fat cereal.

5. **Choose Low-Salt Varieties.** If you are on a very strict low-sodium diet for medical reasons, you should eat cereals with a low-salt content. Almost any cereal is a lower sodium alternative to breakfast pastries, muffins, or biscuits. See table 3.2 and chapter 2 for more sodium information.

CEREAL ALTERNATIVES

Cereal may be one breakfast of champions, but it's not the only one. For you noncereal eaters, rest assured that other breakfasts can fuel you for a high energy day. See the recipes in part IV for some wholesome, high-carbohydrate breakfast breads you might want to enjoy with a glass of low-fat milk and some fruit or juice.

Whatever your choice, always remember that any breakfast is better than no breakfast, and a wholesome, high-carbohydrate breakfast is best for your sports diet.

Table 3.2 Sodium in Cereals	

Although some cereals are higher in sodium than others, their sodium content is within reasonable limits of many low-sodium diets. By eating 200 calories of the highest sodium brands, plus one cup of low-fat milk (125 milligrams sodium), you'll consume only about 700 milligrams sodium, the amount lost through an hour's hard exercise.

Cereal	Sodium (mg/100 calories)
All-Bran (Kellogg's)	350
Corn Flakes (Kellogg's)	300
Cheerios (General Mills)	255
Nutri-Grain Wheat (Kellogg's)	240
Special K (Kellogg's)	225
Wheaties (General Mills)	200
Cap'n Crunch (Quaker)	190
Raisin Bran (Kellogg's)	180
Grape-Nuts (Post)	175
Life (Quaker)	140
Muselix (Kellogg's)	135
100% Natural, lowfat (Quaker)	50
100% Natural (Quaker)	5
Shredded Wheat (Nabisco)	0
Puffed Rice (Quaker)	0

Information taken from the nutrition labels on the cereal boxes, April 1995.

4
chapter

Snacks and Snack Attacks

Many people live on snacks; they energize themselves throughout the day on minimeals. For example, Jan, a teacher, part-time graduate student, and swimmer, typically

- swims between 6:00 and 7:00 in the morning,
- grabs something for breakfast on her way to work,
- has a hectic day at school with little time to stop and eat,
- energizes on emergency food filed in her desk drawer,
- lifts weights at the health club before night school,
- picks up dinner on the way to classes or munches on whatever is around, and
- eats a "real meal" once a week—Sunday dinner with her family.

The rest of the time, she snacks, grazes, and munches.

Jan's eating patterns are common to many Americans. Surveys suggest that snacks can contribute from 20 to 50 percent of daily calories. Because snacking and grazing are replacing the traditional three well-balanced meals, it's important that healthy choices become the backbone of a snacker's diet.

Is Snacking Bad?

Despite popular belief, snacking can be good for you if you make wise choices. Obviously, if you snack on glazed donuts, Twinkies, M&Ms,

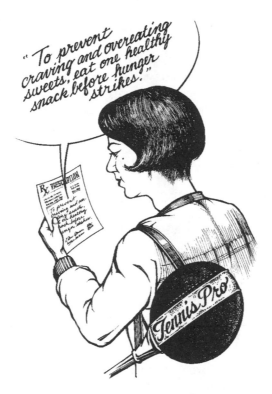

"To prevent craving and overeating sweets, eat one healthy snack before hunger strikes."

chips, and cola, you'll fuel yourself with sweets and fats that lack the nutrients you need for optimal performance. The same way that a car needs gasoline and spark plugs to function, your body needs calories and the vitamins, minerals, and proteins found in wholesome foods.

Wise snack choices include many nutritious and conveniently available items. Jan did a super job of balancing her nutrient intake, despite her hectic schedule and lack of normal meals. Her choices often looked like this:

- **Breakfast:** Pumpernickel bagel and yogurt
- **Lunch at school:** Thick crust pizza with green peppers
- **Emergency munchies:** Peanut butter, crackers, V-8 juice
- **Take-out dinner:** Chinese stir-fry chicken with vegetables and steamed rice
- **Hot dinner at home:** Tomato soup and toasted low-fat cheese sandwich
- **Cold dinner at home:** Cereal with a tall glass of orange juice (the breakfast she never ate that morning)

The following list provides additional ideas for snacks and grazing at home and on the road.

• **Dry cereal.** Mix your favorite cereal with raisins, dried fruits, cinnamon, or nothing! Some good "finger cereals" include Chex, shredded miniwheats, Cheerios, Life, corn bran, and Oat Squares.

• **Popcorn.** Eat plain or sprinkled with spices such as chili powder, garlic powder, onion powder, or soy sauce. If you like, spray with low-calorie butter-flavor sprays so the spices stick (see the recipes in part IV).

• **Pretzels.** Knock off the salt or buy salt free if you wish to reduce your salt intake.

• **Crackers.** Stoned wheat, sesame, bran, RyKrisp and other reduced-fat or fat-free brands.

• **Muffins.** Homemade with little fat are best. If store-bought, choose low-fat muffins; wholesome bran or corn are better than ones made with white flour (see the recipes in part IV).

• **Bagels.** Whole grain varieties provide more vitamins and minerals than do bagels made with white flour.

• **Fruits.** Choose oranges, bananas, apples, or any fresh fruit. When traveling, pack along dried fruit for concentrated carbohydrates. See table 4.1 for some of the best fruits.

• **Frozen fruit bars.** You can slowly savor these pleasant treats in good health.

• **Yogurt.** Low-fat or fat-free are best. By buying quarts of plain yogurt, you'll save money, and have the freedom to flavor it as you choose with vanilla, honey, cinnamon, instant decaffeinated coffee, applesauce, fruit cocktail, berries, or any flavor of the day.

• **Sports bars, breakfast bars, low-fat granola bars.** Prewrapped and portable, these travel well in pockets and gym bags and can be very handy. (See chapter 10 for more details on sports bars.)

• **Nuts, seeds.** Peanuts, pistachios, almonds, sunflower seeds, pumpkin seeds, and other nuts and seeds are excellent for protein, B vitamins, and vitamin E. Because they are high in (healthful) fat, balance them with carbohydrate-rich meals and snacks.

• **Baked potatoes.** Microwave ovens make these a handy snack. They're tasty warm or cold, and because of their high glycemic effect, they are excellent for refueling your muscles after a hard workout. Try sweet potatoes with a dash of nutmeg—mmm! (See chapters 2 and 7.)

SNACK ATTACKS

I always plan for an afternoon snack to boost my energy. This helps me concentrate better by maintaining my blood sugar level; it also takes the edge off my appetite and fuels me for my afterwork bike commute. I pack the snack along with lunch and take the time to eat it.

Table 4.1   The Best Fruits

Vitamin packed and health protective, fruit is a top-notch sports snack. To help you make the best choices, use this list that orders fruits according to their content of nine vitamins and fiber.

Fruit	Nutrition score
Papaya, 1/2	252
Cantaloupe, 1/4	213
Strawberries, 1 cup	186
Oranges, 1 average	169
Tangerines, 2 average	168
Kiwi, 1	154
Mango, 1/2	153
Watermelon, 2 cups	122
Raspberries, 1 cup	117
Grapefruit, 1/2	103
Honeydew, 1/10 melon	81
Apricots, 2 fresh	72
Banana, 1	60
Apple, with skin, 1	58
Pear, 1 average	48
Apple, no skin, 1	42
Peach, 1 average	39
Raisins, 1/4 cup packed	35
Pears, canned, 2 halves	16

Copyright 1995, CSPI. Adapted from *Nutrition Action Healthletter* (1875 Connecticut Ave., N.W., Suite 300, Washington, D.C. 20009-5728. $24.00 for 10 issues).

Not snacking can be a bad practice. You can get too hungry and later overeat. I've learned that if I don't snack on four crackers at the office, I can very easily eat 20 crackers the minute I get home from work!

Snacks prevent not only hunger sensations but also sweets cravings. Snack attacks—not snacks per se—are the nutritional concern. Many athletes think they are hopelessly, and helplessly, addicted to sugary snacks. I believe they are not addicted and that they can change their behavior. In fact, I've helped many clients resolve their problematic sweets cravings easily and painlessly. The solution is simple: Eat before you get too hungry. When you are ravenous, you tend to crave sweets and overeat.

If you frequently experience uncontrollable snack attacks, examine the following case studies and solutions to learn how to tame the cookie monster within you.

Snack Attack #1. The Pre-Dinner Cookie Binge

> "I have the worst sweet tooth. I manage to fight sweet cravings until I get home and then I inevitably attack the chocolate chip cookies. I feel as though I'm powerless and have no control over sweets. I hope you can put me on the straight and narrow."
>
> *David, 47-year-old marathon runner, accountant, and father*

David's story is typical of many of my clients. He came to me feeling guilty about his lack of control over sweets. He required about 3,000 calories per day, but ate zero calories at breakfast and 200 from a yogurt at lunch. No wonder he was uncontrollably ravenous by the time he got home; he had accumulated a 2,800-calorie deficit! Nature took control by encouraging him to eat more than enough so that he would get adequate energy into his system.

I suggested that David eat his 1,600 cookie calories in the form of wholesome meals during the day. He started eating 800 calories for breakfast (cereal, milk, banana, juice, and bagel) and 1,000 calories throughout the afternoon for a snack-like lunch (two yogurts, two large bananas, two juices). Within one day he discovered that he wasn't a cookie monster after all. He could come home, feel untempted by cookies, and have the energy, patience, and desire to cook a wholesome 1,200 calorie meal rather than grab the handiest foods in sight. He also fueled his muscles better with wholesome carbohydrates than with buttery cookies. Most cookies get about half their calories from fat.

Snack Attack #2. Premenstrual Sweet Cravings

> "Once a month I feel driven to devour a bag of chocolate kisses. I can easily tell the time of the month by my eating habits. Premenstrual chocolate cravings do me in."
>
> *Charlene, 20-year-old college cheerleader*

Charlene, like many women, recognized that her eating patterns change with the stages of the menstrual cycle. In the week before her period, she has overwhelming sweet cravings; the week afterward, she tends to crave more protein foods or have very little appetite. Researchers have verified these eating patterns and report that a complex interplay of hormonal changes seems to influence women's food choices.

High levels of estrogen may be linked with the premenstrual carbohydrate cravings.

Women also may crave carbohydrates because they are hungrier. Prior to menstruation, a woman's metabolic rate may increase by 100 to 500 calories (Barr, Janelle, and Prior 1995). That can be the equivalent of another meal! However, when Charlene, like most women, felt bloated and fat due to premenstrual water weight gain, she would put herself on a reducing diet. The result? A double deprivation: The physiological need for extra calories and the calorie-deficient reducing diet. No wonder she experienced overwhelming hunger and craved sweets.

I told Charlene not to diet but instead, when she felt hungry in the week before her period, to give herself permission to eat 200 to 500 additional wholesome calories. She started adding a slice of toast and jam to her standard breakfast, a hot cocoa at lunch, and an afternoon snack of some raisins. She successfully curbed the nagging hunger that had previously plagued her and she was less irritable. Even her friends and family noticed a difference in her moods. She also lost interest in chocolate and was thrilled to survive a menstrual cycle without gaining weight from chocolate gluttony. By reading the nutrition information on the candy bar label, she was able to limit herself to 500 calories of chocolate—no more!

Snack Attack #3. Chocolate Addictions

"Chocolate is my favorite food. I fight the urge to feed myself chocolate bars for lunch, brownies for snacks, and chocolate ice cream for dinner!"

Jocelyn, 17-year-old high school basketball player

Some folks simply love sweets. They need no excuse to indulge in sugary goo. They eat sweets daily, three times if not more, starting with chocolate donuts for breakfast, cookies for lunch, sweet and sour pork for dinner, and then ice cream for dessert. Needless to say, this high consumption of sweets results in a poor diet because these sweets lack vitamins and minerals.

Being a healthy, active teen, Jocelyn's diet had space to fit in some sweets without jeopardizing health. For people eating an overall wholesome diet, 10 percent of the calories can appropriately come from sugar, if desired (American Dietetic Association 1993). Because Jocelyn required 2,800-plus calories per day, she could certainly fit in 280 calories of sugar—a reasonable amount.

Sweets abusers are more at risk for nutritional problems than those who enjoy an occasional treat. There's a big difference between eating a little chocolate as a fun food for dessert after a nourishing meal and eating a box of chocolates to replace that meal.

Chocoholics commonly skip breakfast because they're not hungry in the morning. That's because they ate the whole bag of chocolate chip cookies the night before. They would nourish themselves better by eating one or two cookies for a bedtime snack and then being hungry for a wholesome breakfast the next morning.

In Jocelyn's case, the chocolate problem stemmed from no time for breakfast, dislike of school lunch, and easy access to the vending machine. I encouraged her to eat breakfast on her way to school, which helped her consume less chocolate during the day.

Snack Attack #4. The Pre-Exercise Sugar Fix

"I'm trying very hard to lose weight, and I am careful about what I eat during the day. However, by the time I leave work for my 5:00 aerobics class, I'm drained and searching for a quick energy boost. I choose something light, like a can of soda pop, but I still get light-headed during class. Any suggestions?"

Priscilla, 37-year-old sales clerk, dieter and aerobics dancer

When it comes to needing quick energy for the afternoon workout, be cautioned that eating a high-sugar food during the period 15 to 45 minutes before you exercise might have a negative effect if you are sensitive to swings in blood sugar. The sugar in soft drinks and even fruit juices offers a short term energy boost that later may hinder performance by contributing to hypoglycemia (low blood sugar) shortly after you start to exercise.

A concentrated dose of sugar (either natural sugar in fruit juice or refined sugar in soft drinks and jelly beans) rapidly boosts your blood sugar but simultaneously triggers the pancreas to secrete an abnormally large amount of insulin. Insulin transports excess sugar out of the blood and into the muscles. Exercise, like insulin, similarly enhances this transport. Thus, your blood sugar can drop to an abnormally low level once you start to exercise. Some athletes are more susceptible than others to negative effects caused by this rebound hypoglycemia.

Such was the case with Priscilla. Within 10 to 15 minutes after beginning the aerobics class, she felt light-headed, shaky, uncoordinated, and unmotivated to continue. Some days, she even had to stop for a rest. The rapid drop in blood sugar interfered with her ability to exercise. I

To determine how breakfast and snacks affect energy for exercise, researchers gave ten well-trained men four different exercise trials using four different eating/timing regimens, then measured the men's energy output. Here's what they found:

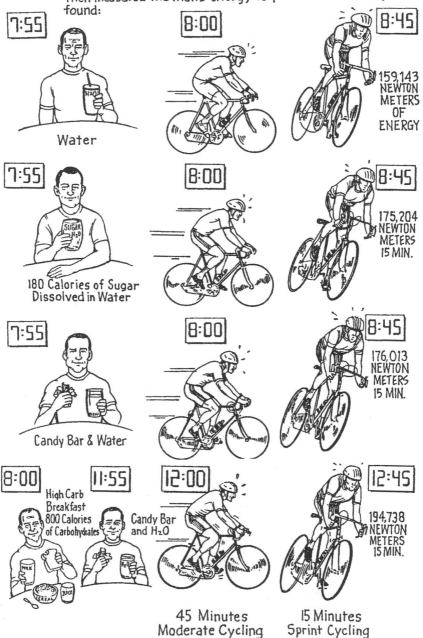

7:55

Water

8:00

8:45

159,143 NEWTON METERS OF ENERGY

7:55

180 Calories of Sugar Dissolved in Water

8:00

8:45

175,204 NEWTON METERS 15 MIN.

7:55

Candy Bar & Water

8:00

8:45

176,013 NEWTON METERS 15 MIN.

8:00

High Carb Breakfast 800 Calories of Carbohydrates

11:55

Candy Bar and H2O

12:00

12:45

194,738 NEWTON METERS 15 MIN.

45 Minutes Moderate Cycling

15 Minutes Sprint Cycling

suggested that she trade her quick-fix calories for more calories at lunch. That did the trick. She had an extra half sandwich at lunch (150 calories) instead of an afternoon can of cola (150 calories), and she enjoyed her higher energy level.

Despite popular belief, most athletes can tolerate a pre-exercise sugar fix without physical problems (Horowitz and Coyle 1993). However, the better solution than pre-exercise sweets is to maintain a high energy level throughout the day by eating adequate calories at breakfast and lunch. Research shows that people who eat a good meal four hours before they exercise perform better than those who eat no snack, and that a meal plus a snack helps them work best.

Without a doubt, breakfast and lunch are the best energy boosters. But if for whatever reason you have skipped breakfast or lunch and are hungry and craving sweets before your afternoon workout, eat the sweets within 10 minutes of exercise if you are concerned about experiencing a "sugar low." This will minimize the risk of a possible hypoglycemic reaction, because the insulin will not have greatly increased in that short period of time. Be aware, however, that the food may talk back!

Snack Attack #5. The Mid-Exercise Sugar Fix

"On weekends, I like to rollerblade for miles. After about 1-1/2 hours, I start to grind away and feel tired and hungry. I really crave sweets and can eat a whole bag of jelly beans."

Chris, a 49-year-old graphic artist

Although eating sugar before exercise may put you at risk of experiencing a hypoglycemic reaction, eating sugar *during* long bouts of exercise has a positive effect. Because sugar feedings during exercise result in smaller increases in both insulin and blood glucose, sugar eaten during exercise is unlikely to cause rebound hypoglycemia. Sugar taken during exercise delays fatigue, a key symptom of low blood sugar. For rollerbladers, cyclists, cross-country skiers, ultrarunners, and others who exercise for more than 60 to 90 minutes, frequent snacks can enhance stamina and enjoyment of endurance exercise.

Some athletes want the natural sugars from fruits and juices, some hit the candy bars or sports bars, and others prefer sports drinks. You need to experiment to determine what foods or fluids work best for you and how much is appropriate. Research suggests that eating 100 to 300 calories per hour of endurance exercise enhances performance

(Murray et al. 1991). A safe range is about 0.5 grams of carbohydrate per pound of body weight, which means about 75 grams (300 calories) if you weigh 150 pounds, or 50 grams (200 calories) if you weigh 100 pounds. (Coyle et al., 1983). Some athletes can tolerate that much or more, others can't. Experiment during training.

Also keep in mind that too much sugar or food taken at once can slow down the rate at which fluids leave the stomach and can be used for replacing sweat losses. Be more conservative with your sugar fixes during endurance exercise in hot weather, when rapid fluid replacement is perhaps more important than carbohydrate replacement. In cold weather, however, when the risks of becoming dehydrated may be lessened, sugar fixes can provide much needed energy. Chapter 10 offers more information on nutrition during exercise.

The Tip of the Pyramid

Snacks can easily be a source of wholesome energy when you choose from the base of the Food Guide Pyramid, and they can be a good in-

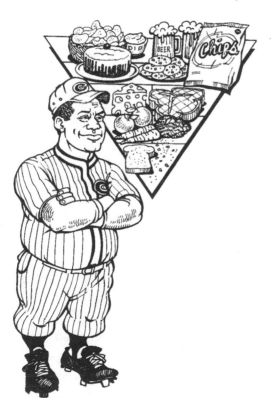

vestment when they prevent hunger. Most active people need and should eat snacks to keep them fueled throughout the day. Enjoy bagels, crackers, fruits, yogurt, and other handy energizers from the base of the Food Guide Pyramid as you desire, knowing they contribute to your nutrient needs for the day. If you choose to snack on sweets and treats, be sure to eat only a small amount from the tip of the pyramid, after you have climbed to the top by first eating basic foods. Otherwise, your diet will end up the shape of an upside down pyramid that topples your health and sports performance!

SNACKS, SWEETS, AND SNACK ATTACKS: THE BOTTOM LINE

Here are the key points you should remember about snacking:

- Snacks can be an important part of your training diet; they help prevent your becoming overwhelmingly hungry. Remember that when you get too hungry, you may not care about what you eat, and you may blow your good intentions on fat and goo.
- A sugary treat can fit into a well-balanced diet. There's nothing wrong with a cookie eaten for dessert after lunch. The nutrition problems arise when you have cookies for lunch.
- If you find yourself craving sweets, determine whether you've eaten adequate calories to support your activities. Chances are you've let yourself get too hungry. Sweet cravings are commonly a sign that you are physiologically ravenous.
- Prevent sweet cravings by eating more calories at breakfast and lunch (and plan an afternoon snack if you will be eating a late dinner) so that you curb the cookie monster that tends to arise in the late afternoon and evening. See chapter 14 for more information about calorie needs.
- Although a sugary snack before exercising may result in hypoglycemia and fatigue for a small percent of the population, pre-exercise sugar actually helps most athletes who need an energy boost.
- Sugar taken during exercise (about 100 to 300 calories per hour) enhances performance if you are working for longer than 60 to 90 minutes.

5
chapter

Super Bowls of Salads

Salads are popular among health-conscious, sports-active people. In summertime, salads are a welcome meal because you can toss almost any food into a bowl and create dinner in a hurry without slaving over a hot stove. Or you can stop by your favorite salad bar and enjoy a heaping, delicious lunch or dinner. Solo cooks often prefer to buy premade salads in a bag at their grocery stores. Although more expensive, these prechopped veggies save preparation time and sometimes money because of less waste from spoiled salad ingredients that linger in the refrigerator.

For Ginger, a traveling salesperson and squash player, salads offer the opportunity for a better-balanced diet. "I choose to eat at restaurants that have a salad bar brimming with all sorts of fresh veggies and fruits. This helps me compensate for my other hit-or-miss meals on the road. I may not get the recommended 5 servings of vegetables every day, but I do munch my way through a big bowl at least four days of the week."

Karin, a collegiate gymnast, also likes salads. "I hate the cafeteria food at my school, so I live on salads. I only wish their salads contained more than pale lettuce and squishy tomatoes." I reminded Karin that any vegetable is better than no vegetable. Salad vegetables do lose some nutritional value as they are exposed to air, but many nutrients remain. I also pointed out that a typical salad-bar meal can easily contain 1,000 calories, with 45 percent of those from fat. Many salad-eating exercisers complain of chronic fatigue because they are eating too few carbohydrates to fuel their muscles and support their sports programs. In a healthy sports salad, 60 to 70 percent of the calories should be from carbohydrates, and at most 25 percent from fat.

A New Leaf on Life

To create a high-energy sports salad that is the mainstay of your meal, use high-carbohydrate foods and limit the fats. The five tips in this section can help you get the most in your salad bowl.

Tip #1. Boost the Salad's Carbohydrate Content

Fill your sport salad with appropriate nutrition by adding

- carbohydrate-dense veggies such as corn, corn relish, peas, beets, and carrots;
- beans and legumes such as chick-peas, kidney beans, and three-bean salad;
- cooked rice, pasta, or potato chunks;
- orange sections, diced apple, raisins, banana slices, and berries;
- toasted croutons (limit your intake of buttered croutons that leave you with greasy fingers); and
- thick slices of whole grain bread and a glass of low-fat milk for accompaniments.

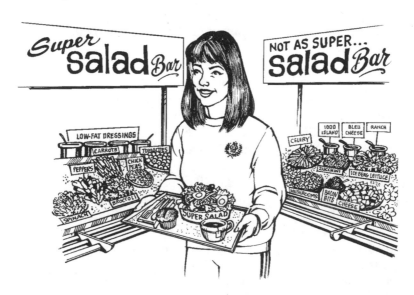

Tip #2. Choose Dark, Colorful Veggies

Salads radiant with red tomatoes, green peppers, orange carrots, and dark lettuces nutritionally surpass those made with paler lettuces, cucumbers, onions, celery, and radishes. For example, a salad made with spinach has seven times the vitamin C as one made with iceberg lettuce; dark romaine has twice the vitamin C. See table 5.1 for ranking salad fixings. Plus, colorful vegetables are brimming with the antioxidant nutrients and phytochemicals that protect your health.

In general, you should choose colorful veggies over pallid ones (see table 1.4). Exceptions include beets and corn; although colorful, they have fewer vitamins than their deeply colored peers. Nevertheless, beets and corn are good choices to boost the carbohydrate value of salads. Cauliflower, although colorless, is a good source of vitamin C (70 milligrams per cup, raw) and the cancer-protective nutrients found in the cruciferous vegetable family to which it belongs.

Tip #3. Reach for the Potassium

Salads easily can heighten your intake of potassium, a mineral that not only is lost in sweat but whose presence also protects against high blood pressure (see chapter 2). You should try to get at least 3,500 milligrams of potassium per day—an easy task for salad lovers. These are some of the veggies richest in potassium:

- Romaine, 4 large leaves (400 milligrams)
- Broccoli, 1 cup chopped, raw (380 milligrams)
- Tomato, 1 medium (370 milligrams)
- Carrot, 1 large (340 milligrams)

Tip #4. Include Adequate Protein

For a well-balanced, main-dish salad, boost the protein value by adding cottage cheese, flaked tuna, canned salmon, sliced turkey, chicken, or other lean meats. Be cautious of salami and cheeses because they can add excess saturated fat. If you prefer vegetarian proteins, include diced tofu, chick-peas, three-bean salad, walnuts, sunflower seeds, almonds, and peanuts.

Do remember that protein is an important part of a sports diet. Too often I counsel athletes who are so busy munching on salad greens and eating carbohydrates that they neglect their protein needs. They often end up anemic, injured, and chronically sick with colds or the flu. (See chapter 8).

Table 5.1   Ranking Salad Fixings

The Center for Science in the Public Interest (CSPI) has developed a system for ranking vegetables in order of their nutritional value and fiber content. In general, notice how the vegetables with more color also have more nutrients. Here's how some popular salad ingredients compare:

Ingredients	Score based on 6 nutrients and fiber
Red pepper, 1/2 medium raw	309
Carrot, 1 medium raw	171
Romaine or cos lettuce, 1 cup	141
Spinach, 1 cup raw	130
Green pepper, 1/2 raw	112
Parsley, 1/4 cup raw	97
Broccoli, 1/2 cup raw	91
Green peas, frozen, 1/2 cup	88
Endive, 1 cup raw	82
Tomato, 1/2 raw	76
Avocado, 1/2 California raw	71
Boston or bibb lettuce, 1 cup	59
Cauliflower, 1/2 cup raw	58
Green beans, 1/2 cup cooked	54
Celery, 1 medium stalk raw	50
Corn, 1/2 cup	50
Cabbage, 1/2 cup raw	43
Iceberg lettuce, 1 cup	40
Beets, 1/2 cup canned	32
Radishes, 1/4 cup raw	18
Cucumber, 1/2 cup raw	14
Onions, 1/4 cup raw	14
Mushrooms, 1/2 cup raw	12
Alfalfa sprouts, 1/2 cup raw	7

Copyright 1996, CSPI. Adapted from *Nutrition Action Healthletter* (1875 Connecticut Ave., N.W., Suite 300, Washington, D.C. 20009-5728. $24.00 for 10 issues).

Tip #5. Remember the Calcium

For calcium (and protein), add grated part skim mozzarella cheese; cubes of tofu; dressing made from plain yogurt seasoned with oregano, basil, and other Italian herbs; or a scoop of low-fat cottage cheese (a better

SUPER SPORTS SALAD VERSUS LOW-IMPACT SALAD

Low-impact salads are primarily pale lettuce drowned in salad dressing. Super sports salads are filled with colorful, vitamin-rich vegetables, carbohydrates, protein-rich beans, and a lite dressing.

Low-impact salad	Calories from carbohydrates	Total calories
3 cups iceberg lettuce	15	20
1/2 large tomato	20	25
5 tablespoons blue cheese dressing	—	400

Total: 445 calories, 10% from carbohydrate, 90% from fat

Sports salad	Calories from carbohydrates	Total calories
3 cups romaine lettuce	15	20
1/2 large tomato	20	25
1/2 green pepper	8	10
1/2 cup broccoli	15	20
1/2 carrot	17	20
1/3 cup chick-peas	80	115
1/2 cup three-bean salad	65	75
1/3 cup toasted croutons	70	80
2 tablespoons lite blue cheese dressing	10	70

Total: 435 calories, 70% from carbohydrate, 10% from fat

source of protein than calcium). Drink low-fat milk or skim milk along with the salad, or have a cup of yogurt for dessert. Do be sure to get a calcium-rich, well-balanced salad if salads are the mainstay of your diet. Don't try to live on lettuce alone!

SALAD SURPRISES

Chef Salad

15% CARBOHYDRATE • 65% FAT

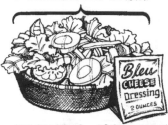

Bleu CHEESE Dressing 2 OUNCES

400 CALORIES • 28 GRAMS OF FAT

Quarter Pound Burger (NO CHEESE)

35% CARBOHYDRATE • 45% FAT

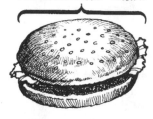

400 CALORIES • 20 GRAMS OF FAT

A bowlful of pale vegetables smothered in dressing offers little more than oil and crunch. A comparison of fat and carbohydrates in common fast foods may surprise you!

SALAD DRESSINGS

Salad dressings are an athlete's nemesis because they appease the appetite with fats rather than fuel the muscles with carbohydrates. A few ladles of blue cheese dressing can drown a small salad's healthfulness in 400 calories of fat. On a large salad, dressing can easily add 800 to 1,000 calories.

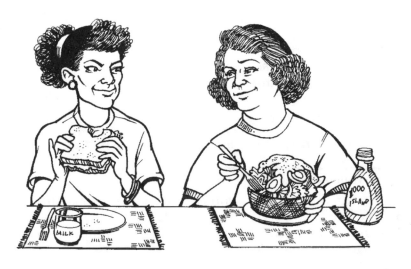

If you want to lose weight, calories from salad dressing can devastate a diet. Salad dressing fooled one gymnast, contributing to weight gain on her so-called reducing diet. When she traded in her supposedly fattening sandwich for a diet salad, she smothered her good intentions in 500 calories of oil. She would have been better off eating the sandwich or using less oil and more calorie-free vinegar.

I often advise my clients to educate themselves about salad dressing calories by measuring out the amount of dressing they normally use on a salad and adjusting it according to their nutrition game plan. Refer to table 5.2 for information about the calories in some popular dressings.

To transform a standard salad dressing into a reduced-fat version, simply dilute the dressing with extra vinegar, lemon juice, water, or milk in creamy dressings. By using only small amounts of this diluted version, you'll get lots of flavor and moistness with fewer calories. Put the dressing in a bottle with a shaker top so that it comes out slowly. One of my clients put it in a spray bottle. At restaurants, always request that the dressing be served on the side so you can control the amount you consume. Add the dressing sparingly, or dip the salad into the dressing before each bite.

Table 5.2   Salad Dressings

A few innocent ladles of salad dressing can transform a potentially healthful salad into a high-fat, nutritional nightmare. Even lite dressings have calories. Use them sparingly! A large salad can easily accommodate 6 tablespoons of dressing—an extra 60 to 650 calories that still count, whether or not it's fat free.

Dressing	Calories in 2 tablespoons	Fat (g)
Plain olive oil	240	26
Plain vinegar	5	—
Herbs, sprinkling	5	—
Blue cheese, Wishbone	170	17
Blue cheese, Wishbone fat-free	50	0
Ranch, Wishbone regular	160	17
Ranch, Wishbone lite	100	9
Ranch, Wishbone fat-free	40	0
Italian, Wishbone regular	100	10
Italian, Wishbone lite	15	.5
Italian, Wishbone fat-free	15	0

Nutrition information from food labels, March 1995.

There are excellent low-fat brands of salad dressing available that can help you reduce your fat and calorie intake without making you feel like a martyr. Diet dressings are very popular, but be forewarned: Even fat-free dressings have calories in them and should be used sparingly. At home you might want to create your own low-calorie, creamy dressing by adding a little blue cheese or Italian seasonings to plain low-fat yogurt. Or adventure into the world of exotic vinegars. Balsamic is one of my favorites.

Replacing these fat calories with more carbohydrates—an extra dinner roll or a baked potato—can improve your body's capacity for exercise. This also holds true for athletes who want to maintain or gain weight. Athletes who are eating generous amounts of olive oil (a heart-healthy fat) to boost their calorie intake should also be eating a foundation of carbohydrates to fuel their muscles.

THE WELL-DRESSED SALAD

Without a doubt, a properly designed and well-dressed salad can boost the nutritional value and healthfulness of your diet. Pile on the colorful veggies, but go easy on even the low-fat dressings. The bigger the bowlful, the more the nutrients. Keep on munching!

6
chapter

Meals Made Quick and Easy

A relaxing dinner—nicely prepared, attractively served, and shared with family and friends—is one of life's pleasures. But if you are like many of my clients, you arrive home after a hard workout, devour the handiest food in sight, and then feel disappointed in yourself for having eaten junk instead of a wholesome meal. Or you get sidetracked into restaurants because you are too tired and too hungry to cook. Restaurant eating, although more expensive, is a tempting alternative to confronting your own kitchen.

Athletes often come to me feeling dissatisfied with their poor dinner choices. They know they should be eating more nutritiously, but they routinely devour the pint of ice cream or frozen yogurt, munch out on pretzels, seek out the closest burger house, or dine on the handiest box of crackers in sight, opting for a quick fix rather than a wholesome, well-balanced meal that grandmother might have cooked.

DINING IN: FOUR TIPS FOR BETTER MEALS

The following tips can help you plan better sports meals at home. Even noncooks can pull together a high-carbohydrate, low-fat sports dinner without much time or effort. The recipes in part IV offer tried-and-true menu suggestions. Here are some additional tips.

Tip #1. Don't Arrive Home Too Hungry

One prerequisite to successful nighttime dining is to eat a hearty lunch or an afternoon snack. As I explained in chapters 3 and 4, this prevents you from attacking the refrigerator the minute you walk in the house in the evening.

> Jack, a triathlete, felt both frustration and a sense of failure because he rarely had energy to prepare a nice dinner. "It's generally eight or nine o'clock by the time I finish my evening workout. At that point, I'm too famished to cook a well-balanced meal. I simply munch on whatever's around. Some days this means a box of crackers. Other days, it's a bag of chips. I know this is bad, but I'm just too hungry to care."

I found a very simple solution to Jack's problem: eat a bigger meal at lunch rather than wait until evening. At that point in his day, he has easy access to good food in the cafeteria, he has time to eat, and he could save himself the hassle of cooking at night by swapping dinner with lunch.

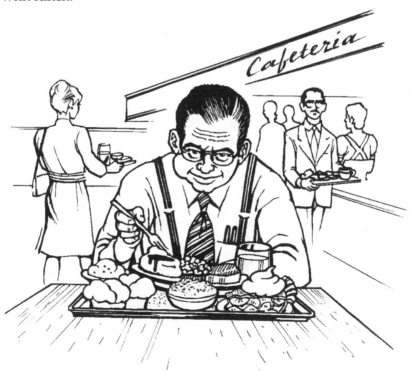

In one day, Jack discovered that the hearty noon meal contributed not only to a higher quality evening workout but also to the energy and mind-set he needed to prepare a more nourishing supper.

Other people have alleviated the I'm-too-hungry-to-cook problem simply by eating a substantial afternoon snack. A four o'clock cup of yogurt for a snack can prevent a six o'clock quart of ice cream for dinner.

Tip #2. Plan Time to Food Shop

Good nutrition starts in the grocery store. By stocking your kitchen shelves and freezer with a variety of wholesome foods that are ready and waiting, you will be more likely to eat a better dinner.

Kirsten, a 24-year-old dental assistant and swimmer, used to spend most of her food budget in restaurants on the way home from work because at home she faced bare cupboards and an empty refrigerator. Although she liked to cook, she rarely did so because she simply didn't plan the time to grocery shop. "Anyway, my schedule is so unpredictable. I often dine out with friends on the spur of the moment. When I do stock up on groceries, the meats and vegetables generally spoil before I get around to cooking them."

I advised Kirsten to stock her freezer with individually wrapped chicken breasts, lean hamburger patties, turkey burgers, and frozen vegetables—particularly vitamin-rich broccoli, spinach, and winter squash. Freezing does not destroy a food's nutritional value, so frozen foods provide quick nutrition with less fuss and waste than fresh items do. The frozen broccoli provides far more nutrients than the wilted, five-day-old stalks that Kirsten occasionally dragged from her refrigerator.

Once she had stocked her kitchen with frozen foods and other staples, Kirsten discovered that she liked to come home for dinner. Her staples included the following items.

Carbohydrates

- Pasta, rice, noodles, and potatoes. Kirsten got into the habit of cooking big batches of rice or pasta. She quickly reheated some the next day by plunging it into boiling water for a minute. She reheated baked potatoes in the microwave.
- Whole grain crackers and breads, including bagels and pita. Kirsten stored the breads in the freezer and quickly thawed them in the toaster or microwave oven.

- Tortillas for making burritos with refried beans and grated low-fat cheese
- Hot and cold cereals for a nontraditional dinner

Vegetables and Fruits

- Frozen broccoli, spinach, and winter squash
- Spaghetti sauce for pasta or for English muffin pizzas
- Salsa for burritos
- Tomato and vegetable juice
- Frozen orange juice

Protein

- Canned clams to toss into pasta. Clams are easy to fix and they are also a great source of zinc. This mineral, important for healing, had been lacking in Kirsten's semivegetarian diet.
- Canned fish for handy, no-cook meals. Tuna sandwiches, salmon on stoned wheat crackers, and sardines with toast provided not only protein but also iron.
- Vegetarian refried beans for burritos and atop baked potatoes
- Tofu for adding to salads, spaghetti sauce, and soups

Dairy Products

- Part skim mozzarella cheese, low-fat cottage and other cheeses, yogurt, and nonfat milk powder. Kirsten could then eat low-fat cheese, wheat crackers, and V-8 juice for a well balanced but lazy meal when she had no desire to cook; or, she could top off a microwaved potato with low-fat cottage cheese; roll up a burrito with beans, cheese, and salsa; mix yogurt with muesli for a main course or dessert.

Table 6.1 lists some of the foods I keep stocked, along with menu suggestions using these staples.

Tip #3. Plan Cook-a-Thons

Laura, a 48-year-old tennis player and stockbroker, enjoyed cooking on the weekends when she had the time. She always created a big batch of something on Sunday so it would be waiting for her when she arrived home tired and hungry after work and workouts.

Table 6.1   Stocking Up on Good Nutrition

I always stock basic foods that won't spoil quickly. On days when I arrive home to an empty refrigerator, I can either pull together a no-cook meal or quickly prepare a hot dinner. Some of my standard menus include these items:

- English muffin pizzas
- Stoned wheat crackers, peanut butter, and milk
- Lentil soup with extra broccoli, leftover pasta, and a sprinkling of Parmesan
- Refried beans and cheese rolled in a tortilla and heated in the microwave
- Tuna sandwich with tomato soup
- Bran cereal with banana and raisins

My standard ingredients:

Cupboard	Refrigerator	Freezer
Spaghetti	Low-fat cheese	English muffins
Rice	Grated Parmesan	Pita bread
Ramen noodles	Low-fat cottage cheese	Multigrain bread
Potatoes	Low-fat yogurt	Bagels
Wheat crackers	Low-fat milk	Broccoli
RyKrisp crackers	Eggs	Winter squash
Pretzels	Oranges	Spinach
Spaghetti sauce	Bananas	Chicken breasts
Minced clams	Carrots	Ground turkey
Tuna	V-8 juice	Extra-lean hamburger
Canned salmon	Tortillas	Orange juice
Kidney beans		concentrate
Vegetarian refried beans		
Soups (lentil, tomato)		
Peanut butter		
Bran flakes		
Oat bran		
Muesli		
Raisins		

When creating a dinner from these staples, I choose items from three of the five food groups, using carbohydrates as the foundation for each meal. The following are sample 650 calorie, 60% carbohydrate, well-balanced meals, with no cooking!

(continued)

Table 6.1 *(continued)*

Food group	Menu #1: Crackers with tuna	Menu #2 Sandwich
1. Grain	8 stoned wheat crackers	2 slices branola bread
2. Protein	1/2 can tuna with 1 tablespoon lite mayo	2 tablespoons peanut butter
3. Fruit		1/4 cup raisins
4. Vegetable	12-ounce can V-8 juice	1 raw carrot
5. Dairy	1 cup fruit yogurt	1 cup low-fat milk

Food group	Menu #3: Pizza	Menu #4 Burrito
1. Grain	2 English muffins	2 flour tortillas
2. Protein	(cheese)	1/2 cup vegetarian refried beans
3. Fruit	1 cup orange juice	Apple
4. Vegetable	3/4 cup spaghetti sauce	Chopped tomatoes
5. Dairy	2 ounces mozzarella cheese	Shredded low-fat cheddar cheese

The portions are appropriate for an active woman who needs about 1,800-2,000 calories per day; a hungry man may want more.

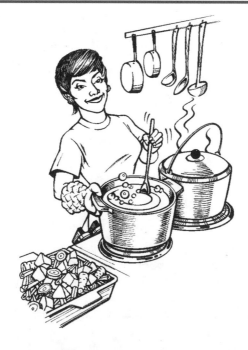

She preferred convenience to variety and thrived well on chili, chili, chili for a week; then curry, curry, curry the next week; goulash, goulash, goulash, and so on. When Laura couldn't face another repetitious dinner, she cooked something else and put the leftovers in the freezer. She preferred this monotonous but nutritious alternative to her previous habit of dining on frozen yogurt by the quart.

Tip #4. Add Variety to Your Pasta Meals

Peter, a 24-year-old runner cooked only one kind of dinner: pasta. He'd eat plain pasta seven days a week, taking pride in his high-carbohydrate, low-fat diet. He thought pasta was a "super food."

Pasta in any shape—spaghetti, ziti, twists, whatever—is without question a very popular meal among sports-active people, even those who dislike cooking. Although carbohydrate-rich pasta does provide muscle fuel ("gas" for your body's engine), pasta is a marginal source of vitamins and minerals (the "spark plugs" needed for top performance). Pasta is made from refined white flour with a few vitamins added back to replace those lost during processing. Whole wheat pastas offer little nutritional superiority, because wheat (and other grains, in general) are better respected for their carbohydrate value than their vitamin density. Even spinach and tomato pastas are overrated; they contain very little of the vegetables.

Pasta becomes a nutritional powerhouse when it is topped with tomato sauce, spinach and garlic sauce, or vegetables. I advised Peter to buy jars of spaghetti sauce to eat on his pasta, and to cook frozen broccoli, spinach, or green peppers to accompany it. He also needed to boost the protein content of his dinner. Canned beans, cottage cheese, or tuna were easy additions. I reminded Peter about the Food Guide Pyramid (chapter 1), and the value of eating at least three out of five food groups with each meal. Peter made the appropriate changes, and a month later reported how much better he felt. "Plus, I'm enjoying the variety. I was getting bored with yet another plate of plain ol' spaghetti."

DINING OUT

Some people enjoy eating in restaurants; others eat in restaurants because they have no choice. Art, a 54-year-old mountain biker and businessman, yearns for homecooked meals, but due to the nature of his work, he spends most of his evenings entertaining clients in the finest restaurants. Professional teams, such as the Boston Celtics, who travel from city to city often struggle with restaurant eating. After a hard evening game, the players may want nothing more than a friendly, homecooked meal, but instead are often stuck in a hotel, challenged to find some healthy food at late hours of the night. Between jet lag, irregular meals, and night games, they have a tough time maintaining a high-carbohydrate sports diet that fuels and refuels their muscles for repeated hard exercise.

Every sports-active person who relies on restaurants for a balanced, high-carbohydrate diet faces the challenge of finding adequate carbohydrates among all the rich temptations, and each has pestered waiters for special requests at one time or another. Unfortunately, many people select whatever's fast and happens to tempt their tastebuds at the moment, particularly when they are tired, hungry, stressed, anxious, or lonely.

Traveling athletes also have the second challenge of keeping themselves well hydrated. Carrying a personal water supply is a good idea, especially on planes, where the environment is very dry and water availability is somewhat limited.

Selecting the Right Restaurant

Here are a few suggestions for successfully selecting high-carbohydrate, low-fat restaurant meals with plenty of fluids. The most important first step is to patronize the restaurants that offer healthful sports foods; don't go to a steak house if you're looking for spaghetti. Study the menu before you sit down to see if the restaurant offers pasta, baked potatoes, bread, juices, and other high-carbohydrate foods. Try to avoid the places that have only fried items. Also check to see if they allow special requests. If the menu clearly states "no substitutions," you might be in the wrong place.

When you're in an appropriate restaurant, choose your foods wisely. In general, you should request foods that are baked, broiled, roasted, or steamed—anything but fried. Low-fat poultry and fish items tend to be better choices than items naturally high in fat, such as prime rib, cheese, sausage, and duck.

Low-Fat and Healthful Restaurant Choices

Keep the following foods in mind as you peruse a menu.

• **Appetizers.** Tomato juice, fruit juice, fruit cocktail, melon, and crackers make great starters for your meal.

• **Breads.** Unbuttered rolls and breads are great; ask for extras! If the standard fare is buttered (as in garlic bread) request some plain bread also, and enjoy the buttery bread in moderation.

• **Soups.** Broth-based soups (such as vegetable, chicken and rice, and Chinese soups) and hearty minestrone, split pea, navy bean, and lentil soups can be good sources of carbohydrates and are more healthful than creamy chowders and bisques. They are also a source of fluids.

• **Salads.** Enjoy the veggies, but limit the chunks of cheese, bacon bits, grated cheese, olives, and other high-fat toppings. Be extra generous with chick-peas and toasted croutons. (For additional information on salads, see chapter 5.)

• **Salad dressings.** Always request that the dressing be served on the side so you can control how much you use. You want to fill up on carbohydrates, not on oily dressings. (See chapter 5.)

• **Seafood and poultry.** Request chicken or fish that's baked, roasted, steamed, stir-fried, or broiled. Because many chefs add a lot of butter when broiling foods such as fish, you might want to request that your entrée be broiled dry—that is, cooked without this extra fat. If the entrée is sautéed, request that the chef sauté it with very little butter or oil and add no extra fat before serving.

• **Beef.** Many restaurants pride themselves on serving huge slabs of beef or one-pound steaks. If you order beef, plan to cut this double portion in half and take the rest home for tomorrow's dinner, share it with a companion (who has ordered accordingly), or simply leave it. Trim all the visible fat, and request that any gravy or sauce be served on the side so that you can use it sparingly, if at all. Your goal is to eat meat as the accompaniment to the meal, not as the focus. Your muscles will perform better if you fuel them with more carbohydrate-rich potatoes, vegetables, breads, and juices.

• **Potatoes.** Order extra to make this the mainstay of your dinner! Baked potatoes are a great source of carbohydrates, unless the chef loads them up with butter or sour cream. Request that these toppings be served on the side so you can control how much you eat. Better yet, trade those fat calories for more carbohydrates. Add moistness by mashing the potato with some milk (special request). This may sound a bit messy, but it's a delicious, low-fat way to enjoy what might otherwise be a dry potato.

• **Pasta.** Pile it on! Pick pasta served with tomato sauces (carbohydrates) rather than the high-fat cheese, oil, or cream sauces. Also be cautious of cheese-filled lasagna, tortellini, and manicotti. They tend to be high-fat choices.

• **Rice.** In a Chinese restaurant, you'll be better off filling up on an extra bowl of plain rice, another good source of carbohydrates, than on eggrolls or other fried appetizers.

INTERNATIONAL CARBOHYDRATES

Ethnic restaurants offer an abundance of carbohydrates in the form of rice, couscous, lentils, beans, and breads. The following list will help you choose high-carbohydrate foods in Mexican and Chinese restaurants.

Carbohydrates Chinese style

1. Request that your food be either steamed or stir-fried with minimal oil.
2. Order extra servings of boiled rice, pancakes (that come with moo shu dishes), lo mein (noodles), with minimal oil.
3. Choose stir-fried rather than deep-fried items (often described as "crispy" or "dipped in batter").
4. Limit oily-looking sauces. Sweet and sour sauce is fine; just request it on stir-fried rather than on deep-fried dishes.

Sample high-carbohydrate meals

Menu #1	Menu #2
Egg drop soup	Wonton soup
Chicken chop suey	Steamed Peking ravioli
Rice, boiled (double serving)	Moo shu chicken with extra pancakes
Fortune cookies	Pineapple chunks

Carbohydrates Mexican style

1. Carbohydrate-rich choices include rice, beans, tortillas, and bean soups.
2. Request plain, not fried, tortillas with tostados.
3. Request less cheese in enchiladas, tacos, and other entrées, when possible.
4. Bean dishes are sometimes loaded with lard. Be cautious!

Sample high-carbohydrate meals	
Menu #1	**Menu #2**
Bean burrito (with less cheese)	Lime soup
Rice, large serving	Chicken enchilada with less cheese
Tortilla chips (only a few!)	Beans and rice
Salsa	Plain tortillas

• **Vegetables.** Request plain, unbuttered veggies with any special sauces (hollandaise, lemon butter) served on the side.

• **Chinese food.** Plain rice with stir-fry combinations such as chicken with veggies, or beef with broccoli are the best choices. You can request that the food be cooked with very little oil.

• **Dessert.** Sherbet, low-fat frozen yogurt, and fruit are among the best choices for your sports diet. Fresh fruit is often available, even if it isn't listed on the menu. If you can't resist a decadent dessert, just be sure that you enjoy it *after* you eat plenty of carbohydrates. That is, don't have a carbohydrate-poor dinner to save room for a high-fat dessert.

Restaurant Savvy

When you are faced with a meal that's all wrong for you, try to make the best of a tough situation. For example, you can scoop the sour cream off the potato, drain the dressing from the salad, scrape off the gravy, or remove the fried batter from the chicken.

You can also top off a carbohydrate-poor meal with your own high-carbohydrate after dinner snacks, such as fig bars, a bagel, pretzels, animal crackers, a banana, graham crackers, dried pineapple, raisins, and juice boxes. Pack these emergency foods along with you. However, also try to make special requests. Remember, you are the boss when it comes to restaurant eating. The restaurant's job is to serve you the high-carbohydrate, low-fat foods that enhance your sports diet. Bon appetit!

FAST FOODS: THE GOOD, THE BAD, AND THE BALANCE

Every day, one out of five Americans takes advantage of the convenience offered by quick-service restaurants. The omnipotence of the fast-food industry has led some kids to believe that the five basic food groups are McDonald's, Wendy's, Taco Bell, Pizza Hut, and KFC! Fortunately for our health, today's quick-service food centers are offering more and more healthful, low-fat options, but the original high-fat fare still has a strong attraction. Fatty foods are best sellers, as confirmed by the strong sales of Big Macs (26 grams fat) but relatively weak sales of the now discontinued McLean Deluxe burgers (12 grams fat).

Eating at a quick-service restaurant is like visiting Fat City. You have an easy opportunity to select a dietary disaster and choose items that are high in saturated fat and calories, but low in carbohydrates, fiber, fruits, and vegetables. The occasional burger and fries meal is of little health concern. But if fast foods are a common part of your sports diet, you must balance out your day's intake with wholesome, nutritious choices. You should also plan in supplemental carbohydrates for fueling up before hard exercise and refueling afterwards.

Fast Foods That Fuel

The trick in eating at quick-service restaurants is to look for the high-carbohydrate cuisine. If you do get sidetracked to the grease, be sure to balance the rest of the day's remaining meals with wholesome, lower fat choices. Here are some suggestions to enhance your sports diet.

Breakfast

• Rather than egg, bacon, sausage, croissant, or biscuit combinations, choose pancakes, hot or cold cereal, juice, unbuttered bagels, English muffins, or other (low-fat) muffins. Spread toast with jelly or jam for extra carbohydrates, but go easy on the butter.

• Because fresh fruits can be hard to find on the menu, remember to carry some with you. An apple or a box of raisins travels well and fits nicely into a pocket.

• Treat yourself to hot cocoa for a higher carbohydrate choice than coffee.

• Find a deli with fresh bagels, fruit, juice, and yogurt.

• If you are staying at a hotel, save yourself time, money, and temptation by bringing your own cereal and raisins (and spoon). Bring powdered milk or buy a half pint of low-fat or skim milk at the corner store. A water glass or milk carton can double as a cereal bowl.

Lunch and Dinner

• Any way you look at them, burgers and french fries have a high-fat content. You'll be better off going to an eatery that offers more than just burgers. Find a menu that offers thick-crust pizza, chili, spaghetti, soups (brothy or beany ones), roast or grilled chicken meals with mashed potatoes, rice, vegetables, and salad bars complete with kidney beans, chick-peas, and bread.

• If you do order a burger, request a second roll or extra bread. Squish the grease into the first roll, then replace it with the fat-free roll. Boost carbohydrates with beverages such as juice, soft drinks, or low-fat shakes. Pack supplemental carbohydrates, such as pretzels or fig bars.

• Better than a burger, satisfy your hankering for red meat with a lean roast beef sandwich from a deli, Arby's, or Roy Rogers. For 260 calories, you can buy a Burger King hamburger (10 grams of fat) or a Roy Rogers Roast Beef sandwich (only 4 grams of fat).

• Beware of grilled chicken sandwiches if they come with a special sauce. The 29 grams of fat in the BK Broiler sandwich makes it as fatty as a fried chicken sandwich. Wipe that mayo off!

• Meals with chicken that is roasted or grilled are generally preferable to fried chicken meals. If you do order fried chicken, get the larger pieces, remove all the skin, and eat just the meat. Order extra rolls, biscuits with honey or jam, corn on the cob, and other vegetables for more carbohydrates.

Even though roasted chicken is preferable to fried, be aware that the skin is still very fatty. For example, by removing the skin and wing from a KFC Rotisserie Gold quarter breast, you remove 13 grams of fat and 115 calories. Although many of the accompaniments are butter ladened, any vegetable tends to be better than no vegetable. A 2/3-cup serving of Boston Market's mashed potatoes has 8 grams of fat, the creamed spinach is 75 percent fat, and the squash is 38 percent fat. The gravy, on the other hand, is relatively low in fat (1 gram per 2 tablespoons gravy). Surprise!

• At a salad bar, be generous with the colorful vegetables and hearty breads, but be careful to choose fat-free or lite dressings. (See chapter 5 for more salad information). Also note that a Caesar salad is not a dieter's delight. For example, Boston Market's Chicken Caesar Salad with 4 tablespoons of dressing totals 670 calories; two-thirds are from fat (47 grams). You'd have been better off eating a chicken breast (remove the skin and wing), corn bread, steamed vegetables, and whole kernel corn for 80 fewer calories and only 15 grams of fat.

• Resist the temptation to choose baked potatoes smothered with cheese sauce and high-fat toppings. Wendy's cheese-stuffed potato, for example, gets 35 percent of its calories from fat (23 grams, almost 6 teaspoons of butter). The chili and cheese topping isn't any better at 36 percent fat (24 grams).

Your best bet is to order an extra plain potato and split the broccoli and cheese topping (14 grams of fat) between the two. That way, you end up with a hearty 770 calorie, high-carbohydrate meal, with only 15 percent of the calories from fat. For additional protein, drink a glass of low-fat milk.

• Order thick-crust pizza that has extra crust rather than extra cheese. The more dough, the more carbohydrates. For example, a slice of Pizza Hut's pan pizza has 10 grams more carbohydrates than a slice of their thin pizza does. Pile on veggies (green peppers, mushrooms, onions) but shy away from the pepperoni, sausage, and hamburger.

• Seek out the deli that offers wholesome breads. Request a sandwich that emphasizes the bread rather than the filling. A large submarine roll provides far more carbohydrates than half a small pita. Hold the mayo, and add moistness with lite salad dressings (if available), mustard or ketchup, sliced tomatoes, and lettuce. The lowest fat fillings are turkey, ham, and lean roast beef.

• Hearty bean soups accompanied by crackers, plain bread, an English muffin, or corn bread provide a satisfying, carbohydrate-rich, low-fat meal. Chili, if not glistening with a layer of grease, can be a good choice. For example, a Wendy's large chili with eight saltines provides a satisfying 400 calories, and only 25 percent are from fat (11 grams). Taco Bell's bean burritos are another bargain.

Yes, you can eat a high-carbohydrate sports diet, even if you are eating fast foods. You simply need to balance the fats with the carbohydrates. Table 6.2 provides some appropriate choices.

CARBS TO CARRY

Whether you are on the team bus or on a budget that requires you to eat at quick-service restaurants, be sure to pack your gym bag with portable carbohydrates to supplement the fattier fare. Some easy-to-tote choices include:

Bagels	Dried apricots
Crackers	Raisins
Pretzels	Fresh fruit (apples, oranges, bananas)
Fig Newtons	Juices (single serving
Pop-Tarts	containers)
Breakfast cereals	Trail mix or granola
(single-servings)	with dried fruits

Table 6.2   Sample High-Carbohydrate Fast-Food Menus

The optimal sports diet gets 60 to 70 percent of its calories from carbohydrates. At quick-service restaurants, you can very easily consume a suboptimal 40- to 50-percent carbohydrate diet, because fatty foods are readily available, inexpensive, and often tempting. Hence, you have to plan ahead, bring wholesome snacks with you, and make special requests when possible.

The following menus are sample sports meals that offer at least 60 percent carbohydrates. Some of the food items (such as soft drinks) are not generally recommended as a part of an optimal daily diet, but they can be incorporated into a meal on the road from time to time.

The purpose of these sample meals is simply to give you an idea of what a 60-percent carbohydrate diet looks like, so you can use it to guide your food choices. The menus are appropriate for active women and men who need 2,000 to 2,600 or more calories per day. *For extra carbohydrates, eat more of the foods in italics.*

Meal	Item	Total calories
Breakfast		
McDonald's	*Orange juice*, 6 ounces	85
	Pancakes with syrup	420
	English muffin with jelly	155
Total: 660 calories, 85% carbohydrates		
Dunkin' Donuts	*Bran muffin, large*	300
	Chocolate milk	150
Total: 450 calories, 70% carbohydrates		
Family restaurant	*Apple juice*, large (10 ounces)	145
	Raisin bran, 2 small boxes	220
	1% milk, 8 ounces	110
	Sliced banana, medium-large	135
Total: 610 calories, 90% carbohydrates		
Lunch		
Sub shop	Turkey sub, no mayo	590
	Cranapple juice (8 ounces)	160
Total: 750 calories, 60% carbohydrates		
Wendy's	*Baked potato*, plain	310
	Chili, large (12 ounces)	300
	Frosty Dairy Dessert, small	340
Total: 950 calories, 70% carbohydrates		
Salad bar	Lettuce, 1 cup	15
	Green pepper, 1/2	10
	Broccoli, 1/2 cup	20
	Carrots, 1/2 cup	20

(continued)

Table 6.3   *(continued)*

Meal	Item	Total calories
	Tomato, large	50
	Chick-peas, 1/2 cup	160
	Feta cheese, 1 ounce	75
	Italian dressing, 2 tablespoons	100
	Bread, 1-inch slice	200
Total: 650 calories, 60% carbohydrates		
Dinner		
Pizza	Cheese pan pizza, 2 slices	500
	Large cola, 12 ounces (no ice)	150
Total: 650 calories, 60% carbohydrates		
Italian restaurant	*Minestrone soup*, 1 cup	90
	Spaghetti, 2 cups	400
	Tomato sauce, 2/3 cup	120
	Parmesan cheese, 1 tablespoon	30
	Rolls, 2 large	280
Total: 920 calories, 75% carbohydrates		
Family restaurant	Turkey, 5 ounces white meat	250
	Stuffing, 1 cup	200
	Mashed potato, 1/2 cup	100
	Peas, 2/3 cup	70
	Cranberry sauce, 1/4 cup	100
	Orange juice, 8 ounces	110
	Sherbet, 1 scoop	120
Total: 950 calories, 65% carbohydrates		

Some Last Words About Supper

Active people commonly eat a huge dinner as a result of having eaten too little during the day. If this sounds familiar, experiment with reorganizing your good nutrition game plan so that you put more emphasis on breakfast and lunch as a means of fueling up and remaining fueled throughout the busy day. Use the evening meal as a time to refuel, but whenever possible keep it relatively equal in size to breakfast and lunch. As Hank, a college basketball player said, "I used to stuff myself at night and feel lousy. Now I eat breakfast like a king, lunch like a prince, and dinner like a pauper. I've found that by eating this way, I have lots of energy for basketball practice in the afternoon, and I'm not that hungry afterward. I eat a lighter dinner and sleep much better. I feel much better overall."

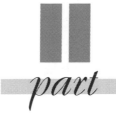

part

Sports Nutrition for Success

chapter

Carbs to Go
and Keep Going

Without question, carbohydrates are the best choices for fueling your muscles and promoting good health. People of all ages and athletic abilities, from elite runners to spectators, should nourish themselves with a wholesome, high-carbohydrate, adequate protein, low-fat diet.

Unfortunately, confusion about carbohydrates, what they are and how much to eat, keep people from properly balancing their sports diet. As one runner put it, "I know I should eat carbohydrates for muscle fuel, but which are best? How much is too much? Does it matter if I choose fruits, vegetables, sugar, refined flour, or brown rice?" Like many active people, he was confused by this seemingly complex subject.

The purpose of this chapter is to eliminate this confusion so you can make choices that best promote your health, desired weight, and performance.

SIMPLE SUGARS

The carbohydrate family includes both simple and complex carbohydrates. The simple ones are monosaccharides and disaccharides (single and double sugar molecules). Glucose, fructose, and galactose are the simplest sugars and can be symbolized like this:

The disaccharides can be symbolized like this:

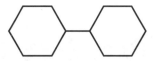

Three common disaccharides include table sugar (sucrose, a combination of glucose and fructose), milk sugar (lactose, a combination of glucose and galactose), and corn syrup (a combination of glucose and fructose commonly used in soft drinks). These are converted into glucose molecules before entering the bloodstream to provide fuel for the body.

Table sugar, honey, and corn syrup contain glucose and fructose but in different forms. Table sugar is a disaccharide that is converted into monosaccharides: 50 percent glucose and 50 percent fructose. The high fructose type of corn syrup used in soft drinks breaks down to about 55 percent fructose and 45 percent glucose. Honey coverts into 31 percent glucose, 38 percent fructose, 10 percent other sugars, 17 percent water, and 4 percent miscellaneous particles. Table 7.1 describes the types of sugars found in some fruits and vegetables.

Table 7.1   Natural Sugars in Some Fruits and Vegetables

Fruits and vegetables contain mixtures of different types of sugars. All sugars are converted into glucose before being used for energy.

Food	Glucose	Fructose (% of total solids)	Sucrose
Apple	7	40	25
Grape	35	40	12
Peach	7	10	55
Carrot	7	7	35
Green bean	15	15	3
Tomato	20	25	—

Data from E. Sweeney (Ed.), 1977, *The food that stays: An update on nutrition, diet, sugar and calories.* (New York: Med Com, Inc.)

Some athletes mistakenly think that honey is nutritionally superior to refined white sugar. If you prefer honey because of the pleasant taste, fine. But it's not superior for health or performance. Sugar in any form—honey, brown sugar, raw sugar, maple syrup, or jelly—has insignificant amounts of vitamins or minerals, and your body digests any type of sugar or carbohydrate into glucose before using it for fuel. Table 7.2 compares the nutritional value of some sugars.

A third type of sugar that has entered the sports market is the glucose polymer. Polymers are chains of about five glucose molecules. Sports drinks sweetened with polymers can provide more energy value with less sweetness than regular sugar provides.

Table 7.2   Nutritional Value of Sugar

Although natural sugars may have a bit more nutritional value than refined white sugar, sugars are insignificant sources of vitamins or minerals. The exception would be molasses in large amounts.

	Calories (per Tbsp)	Calcium (mg)	Iron (mg)	Riboflavin (mg)
White	48	—	—	—
Brown	52	12	0.3	trace
Honey	64	—	0.1	—
Molasses	53	40	0.6	trace
RDI		1,000	18	1.7

Nutrient data from J. Pennington, 1992, *Bowes & Church's Food Values of Portions Commonly Used*, 16th ed. (Philadelphia: Lippincott).

COMPLEX CARBOHYDRATES

Complex carbohydrates, such as starch in plant foods and glycogen in muscles, are formed when sugars link together to form long, complex chains, similar to a string of hundreds of pearls. They can be symbolized like this:

Plants store extra sugars in the form of starch. For example, corn, which is sweet when it's young, becomes starchy as it gets older. Its

Steps of Digestion: Food Into Fuel

Mouth: Starches are partially digested by saliva in the mouth. The swallowed food goes down the esophagus into the stomach.

START

Liver: Receives digested food components and stores extra glucose to be released into the bloodstream for future use.

Stomach: The chewed food is liquified with gastric juices and ground down into smaller particles. Protein is broken into amino acids. The food gradually empties into the small intestine, where the nutrients become available to the body. Water can empty from the stomach at the rate of about 1 quart per hour; solid foods take longer. Emptying time depends on caloric density.

Small intestine: Starches break into simple sugars; protein is further digested into amino acids, and fat into fatty acids. These digestive products are then absorbed into the blood—stream and either used or transported to the liver. The indigestible waste products move into the large intestine.

Large intestine: Receives indigestible waste products, reabsorbs water and minerals, and excretes waste as feces.

extra sugar converts into starch. In contrast to corn and other vegetables, fruits tend to convert starches into sugars as they ripen. A good example is the banana:

- A green banana with some yellow is 80 percent starch and 7 percent sugar.
- A mostly yellow banana is 25 percent starch and 65 percent sugar.
- A spotted and speckled banana is 5 percent starch and 90 percent sugar.

The potatoes, rice, bread, and other starches that you eat get digested into glucose, then either burned for energy or stored for future use. Humans store extra glucose mostly in the form of muscle glycogen and liver glycogen. This glycogen is readily available for energy during exercise.

Sugars and starches have similar abilities to fuel muscles but different abilities to nourish them with vitamins and minerals:

- The carbohydrates in sugary soft drinks provide energy but no vitamins or minerals.
- The carbohydrates in polymer drinks provide energy but no vitamins or minerals, unless the drink is fortified.
- The carbohydrates in wholesome fruits, vegetables, and grains provide energy, vitamins, and minerals—the fuel and spark plugs that your engine needs to function best.

QUICK AND SLOW CARBS

Athletes used to be told to choose starchy complex carbohydrates such as bagels, potatoes, and bread for pre-exercise snacks because these foods were thought to contribute to a stable blood sugar level. Sugary simple carbohydrates, in contrast, were thought to trigger a "sugar high" followed by a "sugar low" and a debilitating hypoglycemic reaction. (See chapter 4 to learn how this is not usually the case.)

Today we know that a carbohydrate's effect on blood sugar cannot be determined by whether it is a simple or complex carbohydrate. Instead, it's determined by its glycemic response, or the food's ability to contribute glucose to the bloodstream. A food's glycemic response is influenced by many factors, including the amount eaten, fiber content, amount of added fat, and the way the food is prepared. By ranking foods according to their ability to elevate blood sugar, nutrition professionals have developed a glycemic index. A baked potato has a higher glycemic effect than a boiled potato; wheat made into bread has a higher glycemic effect than wheat made into pasta; plain sugar has a higher glycemic effect than sugar combined with fat, such as ice cream or cookies.

The glycemic index was originally designed to help people with diabetes closely control their blood sugars. Because people with diabetes tend to eat foods in meal combinations that buffer the individual glycemic responses, the glycemic index becomes less predictive for them. Athletes, however, tend to eat a singular food for a sports snack and can perhaps gain greater benefit from this ranking system that determines whether you should eat a food before, during, or after exercise.

High-glycemic-index carbohydrates (potatoes, corn flakes, honey) quickly enter the bloodstream, and are best to eat during or after exercise. Low-to-moderate glycemic-index foods (rice, pasta, bananas) slowly enter the bloodstream and are desirable before exercise because they provide sustained energy. Low-glycemic foods may eliminate the need for consuming carbohydrates during long-term exercise to maintain normal blood sugar levels.

Table 7.3 lists the glycemic index of some popular sports foods. See chapters 10 and 11 for additional information about foods before, during, and after exercise.

Table 7.3   Glycemic Index of Some Popular Foods

Food*	GI	Food*	GI
High			
Glucose	100	Mars Bar	68
Gatorade	91	Grape-Nuts	67
Potato, baked	85	Stoned wheat thins	67
Corn flakes	84	Cream of Wheat,	
Rice cakes	82	regular	66
Potato, microwaved	82	Couscous	65
Jelly beans	80	Table sugar (sucrose)	65
Vanilla wafers,		Raisins	64
Nabisco	77	Oatmeal	61
Cheerios	74		(42-75)
Cream of Wheat,		Ice cream	61
instant	74		(36-80)
Graham crackers	74	**Moderate**	
Honey	73	Muffin, bran	60
Watermelon	72	Bran Chex	58
Bagel, Lender's white	72	Orange juice	57
Bread, white	70	Potato, boiled	56
Bread, whole wheat	69	Rice, white long grain	56
	(65-75)	Rice, brown	55
Shredded wheat	69	Popcorn	55
Soft drink, Fanta	68	Corn	55

Food*	GI	Food*	GI
Moderate, *continued*			
Sweet potato	54	PowerBar	30-35
Pound cake, Sara Lee	54	Chocolate milk	34
Banana, overripe	52	Fruit yogurt, low-fat	33
Peas, green	48	Chick-peas	33
Bulgur	48	P R Bar	33
Baked beans	48	Lima beans, frozen	32
Rice, white parboiled	47	Split peas, yellow	32
Lentil soup	44	Milk, skim	32
Orange	43	Apricots, dried	31
All-Bran cereal	42	Green beans	30
Spaghetti (no sauce)	41	Banana, underripe	30
Pumpernickel bread	41	Lentils	29
Apple juice, unsweetened	41	Kidney beans	27
		Milk, whole	27
Low		Barley	25
Apple	36	Grapefruit	25
Pear	36	Fructose	23

*Amount based on 50 grams of carbohydrate per serving

Foods with a high glycemic response have a value above 60; foods with a moderate glycemic response have a value between 40 to 60; and foods with a low glycemic response have a value less than 40.

Data from food companies and K. Foster-Powell and J. Brand Miller, 1995, "International tables of glycemic index," *Am J Clin Nutr* 62: 871S-893S.

STORED GLUCOSE AND GLYCOGEN

The average 150-pound male has about 1,800 calories of carbohydrates stored in the liver, muscles, and blood in approximately the following distribution:

Muscle glycogen	1,400 calories
Liver glycogen	320 calories
Blood glucose	80 calories
Total:	1,800 calories

These limited carbohydrate stores influence how long you can enjoy exercising. When your glycogen stores get too low, you hit the wall—that is, you feel overwhelmingly fatigued and yearn to quit.

FOOD CHOICES BEFORE ENDURANCE EXERCISE

Does the glycemic effect of a food really influence exercise performance? Yes, according to research with endurance athletes who ate different types of foods one hour before exercising to exhaustion (Thomas, Brotherhood, and Brand 1991).

Cyclists ate 0.5 grams of carbohydrate per pound of body weight (about 70 grams or 280 calories) of either lentils, a low-glycemic index (GI) food (GI 29); baked potato or sugar water (GI 100), two high-glycemic index foods; or plain water (GI 0). They then exercised until they were exhausted; the average minutes to exhaustion follow.

Pre-exercise food	Minutes of exercise
Lentils	117
Glucose	108
Water	99
Potato	97

Lentils, the low-glycemic-index meal, prolonged exercise time by 20 minutes compared to the potato meal! Both potato and glucose, the high-glycemic-index foods, were associated with shorter exercise times.

Because the study included only seven subjects, the results are somewhat limited. But it is interesting to note these points:

• Every subject did better with the low-glycemic lentil meal as compared to the high-glycemic potato meal and exercised about 20 minutes longer (times varied greatly, with one person improving 6 seconds, another 52 minutes).

• Five subjects did better with about 280 calories of high-glycemic glucose as compared to zero calories of plain water by about 9 minutes (range: 5 to 20 minutes longer). Two subjects did worse with glucose by about 13.5 minutes.

• Four subjects did worse (3 to 46 minutes) with the high-glycemic potato as compared to high-glycemic glucose.

Clearly, each subject experienced a different exercise response with the four tests. The overall message is that what you eat before your exercise can affect your performance. Choose wisely!

In comparison to the approximately 1,800 calories of stored carbohydrates, the average, lean 150-pound man also has about 60,000 to 100,000 calories of stored fat—enough to run hundreds of miles! Unfortunately for endurance athletes, fat cannot be used exclusively as fuel because the muscles need a certain amount of carbohydrates to function well; carbohydrates are a limiting factor for endurance athletes.

During low-level exercise such as walking, the muscles burn primarily fats for energy. During light to moderate aerobic exercise, such as jogging, stored fat provides 50 to 60 percent of the fuel. When you exercise hard, as in sprinting or racing or other intense exercise, you rely primarily on the glycogen stores.

Biochemical changes that occur during training influence the amount of glycogen you can store in your muscles. The figures below indicate that well-trained muscles develop the ability to store about 20 to 50 percent more glycogen than untrained muscles (Costill et al. 1981; Sherman et al. 1981). This enhances endurance capacity and is one reason why a novice runner can't just carbo-load and run a top-quality marathon.

Muscle glycogen per 100 grams (3.5 ounces) of muscle:

Untrained muscle	13 grams
Trained muscle	32 grams
Carbo-loaded	35-40 grams

BONKING

Whereas depleted muscle glycogen causes athletes to hit the wall, depleted liver glycogen causes them to "bonk" or "crash." Liver glycogen is fed into the bloodstream to maintain a normal blood sugar level essential for "brain food." Despite adequate muscle glycogen, an athlete may feel uncoordinated, light-headed, unable to concentrate, and weakened because the liver is releasing inadequate sugar into the bloodstream.

You already know that your muscles and brain require glucose for energy. What you may not be aware of is that although the muscles can store glucose and burn fat, the brain does neither. This means that food must be consumed close enough to strenuous events to supply sugar to the blood, or the brain will not function optimally. Athletes with low blood sugar tend to perform poorly because the poorly fueled brain limits muscular function and mental drive.

John, a 28-year-old runner and banker, faithfully carbo-loaded his muscles for three days prior to his first Boston Marathon. On the evening before the marathon, he ate dinner at 5:00, then went to bed at 8:30 to ensure himself a good night's rest. But, as often happens with anxious athletes, he tossed and turned all night (which burned off a significant amount of calories), got up early the next morning, and chose not to eat breakfast, even though the marathon didn't start until noon. By noon, he had depleted his limited liver glycogen stores. He lost his mental drive about 8 miles into the race, and quit at 12 miles. His muscles were well-fueled, but that energy was unavailable to his brain, so he lacked the mental stamina to endure the marathon.

John could have prevented this needless fatigue by eating some oatmeal, cereal, or other carbohydrate at breakfast to refuel his liver glycogen stores. Athletic success depends on both well-fueled muscles and a well-fueled mind. (See chapter 10 for more information.)

RUNNERS AND BODYBUILDERS: SIMILAR DIETS?

"I know that for running I should eat carbohydrates to fuel my muscles. But for weight lifting, shouldn't I eat a lot of protein to build them up?"

Perhaps, like Julie, a 34-year-old runner who lifts weights, you are confused about what to eat for energy, strength, and top performance: carbohydrates or protein. I recommend this:

- Eat carbohydrate-rich breakfasts, such as oatmeal, rather than eggs.
- Focus your lunches and dinners on breads, potatoes, pasta, rice, fruits, and vegetables. Two-thirds of your plate should be covered with these carbohydrates.
- Eat fish, chicken, lean meats, low-fat cheeses, and other proteins as an accompaniment to lunch and dinner, not as the main focus. Or eat carbohydrate-rich protein alternatives such as beans and rice, lentil soup, chili, hummus, and other vegetarian choices.

Carbohydrates are fundamental for both runners and bodybuilders, because unlike protein or fat, carbs are readily stored in your muscles for fuel during exercise. Adequate protein is important for building and protecting your muscles—do not undereat protein—but you should dedicate only one-third of your dinner plate to protein-rich foods. The

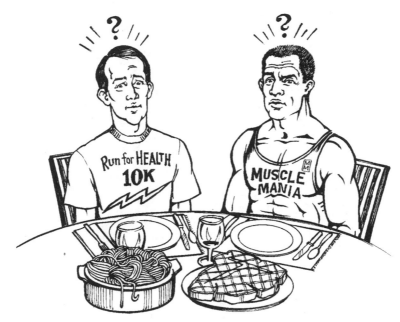

rest of your plate should be filled with carbohydrates. (See chapter 8 for more information about protein requirements).

A landmark study by exercise physiologist Dr. J. Bergstrom and his colleagues (1967) explains why carbohydrates are essential for high-energy athletic performance. The researchers compared the rate at which muscle glycogen was replaced in subjects who exercised to exhaustion and then ate either a high-protein and high-fat diet, or a high-carbohydrate diet (see figure on page 116).

The subjects on the high-protein and high-fat diet (similar to the diet of folks who live on steak, eggs, hamburgers, tuna salad, peanut butter, and cheese) remained glycogen depleted for five days. The subjects on a high-carbohydrate diet totally replenished their muscle glycogen in two days. Conclusion: Protein and fats don't get stored as muscle fuel; carbohydrates are important to replace depleted glycogen stores.

CARBOHYDRATES FOR DAILY RECOVERY

Carbohydrates are important for not only endurance athletes but also those who train hard day after day and want to maintain high energy. If you eat a low-carbohydrate diet, your muscles will feel chronically fatigued. You'll train, but not at your best.

The figure on page 117 illustrates the glycogen depletion that can occur when athletes eat an inadequate amount of carbohydrates and still try to exercise hard day after day (Costill et al. 1971). On three

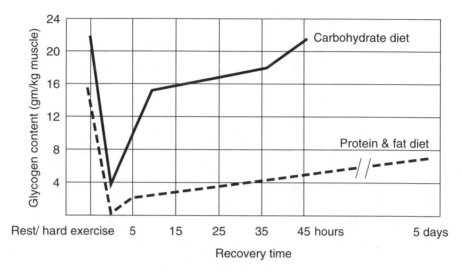

Carbohydrates are the best sources of glycogen.

Reprinted, by permission, from J. Bergstrom et al., 1967, "Diet, muscle glycogen and physical performance," *Acta Physiologica Scandinavica* 71: 140.

consecutive days, the subjects in this study ran hard for 10 miles (at a pace of 6 to 8 minutes per mile). They ate their standard meals: a diet that provided about 45 to 50 percent of calories from carbohydrates, not the 60 to 70 percent required in a top-performance sports diet. The subjects' muscles became increasingly glycogen depleted. Had the runners eaten larger portions of carbohydrates (and smaller portions of proteins and fats), they would have better replaced their glycogen stores and better invested in top performance.

This study emphasizes the need not only for a daily carbohydrate-rich diet but also for rest days with light or no training. The runners required extra rest time for their muscles to replace the burned-up glycogen. Depleted muscles may need two days to refuel after exhaustive exercise. An adequate recovery program is particularly important if you are an endurance athlete or a person who does daily hard workouts; you deplete significantly more glycogen during your intense workouts than does the casual exerciser who has glycogen to spare.

Pat, a 33-year-old computer programmer and former compulsive runner, learned the importance of rest days and adequate carbohydrates through a sports nutrition experiment. She insisted on training every day to get in shape for the Boston Marathon. I invited her to vary her training and recovery diet to determine whether her running improved with running less and eating better.

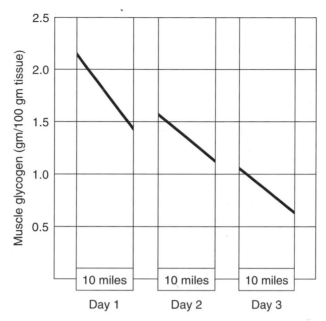

Glycogen depletion occurs with repeated days of exercise when carbohydrate intake is inadequate (45%-50%).

Data from D. Costill, R. Bowers, G. Branam, et al., 1971, "Muscle glycogen utilization during prolonged exercise on successive days," *J Appl Physiol* 31: 834-838.

Pat accepted the invitation and started to experiment with her two-hour Sunday run.

• **Experiment #1**. After her workout, she ate her favorite brunch: a high-protein, high-fat three-egg cheese omelette. When she ran on Monday, her legs were "dead"—tired, heavy, and unrecovered from Sunday's hard effort.

• **Experiment #2**. The next Sunday, Pat ate a high-carbohydrate recovery meal: pancakes, maple syrup, orange juice, and fresh fruit. She ran on Monday and felt much better than the previous week, but not great. She still needed more time to recover from Sunday's depleting workout.

• **Experiment #3**. The third Sunday, Pat ate the same breakfast as in experiment #2, but she took a rest day on Monday. On Tuesday, she ran effortlessly. "I felt super—lots of energy, totally recovered, and ready for action. I haven't done a high-quality Tuesday workout like that for a long time."

Based on this experience, Pat concluded that a rest day for refueling after a hard workout was a worthwhile investment in high-quality

Rest and Athletic Performance

Many athletes hesitate to cut back on exercise before a competition because they are afraid of getting out of shape. If this sounds like you, remember that rest will enhance, not hurt, your performance! You won't lose fitness, but rather will gain strength and endurance with better-fueled muscles.

Rest days are a very important part of an exercise program, because tired muscles require time to heal the tiny injuries that occur during training and refuel depleted glycogen stores. Athletes who underestimate the value of rest, and instead train relentlessly, set the stage for injuries, chronic glycogen depletion, chronic fatigue, and reduced performance. These same athletes often hope that vitamin supplements, special sports foods, and other pills and potions will boost their energy. All they really need to perform better is less exercise.

Cyclists who intensely trained for six weeks then tapered their exercise for up to two weeks improved by about 9 percent. Marathon runners (training 45 to 50 miles per week) showed the best improvement when they ran only 6 miles during a one-week taper and included some speed workouts (500-meter intervals) as compared to a taper with no running or about 20 miles per week of slow running (Houmard et al. 1990). If you are severely overtrained, you may need weeks, if not months, to recover. One study with swimmers showed that a two-and-a-half-week taper was inadequate to recover from the staleness acquired during a six-month season (Hooper et al. 1995). The bottom line: Don't underestimate the value of rest!

training. She stopped forcing herself to do the obligatory daily training run on the days when her muscles felt fatigued. Instead, she planned at least one rest day per week into her training schedule and started focusing on quality rather than quantity training. Her running improved, as did her mental outlook and enthusiasm for her sport. She ran a personal best in the marathon, cutting 8 minutes off her time.

GETTING CARBO-LOADED

When it comes to preparing for a marathon, triathlon, long-distance bike race, or other endurance event that will last for more than 90 minutes of intense exercise, you should gradually reduce your training for the two weeks prior, to rest your muscles to allow them to become saturated with carbohydrates, and continue to eat your tried-and-true, high-carbohydrate (60 to 70 percent) training diet. Your diet the three days prior to the event should be the same as your daily training diet, assuming you eat appropriately for your day-to-day training.

In times past, some athletes followed a week-long regimen that involved an exhaustive bout of exercise followed by three depletion days of a low-carbohydrate diet, then three loading days of a high-carbohydrate intake. Research indicates that the depletion phase offers no benefits (Sherman et al. 1981).

Today, exercise physiologists agree that the most effective way to prepare for a major endurance event is to change your training, not your diet, and to be sure your training diet is 60 to 70 percent carbohydrates. Read chapter 10 for more information about carbohydrate loading.

ARE CARBOHYDRATES FATTENING?

Some athletes eat too few carbohydrates because they believe them to be fattening.

> Jamie, a 17-year-old gymnast, wanted to eat carbohydrates for fuel, yet also wanted to lose weight for gymnastics. Like many dieters, Jamie considered carbohydrates to be forbidden foods, and she was frustrated. "I don't keep crackers, bread, cereal, or bagels in the house, because when they are there, I eat them—too many of them! I want to lose weight, not gain it from all those fattening carbohydrates."

The inaccurate advice from diet gurus of years past still lingers among dieters who fear bread as being fattening. Carbohydrates are *not* fattening! Excess fats are fattening—butter on bread, oil on pasta, mayonnaise in sandwiches, cheese on crackers. Fats provide 36 calories per teaspoon, as compared to 16 for carbohydrates. But the conversion of excess carbohydrates into body fat is limited because you burn the carbs when you exercise. Your body burns carbohydrates and stores the fats;

the metabolic cost of converting excess carbohydrates into body fat is 23 percent. Excess dietary fats, on the other hand, are easily stored as body fat; the metabolic cost of converting excess dietary fat into body fat is only 3 percent of ingested calories (Sims and Danforth 1987).

If you are destined to be gluttonous, your better bet is to overeat pretzels (carbohydrates) rather than peanuts (fats). You'll fuel your muscles better and the next day you'll have a high-energy workout with well carbo-loaded muscles. But do be aware that a continuous intake of excess carbohydrates will eventually contribute to weight gain. When your glycogen stores are filled, the excess calories will get stored as body fat (Hill et al. 1992).

Rather than trying to stay away from breads and bagels and other grains, remember these points:

- Carbohydrates are less fattening than fatty foods.
- You need carbs to fuel your muscles.
- You burn carbs off during hard exercise.
- Carbohydrates are a friendly fuel; the enemy is too many fats.
- When dieting to lose weight, you should energize with cereal, bread, pasta, and potato, but reduce your intake of the butter, margarine, and mayonnaise that often accompany them.

Some advertisements for sports foods claim that athletes should eat fewer carbs and more fat to burn more body fat and lose weight. Not true! No research to date shows that burning fat results in losing body fat. The only way to lose body fat is to create a calorie deficit. Chapter 14 has more information on carbohydrates and weight reduction.

FOODS HIGHEST IN CARBOHYDRATES

All too often I talk with athletes who think they eat a carbohydrate-rich diet when in reality they don't.

Jim, a 19-year-old college student, intended to carbo-load the night before the Newport Marathon. Due to inadequate nutrition knowledge, he "carbo-loaded" with a pizza supreme. Little did he know that of the 1,800 calories in the large pizza, 1,200 were from the protein and fat in the double cheese, sausage, and pepperoni. Only 35 percent of the calories from the thin crust and tomato sauce were from carbohydrates. No wonder he felt sluggish during the race!

I gave Jim a list, "Carbohydrates in Commonly Eaten Foods" (table 7.4), to post on his refrigerator. With this tool, he learned to select high-carbohydrate foods.

In addition, I taught him how to make better selections based on the nutrition facts panel on food labels. You, too, can use labels to guide your selections.

The nutrition facts panel lists the number of grams of carbohydrate, protein, fat, and alcohol (if present) per serving, as well as the calories per gram:

- 1 gram carbohydrate = 4 calories
- 1 gram protein = 4 calories
- 1 gram fat = 9 calories
- 1 gram alcohol = 7 calories

Using this information, you can make some simple calculations. To determine the number of carbohydrate calories in a food item, multiply the number of grams of carbohydrate by 4 (calories per gram). Next, compare the carbohydrate calories to the total calories per serving to determine the percentage of calories that are from carbohydrates.

Nutrition Facts
Serving Size 1oz. (About 27 peanuts)
Servings Per Container About 14

Amount Per Serving

Calories 170   Calories from Fat 130

%Daily Value+

Total Fat 15g	24%
Saturated Fat 2g	11%
Polyunsaturated Fat 4g	
Monounsaturated Fat 9g	
Cholesterol 0mg	0%
Sodium 55mg	2%
Potassium 160mg	5%
Total Carbohydrate 6g	2%
Dietary Fiber 2g	9%
Sugars 0g	
Protein 6g	

Table 7.4   Carbohydrates in Commonly Eaten Foods

To fuel your muscles, the foundation of every meal should be carbo-hydrate-rich foods. To precisely determine your carbohydrate needs, do one of these two things:

1. **Eat 3 to 5 grams of carbohydrates per pound of body weight** (Applegate 1991).

Example: If you weigh 160 pounds, this comes to 480 to 800 grams, or about 60 percent of a 3,200 to 5,300 calorie diet—a range of fuel appropriate for an active 160-pound person. *Note.* This method of calculating carbohydrate needs works best for very active athletes with high calorie needs, not for sedentary people.

2. **Determine your calorie needs (see chapter 14) and multiply by 60 percent.**

Example: If you need about 3,200 calories, at least 60 percent of them (60% × 3,200 = 1,920) should be from carbohydrates. There are 4 calories per gram of carbohydrate, so this translates into 480 grams—your target.

Food labels are the handiest source of carbohydrate information. The following list of carbohydrate-rich foods can also help you keep a tally.

Food	Amount	Carbohydrates (g)	Total calories
Fruits			
Apple	1 medium	20	80
Orange	1 medium	15	65
Banana	1 medium	25	105
Raisins	1/3 cup	40	150
Apricots, dried	10 halves	20	85
Vegetables			
Corn, canned	1/2 cup	15	70
Winter squash	1/2 cup	15	60
Tomato sauce, Prego	1/2 cup	10	95
Peas	1/2 cup	10	60
Carrot	1 medium	10	40
Green beans	1/2 cup	5	20
Broccoli	1/2 cup	5	20
Zucchini	1/2 cup	2	10
Bread-type foods			
Hoagie roll	1	75	400
Branola bread	1 slice	20	85
Bagel	1 small	31	165
English muffin	1	25	130
Pita	1 small	21	105
Pancakes	3- to 4-inch	35	185

Food	Amount	Carbohydrates (g)	Total calories
Waffle, Eggo	1	15	120
Saltines	5	10	60
Graham crackers	2 squares	10	70
Breakfast cereals			
Grape-Nuts	1/4 cup	25	105
Raisin Bran, Kellogg's	3/4 cup	30	120
Granola, low-fat	1/2 cup	45	210
Oatmeal, maple instant	1 packet	30	165
Cream of wheat, cooked	3/4 cup	24	115
Beverages			
Apricot nectar	8 ounces	35	140
Cranraspberry juice	8 ounces	36	145
Apple juice	8 ounces	30	120
Orange juice	8 ounces	25	105
Gatorade	8 ounces	14	50
Cola	12 ounces	39	155
Beer	12 ounces	13	145
Milk, chocolate	8 ounces	25	180
Milk, 2%	8 ounces	12	120
Grains, pasta, starches			
Baked potato	1 large	50	220
Baked beans	1 cup	50	260
Lentils, cooked	1 cup	40	230
Stuffing, bread	1 cup	40	340
Spaghetti, cooked	1 cup	40	200
Rice, cooked	1 cup	45	200
Ramen noodles	1/2 package	25	180
Entrees, convenience foods			
Lentil soup	10.5 ounces	27	170
Bean burrito, frozen	5 ounces	45	370
Refried beans, canned	1 cup	32	200
Spaghettios	1 cup	36	200
Macaroni and cheese, canned	1 cup	29	210
Sweets, snacks, desserts			
Cranberry sauce	1 tablespoon	7	30
Maple syrup	1 tablespoon	13	50
Strawberry jam	1 tablespoon	13	50
Honey	1 tablespoon	15	60
Oreo	1	8	50
Fig Newton	1	11	60
Pop-Tart, blueberry	1	30	195
Fruit yogurt	1 cup	50	225
Frozen yogurt	1 cup	44	240

Nutrient data from food labels and J. Pennington, 1992, *Bowes & Church's Food Values of Portions Commonly Used*, 16th ed. (Philadelphia: Lippincott.)

For example, vanilla Häagen-Dazs ice cream has 270 total calories per half-cup serving and 21 grams of carbohydrates.

$$21 \text{ g carb} \times 4 \text{ cal/g} = 84 \text{ calories from carbohydrates}$$

$$84 \text{ cals carb divided by } 270 \text{ total cals} = 32\% \text{ carbohydrates}$$

Using food label information, you can determine that ice cream contains relatively fewer carbohydrates than frozen yogurt does.

- For every 100 calories of vanilla Häagen-Dazs (3 tablespoons), you get only 8 grams of carbohydrates = 32 calories of carbohydrates = 32% of total calories.
- For every 100 calories of frozen yogurt (1/2 cup), you get about 18 grams of carbohydrates = 72 calories carbohydrates = 72% of total calories.

COUNTING CARBOHYDRATES

Your diet should be at least 60 percent carbohydrate for daily training, and 65 to 70 percent carbohydrate before an endurance event. You can achieve a diet that is 60 to 70 percent carbohydrate by opting for more starches and grains and fewer fatty, greasy foods: Replace muffins with bagels, granola with muesli, pesto sauce with tomato sauce on pasta. See table 7.5 for additional examples. Note that a high-carbohydrate diet can, and should, include a small amount of fat. If you try to eat carbohydrates exclusively, you may end up with an unbalanced intake, a linear diet that differs from the balance and variety found with the Food Guide Pyramid (see chapter 1).

Like many registered dietitans and sports nutritionists, I use a computer program that calculates the percent of carbohydrate and fat in a diet so athletes can see how their intake compares to the target goals of 60 percent carbohydrate, 25 percent fat and 15 percent protein.

Dave, a 27-year-old nutrition fanatic, was flabbergasted to discover that his diet was only 50 percent carbohydrates. "I've been eating many more carbohydrates than I used to! And I really don't eat any extra fats. I've stopped using butter, mayonnaise, and salad dressing. Are you sure that your computer is working properly?"

The computer was fine. Dave simply indulged in too many helpings of peanuts, almonds, granola, and sunflower seeds, his favorite snacks. Upon trading them in for higher carbohydrate items—pretzels, raisins,

Table 7.5   Calculated Carbohydrates

When you are reading food labels, you can translate *grams* of fat and carbohydrates into *calories*. One gram of fat = 9 calories, 1 gram of carbohydrate = 4 calories.

For the best sports diet, you want to choose foods rich in calories from carbohydrates, but limited in fat. Be aware that some popular high-carbohydrate foods, such as fruit-flavored yogurts and many fat-free desserts, are filled with carbohydrates from nutritionally empty sugar calories. Balance them with carbohydrates from wholesome foods.

Food	Total calories	% calories from carb	% calories from fat
1 blueberry muffin, Weight Watchers	170	75	25
1 blueberry muffin, Sara Lee	220	45	50
2 small bagels, Lenders	320	75	5
1 bagel and 3 tablespoons cream cheese	310	40	47
1 cup cream of mushroom soup, Healthy Choice	60	60	30
1 cup cream of mushroom soup, Campbell's	100	35	65
1 serving Stouffer's Macaroni and Cheese	310	37	47
1 serving Lean Cuisine Macaroni and Cheese	270	58	23

Nutrient data from food labels, May 1995.

dried apricots, and bananas—he easily boosted his carbohydrate intake to 68 percent. "You know, my training has improved since I made that switch. My muscles feel springier and I have greater endurance. I feel great; I'm glad I learned this simple solution to my needless fatigue!"

Learning about the composition of your training diet is very important. I generally see more athletes carbohydrate depleted during training periods than before competitions. They take good care of their diets prior to an important event, but often neglect it in the hubbub of daily life. Unfortunately they can't compete at their best if they don't train at their best.

If you want to feel completely at peace with your diet and verify that you are eating the right balance of carbohydrates, protein, and fat, consult with a registered dietitian, evaluate your diet using a computer program (see appendix A), or count grams of carbohydrates (and protein and fat) based on your body's needs. Some simple meals based on store-bought foods with nutrition labeling might be cereal, milk, and juice; a peanut butter and jelly sandwich and a yogurt; spaghetti with jarred tomato sauce, cottage cheese and frozen vegetables. Although gathering food label information may seem a huge project, it actually can be very interesting. It can also provide the peace of mind from knowing you're making wise choices that invest in both health and performance.

CARBOHYDRATES VERSUS FATS: A DELICATE BALANCE

As I've mentioned before, although you want to maximize your intake of carbohydrates and limit your intake of fats, you shouldn't cut out all fats from your sports diet. I overheard one runner advising her buddy, "Be sure to stay away from *all* fats before the race. Fatty foods prevent you from storing the glycogen in your muscles." This simply is false. Fat does not interfere with glycogen storage.

However, if you want to fuel your muscles, don't stuff yourself with too much fat and then eat inadequate carbohydrates. You'll be better off eating pasta with carbohydrate-filled tomato sauce than with fettucini Alfredo's butter and cheese sauce. After you have carbo-loaded, you can splurge on dessert, if you like. The point is, first fuel up on carbs, then (if you still have the yen) fill in the cracks with fats.

Another mistake dedicated athletes commonly make is reducing their fat intake without replacing those calories with adequate carbohydrates. Don, a basketball player, cut butter, mayonnaise, and salad dressing from his diet and lost 2 pounds within a week of this nutrition change; he neglected to replace the deleted fat calories with adequate carbohydrates. He should, for example, have eaten two potatoes to get the same amount of calories in the one potato drenched with butter and sour cream.

Athletes who choose very low-fat diets must eat large quantities of carbohydrates to get adequate calories. If they have big appetites, as do six-foot, ten-inch basketball players, they often tire of chewing before they are adequately fed! The main focus of the diet should be on carbohydrates, but some fats can still be included. Eating 3 to 5 grams of

CARBOHYDRATES WITH HIDDEN FATS

The following foods have fooled many unsuspicious athletes into thinking they are fueling up on carbohydrates when they are actually filling up on hidden fats. Your target fat intake for the day should be about 25 percent of your total calories (see chapter 2).

Food	Percent calories from fat	Higher carbohydrate alternative	Percent calories from fat
Granola	35	Grape-Nuts	1
Muffin, homemade	25	Bagel, plain	1
Ritz crackers	50	Saltines	15
Pizza, thin crust	40	Pizza, thick crust	30
Macaroni and cheese	45	Spaghetti, tomato sauce	10
Ice cream, gourmet	55	Frozen yogurt, fat-free	0

Note: Nutrient data from food labels and J. Pennington, 1992, *Bowes and Church's Food Values of Portions Commonly Used*, 16th ed. (Philadelphia: Lippincott).

carbohydrate per pound of body weight will saturate your muscles with carbohydrates. After that, you can eat the balance of the calories in protein and fat.

The Base of the Pyramid

Any way you look at them, carbohydrates of any type are important for athletes. If you're wise, you'll choose to eat primarily wholesome breads, grains, and cereals from the base of the Food Guide Pyramid, along with a strong intake of carbohydrate-rich fruits, vegetables, and beans. Save the sugary carbohydrates from the tip of the pyramid for occasional treats.

8
chapter

Protein to Promote Training

Protein-rich foods used to be the mainstay of athletes' diets. Traditionally, athletes devoured plates of beef, eggs, tuna, chicken, and other protein-rich foods. The theory was that if they ate a lot of protein, they would build a lot of muscle. But extra protein does not build muscle bulk; exercise does. To build and strengthen muscles, you have to include in your training routine strengthening exercises such as weight lifting, push-ups, and other forms of resistance exercise.

Mike, a national-class power lifter, was very confused by conflicting stories about the best foods for building muscles. His buddies at the gym would tell him to bulk up on steak, tuna, turkey, and egg whites and to chug protein drinks. But his neighbor, a marathon runner, encouraged him to carbo-load with lots of spaghetti. Mike's mother, an Italian, fed him what she thought was best: pasta. I reassured Mike that pasta was indeed the best choice to combine with his training program. He exclaimed, "I knew that pasta power helped me to become a winner!"

As I explained in chapter 7, bodybuilders need a carbohydrate-based diet because carbohydrates are stored in the muscles for energy. You can't lift weights and demand a lot from your workout sessions if your muscles are carbo-depleted. High-protein diets don't provide enough

Do Runners Need Less Protein Than Weight Lifters?

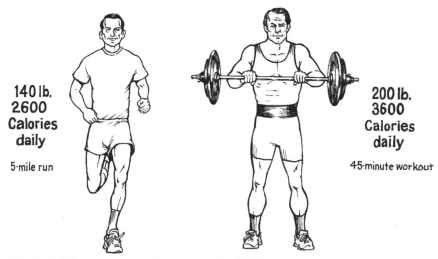

140 lb.
2600
Calories
daily

5-mile run

200 lb.
3600
Calories
daily

45-minute workout

15% X 2600 = 390 protein calories = 98 g protein   15% X 3600 = 540 protein calories = 135 g protein

muscle fuel to let you exercise hard enough to build to your potential. Refer back to page 116 for more details.

The best sports diet contains adequate, but not excess, protein to build and repair muscle tissue, grow hair and fingernails, produce hormones, boost your immune system, and replace red blood cells. Most athletes who eat moderate portions of protein-rich foods daily get more protein than they need. Any excess protein is burned for energy or stored as glycogen or fat. Humans do not store excess protein as protein, so we need to consume adequate protein daily. This is particularly important for active people who are restricting calories, because protein is burned for energy when carbohydrates are scarce.

HOW MUCH PROTEIN DO YOU NEED?

When it comes to protein intake, athletes seem to fall into two categories: protein pushers—the bodybuilders, weight lifters, and football players who can't seem to get enough of the stuff—or protein avoiders—the runners, triathletes, dancers, and weight-conscious athletes who never touch meat and trade most protein calories for more carbohydrates. Both groups can perform poorly due to dietary imbalances.

Doug, for example, was a protein pusher. A high school football player, he routinely snacked after practice on a few large burgers and a quart of milk. That one snack satisfied his protein needs for the whole day! As an athlete, he has a slightly higher protein need than a sedentary person, but he overcompensated for that need with the big portions he devoured at meals alone, never mind his high-protein snack.

John, a triathlete who boasted about the high quality of his high-carbohydrate, low-fat, low-protein sports diet, was a protein avoider. He was humbled when he learned that his food intake was deficient in not only protein, but also in iron (for red blood cells), zinc (for healing), calcium (for bones), and several other nutrients. No wonder he became anemic, suffered a lingering cold and flu, and performed poorly despite consistent training.

Defining Protein Needs

Research has yet to define the exact protein needs of sports-active people because their needs vary. All active people need more protein than the current Recommended Dietary Allowance of 0.4 grams of protein per pound of body weight (0.8 g/kg). These are the people with the highest protein needs:

• **Endurance athletes and others doing intense exercise.** About 5 to 10 percent of energy can come from protein during endurance exercise, particularly if muscle glycogen stores are depleted.

• **Dieters consuming too few calories.** The protein is burned for energy instead of to build and repair muscles.

• **Untrained people starting an exercise program.** Extra protein is needed to build muscles.

• **Growing teenage athletes.** They need enough protein for both growth and sports.

Although people starting an intensive weight training program need more protein than the current RDA, excessive amounts do not enhance gains in muscle strength. In Dr. Lemon's study (Lemon et al. 1992), 22-year-old men lifted weights for 90 minutes a day, six days a week. These subjects required about 0.7 grams of protein per pound of body weight per day to stay in protein balance. For the 150-pound man, this is about 102 grams of protein per day—far less than most bodybuilders typically eat. Hence, protein requirements become a moot point.

In general, 0.6 to 0.8 grams of protein per pound of body weight (1.4 to 1.8 g Pro/kg) seems to be appropriate for strength athletes. Endurance athletes, who use protein as a fuel source, need about 0.55 to 0.6 grams of protein per pound of body weight (1.2 to 1.4 g Pro/kg). In contrast to the belief that if a little more protein is good, a lot more will be better, there is to date no scientific evidence suggesting that protein intakes exceeding 0.9 grams protein per pound (2.0 g Pro/kg) will provide an additional advantage (Lemon 1995). But many athletes eat that plus more in their quest for enhanced performance.

Because individuals have a range of protein needs, the following are some safe and adequate recommendations for protein intake. These recommendations include a margin of safety and are not minimal amounts (Lemon 1995; Lemon et al. 1992; Walberg et al. 1988):

	Grams of protein per pound of body weight
Current RDA for sedentary adult	0.4
Recreational exerciser, adult	0.5-0.75
Competitive athlete, adult	0.6-0.9
Growing teenage athlete	0.8-0.9
Adult building muscle mass	0.7-0.9
Athlete restricting calories	0.8-0.9
Maximum useable amount for adults	0.9

Calculating Your Protein Needs

It's easy to figure out your protein needs. To learn if you are meeting your protein needs in your current diet, follow two easy steps.

First, identify yourself in the categories listed in the list above that recommends the amount of protein needed by a variety of people. A 120-pound bike racer, for example, categorized as a "competitive athlete, adult," would need about 72 to 108 grams of protein per day:

$$120 \text{ lb} \times 0.6 \text{ g/lb} = 72 \text{ g protein}$$

$$120 \text{ lb} \times 0.9 \text{ g/lb} = 108 \text{ g protein}$$

A 150-pound teenage swimmer in the category of "growing athlete" would need about 120 to 135 grams of protein per day:

$$150 \text{ lb} \times 0.8 \text{ g/lb} = 120 \text{ g protein}$$

$$150 \text{ lb} \times 0.9 \text{ g/lb} = 135 \text{ g protein}$$

Then, keep track of your protein intake by listing everything you eat and drink for one 24-hour period. Use the nutrition information on food labels to keep a tally of the protein you consumed. For example, the nutrition facts on the label of a 6-ounce can of tuna might tell you it contains 15 grams of protein and 2-1/2 servings per can. So, if you eat the whole can, you get about 40 grams of protein.

Table 8.1 lists the amount of protein in some common foods; the information on food labels can provide additional information (table 1.5 does, too).

Most fruits and vegetables have only small amounts of protein that may contribute a total of 5 to 10 grams of protein per day, depending on how much you eat. Butter, margarine, oil, sugar, candy, soda, alcohol, and coffee contain no protein, and most desserts contain very little.

Table 8.1   Protein in Commonly Eaten Foods

Although animal products generally provide the highest quality protein, you don't have to eat beef to get plenty of protein. You can eat a variety of plant proteins. Note that you need to eat a generous portion (more calories) of beans and other plant protein to equal the protein in animal foods. (See chapter 1 for more protein information.)

	Grams of protein/ standard serving		Grams of protein/ 100 calories (amount)	
Animal source				
Egg white	3.5	from 1 large egg	20	6 egg whites
Egg	6	1 large	8	1.3 eggs
Cheddar cheese	7	1 ounce	6	0.9 ounces
Milk, 1%	8	8 ounces	8	8 ounces
Yogurt	11	1 cup	8	6 ounces
Cottage cheese	15	1/2 cup	15	1/2 cup
Haddock	27	4 ounces cooked	21	3 ounces
Hamburger	30	4 ounces broiled	10	1.5 ounces
Pork loin	30	4 ounces roasted	10	1.5 ounces
Chicken breast	35	4 ounces roasted	18	2 ounces
Tuna	40	6 ounces	20	3 ounces
Plant sources				
Almonds, dried	3	12 nuts	3.5	14 nuts
Peanut butter	4.5	1 tablespoon	4.5	1 tablespoon
Kidney beans	6	1/2 cup	6	1/2 cup
Hummus	6	1/2 cup	3	1/4 cup
Refried beans	7	1/2 cup	7	1/2 cup
Lentil soup, Progresso	11	10.5 ounces	6.5	6 ounces
Tofu, extra firm	11	3.5 ounces	12	4 ounces
Baked beans	14	1 cup	7	1/2 cup

Data from food labels and J. Pennington, 1992, *Bowes & Church's Food Values of Portions Commonly Used*, 16th ed. (Philadelphia: Lippincott).

Healthfully Including Meat in Your Diet

"I eat very little meat because I rarely buy it," commented Sue, a single woman who lived alone and rarely cooked. "I wonder if this hurts my diet?"

If you, like Sue, think you eat too little protein, iron, and zinc—and you are willing to eat animal proteins—including a small amount of lean red meat into your sports diet two to four times per week can actually help improve the quality of your sports diet. Here are some tips to keep in mind for health-promoting, low-fat meat eatery:

• **Buy extra-lean cuts of beef, pork, and lamb to reduce your intake of saturated fats.** Forego cuts with a marbled appearance, and trim the fat off steaks and chops before cooking them.

• **Get rid of more fat.** After browning hamburger, drain it in a colander and rinse it with hot water to remove the fat before adding it to spaghetti sauce.

• **At a cafeteria, request two rolls when you order one hamburger.** Use one roll to absorb the grease; throw it away, and then eat the second roll with the degreased burger.

• **Use meat as the accompaniment to a meal.** Add a little extra-lean hamburger to spaghetti sauce, stir-fry a small piece of steak with lots of veggies, serve a pile of rice along with one lean pork chop, make a savory potato-rich stew with a little lean lamb, buy deli roast beef for sandwiches made on hearty bread.

The easier way to assess if you are getting adequate, but not excess, protein in your daily diet is to use this rule of thumb: *16 ounces (2 cups) of milk or yogurt + 4 to 6 ounces (1 moderate serving about the size of a woman's palm) of protein-rich foods = daily protein requirement.* Combined with the small amounts of protein in other foods that round out the meals, this should suit the needs of a healthy adult. Here's a sample of one day's worth of protein-rich foods for an active adult; of course, you'll need to eat other foods to round out your nutritional requirements.

Breakfast	1 cup milk on cereal
Lunch	2 ounces sandwich filling (tuna, roast beef, turkey)
	1 cup yogurt
Dinner	4 ounces meat, fish, poultry, or the equivalent in lentils or other beans and legumes

Growing teens and others with high-protein needs can get additional protein and calcium by drinking another 2 cups of milk.

Note that you have a daily need for protein. As I mentioned before, some athletes eat protein-rich foods only once or twice per week, and live on bagels and pasta for most of their meals. They cheat themselves of an optimal sports diet (see chapter 1). Eating a proper meat-free diet can be simple, even for people who dislike cooking. See table 8.2 for a sample cook-free, vegetarian meal plan.

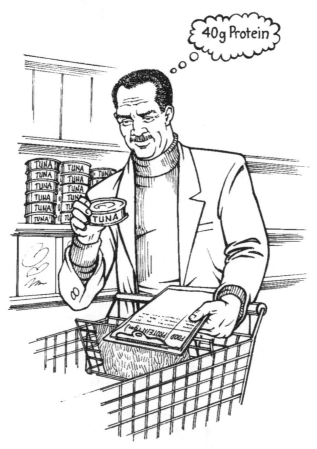

Table 8.2   Simple Vegetarian Meals

This cook-free menu is appropriate for an active, 150-pound lactoveg-etarian (that is, a vegetarian who drinks milk and eats dairy foods) who might need about 2,800 calories per day. Including low-fat dairy foods is one trick for balancing a simple vegetarian diet. Low-fat milk, yogurt, and cheeses are convenient, quick, easy, and popular protein sources.

Food	Protein (g)	Calories
Breakfast		
1 cup orange juice	2	110
2 cups bran flakes	8	240
1 medium banana	1	100
1.5 cups low-fat milk	12	150
Lunch		
2 peanut butter sandwiches	30	700
1 apple	1	100
2 cups milk	16	200
Snack		
1 cup fruit yogurt	10	250
Dinner		
1 medium pizza	70	1,000
Totals:	*150*	*2,850*

Note. The 150 grams of protein accounts for 20 percent of the 2,850 calories, and allows 1 gram of protein per pound of body weight. This is slightly higher than the recommended sports diet with 15 percent of calories from protein, or 0.6 to 0.9 grams of protein per pound of body weight. This demonstrates that lactovegetarians can easily get adequate protein with wise food choices.

Too Much Protein

Contrary to what most people think, too much protein can be a real health and performance problem.

Luke, an aspiring basketball champ, called himself a meat and pota-toes man. He'd chow down on burgers and thick steaks and barely nibble on the spuds, much to the detriment of his athletic aspirations. He tired easily and asked me if this high-protein diet might be hurting his performance. Here's what I told him:

• If you fill your stomach with too much protein, you won't be fuel-ing your muscles with carbohydrates.

- Anyone who eats excess protein may need to urinate more frequently, because protein breaks down into urea, a waste product eliminated in the urine. Frequent trips to the bathroom may be an inconvenience during training and competition, to say nothing of increasing the risk of becoming dehydrated and burdening the kidneys.

- You can save money by eating smaller portions of beef, lamb, pork, and other animal proteins that tend to be expensive. Use that money to buy more plant proteins (beans, lentils, tofu) and more fruits, vegetables, grains, and potatoes.

- A diet high in protein tends to be high in fat (juicy steaks, bacon and eggs, pepperoni pizza, and so on). For your heart's sake and for improved athletic performance, you should reduce your intake of the saturated fats found in animal proteins. This may also reduce your risk of certain cancers.

I encouraged Luke to reduce his meat portions at dinner to one-third of his plate and to fill two-thirds with potatoes, vegetables, and bread. Within two days, he noticed an improvement in his energy level. He then changed his breakfast from ham and eggs to cereal and a banana, and lunch became chili or pasta rather than burgers. His diet gradually became a winner. "You know, " he now says, "food works. The right foods definitely enhance my sports performance!"

PROTEIN AND THE VEGETARIAN

There are many kinds of vegetarians. Some eat just no red meat, others eat no chicken, fish, eggs, or dairy foods. Most people who eliminate animal proteins make the effort to replace beef with beans; that is, they include kidney beans, chick-peas, peanut butter, tofu, and other plant proteins in their daily diet. They get adequate protein to support their sports program. Some nonmeat eaters, however, simply fuel up on only carbohydrates and neglect their protein needs. They may think meat is hard to digest or bad for the heart, or they may believe it is unethical to eat meat.

Whatever their reason for abstaining from meat, they often overlook the fact they still need to eat adequate protein to maintain good health. The following is a typical example of one athlete's protein deficient diet.

Jim, a 150-pound runner, consumed only 6 percent of his calories from protein. That was equal to 0.3 grams of protein per pound, or half the recommended intake. A normal day's eating for Jim looked something like this:

Meal	Protein (g)*	Approximate calories
Breakfast		
2 bagels, plain	4	400
2 cups orange juice	2	220
Lunch		
2 large bananas	3	300
2 cups apple juice	—	240
1 large muffin	4	300
Dinner		
3 cups cooked pasta	20	660
1 cup tomato sauce	2	100
2 cups cranberry juice	—	300
Snack		
1 cup dried fruit	5	480
Total	40	3,000

Recommended protein intake*: 90 to 135 grams protein

*0.6 to 0.9 grams of protein per pound of body weight = 90 to 135 grams

"Vegetarian" Female Athletes

Female athletes often refer to themselves as vegetarians but they fit into the nonmeat eater category. Those who consume a low-calorie and a low-protein diet are often found to be amenorrheic; that is, they stop having regular menstrual periods. Research suggests that amenorrheic athletes have a 4.5-times higher risk for suffering a stress fracture than regularly menstruating athletes do (Clark, Nelson, and Evans 1988; Nelson et al. 1986). Eating a balanced diet with adequate protein and calories can enhance resumption of menses and enhance overall health.

Sue, now a healthy dancer, used to live on fruit for breakfast, a salad for lunch, and stir-fried vegetables with brown rice for dinner. Once or twice a week, she'd sprinkle a few garbanzo beans on a salad or add some tofu to the stir-fry. She thought her diet was great, when in fact it was deficient in several nutrients. At one point she suffered a stress fracture that healed very slowly. She had spindly arms and legs, the "anorexic look," and her menstrual period was absent, another sign of an unhealthy body. See chapter 15 for more information on amenorrhea.

Sue needed to be reminded that a well-balanced sports diet includes adequate protein and that small portions of lean beef, pork, and lamb can appropriately fit into the heart-healthy diet of those who have no

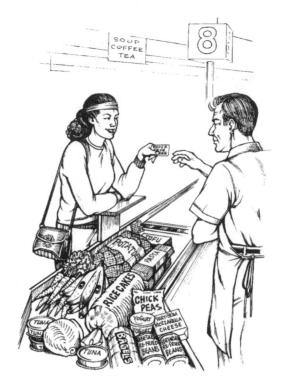

ethical objections to eating animal foods. Dark meats are important sources of the minerals iron and zinc. See table 12.4 and read chapter 12 to further learn how vegetarians and meat eaters can boost their intake of these two minerals.

The Balanced Vegetarian Diet

Without question, a diet based on plant foods can contribute to good health. A plant-based diet tends to have more fiber, less saturated fat and cholesterol, and more phytochemicals—active compounds that may play an important role in preventing and treating diseases such as cancer (see chapter 2). Foods rich in phytochemicals include not only fruits and vegetables, but also the protein-rich foods common to a plant-based diet: legumes, dried beans, and peas.

If you want to omit animal protein from your diet, or if you already do, you are making a potentially healthful lifestyle change. The trick is to choose a balanced vegetarian diet and choose enough vegetable proteins to satisfy your protein requirements. This can be easier for a man who is eating 3,000 or more calories to do than for a woman dieter who eats half that amount.

Ann, a vegetarian dieter and personal trainer, thought she was eating adequate protein when she included 1 tablespoon of peanut butter (only 4 grams of protein) on a bagel for breakfast, a half cup of garbanzo beans (only 6 grams of protein) on a lunchtime salad, and one-quarter cake of tofu (only 9 grams of protein) at dinner. These 19 grams of protein fell short of the daily 50 to 70 grams of protein she needed. No wonder she wasn't building muscle the way she wanted!

When Ann recognized her diet was deficient in plant proteins, she traded in calories from protein-poor bagels, pasta, and fruits for more calories from protein-rich beans. This boosted her intake of the amino acids she needed to build muscles. She had better workouts and felt better overall.

The need for protein is actually a need for amino acids. All proteins are made up of amino acids that your body needs to build tissue; hence, their nickname "building blocks." There are 21 of these amino acids, and every protein in your body is made up of some combination of them. Your body can make some amino acids itself; eight of them (nine for children), however, called the *essential amino acids*, must come from the foods you eat (see table 8.3).

Milk, other dairy foods, fish, poultry, meat, and all animal sources of protein contain all eight or nine essential amino acids and are often referred to as *complete proteins*. So is the protein in soy foods such as

---

Table 8.3   Amino Acids: The Building Blocks of Life

The following nine amino acids are essential to eat in your diet because your body cannot make them. Histidine is essential for infants because they cannot synthesize it, but adults can.

histidine	lysine[1]	tryptophan[4]
phenylalanine	methionine[2]	valine
isoleucine	threonine[3]	leucine

Your body can make these 12 nonessential amino acids that are also building blocks of protein:

alanine	asparagine	aspartic acid
cysteine	cystine	glutamic acid
glycine	proline	glutamine
arginine	serine	tyrosine

[1]This amino acid is low in wheat, rice, and corn and limits these grains' abilities to make complete proteins unless they are eaten in combination with another food rich in lysine; [2]Low in beans; [3]low in rice; [4]low in corn

tofu, tempeh, and soy milk. The protein in rice, beans, pasta, lentils, nuts, fruits, vegetables, and other plant foods are *incomplete* because they have low levels of some of the essential amino acids. Therefore, vegetarians must know how to combine incomplete proteins to make them complete. Vegetarians who drink milk can easily do this by adding dairy to each meal, such as by combining milk with oatmeal, or sprinkling grated low-fat cheese on beans. The strict vegetarian needs to choose complementary vegetable proteins that are high in the particular limiting amino acid.

In times past, vegetarians were told to eat the complementary proteins together at each meal. We now know that eating them over the course of the day is equally effective. Nevertheless, the following combinations work well together:

Grains and milk products (for lactovegetarians)

- Cereal + milk
- Pasta + cheese
- Bread + cheese
- Grains + beans and legumes (such as peanuts and kidney, pinto, lima, and navy beans)
- Rice + beans
- Pita + split pea soup
- Tortillas + beans
- Corn bread + chili with kidney beans
- Brown bread + baked beans

Legumes and seeds

- Chick-peas + tahini (as in hummus)
- Tofu + sesame seeds

Following these guidelines, vegetarian athletes can plan their diets to be sure they consume an adequate amount of complete protein every day. One key is to eat a wide variety of foods to optimize the intake of a wide variety of amino acids.

Some vegetarians who avoid red meat for health reasons often turn to eggs and cheese for protein. They thrive on omelets, cheesy lasagna, salads frosted with shredded cheese, and slices of whole grain bread piled high with cheese. They are unaware, though, that cheese and eggs have far more fat and cholesterol than lean meats, and that eating a grilled cheese or egg salad sandwich is, in that respect, worse than a lean roast beef sandwich without mayonnaise. As I have mentioned before, lean meat, eaten in small portions as the accompaniment to lots of carbohydrates, is not the health culprit it is deemed to be. Refer to table 2.4, for the amount of fat and cholesterol in some meats.

Tofu (soybean curd) and other soy products such as soy milk are excellent additions to a meat-free diet. Not only do they contain a source of high-quality protein that is equivalent in value to animal protein, but they also have properties that may protect against heart disease and cancer. The more often you include soy foods in your diet, the more likely you are to lower the bad cholesterol, increase the good cholesterol, and delay cancer tumor growth. As little as 1/2 cup of tofu, 1/3 cup of soy flour, or 1 cup of soy milk per day can bring positive health changes.

For women, soy may have additional benefits. Soy protein contains a plant estrogen called genistein that has been shown to reduce the risk of breast cancer. The addition of just 1 serving a day of soy foods has also been shown to lengthen the menstrual cycle for up to five days (Cassidy, Bingham, and Setchell 1994). This reduced exposure to estrogen may explain why soy protein is associated with reduced risk of breast cancer.

Even though most vegetarians can get the right amount of protein, they may lack iron and zinc, minerals found primarily in meats and other animal products. As I've mentioned before, iron is a vital component in red blood cells, and zinc plays an important role in tissue growth and maintenance. Chapter 12 explains how vegetarians (and meat eaters) can ensure a proper intake of these two nutrients. Pure vegans, who eat only plant foods, need to be sure they get adequate riboflavin, calcium, and vitamin B-12, either through a supplement or carefully selected food sources. Appendix B lists resources to help vegans achieve a balanced diet.

PROTEIN SUPPLEMENTS AND AMINO ACIDS

According to the advertisements in bodybuilding magazines, protein powders and amino acid pills are essential for optimal muscle development. If you have been hanging around the power gyms, you've undoubtedly heard intense conversations about some of these products, such as arginine, ornithine and free-form amino acids. The protein-praising bodybuilders who come to me for advice often lug gym bags bulging with assorted pills, powders, and potions. They wonder if these supplements are worth the price and if they work. Some are avid believers in the stuff, and others are skeptical.

Joseph, a 21-year-old college student, marveled at the 6 pounds he had gained in two months with protein powders and amino acid supplements. However, he had simultaneously improved his eating and exercise program. I suspect that the wholesome meals and consistent training make more of a difference than the protein supplements.

AMINO ACIDS: FOOD VERSUS PILLS

Bodybuilders commonly spend a lot of money on special amino acid supplements that claim to provide more energy, stamina, and muscle mass. These folks could have gotten more amino acids if they'd spent that money on wholesome foods! This chart shows the amounts of two popular amino acids, arginine and leucine, that occur naturally in food and how they compare to the amounts found in commercial supplements.

Amount	Arginine (mg)	Leucine (mg)
Food		
2 egg whites	380	600
1 cup skim milk	350	950
4 ounces chicken breast		
(1 small)	2,100	2,650
6 ounces tuna (1 can)	2,700	3,700
Supplement		
1 serving Twin Labs		
Amino Fuel	85	320
1 serving Ultimate Nutrition's		
Amino Gold	350	1,260
1 serving Nature's Best		
Amino Acids	440	1,300

When compared according to milligrams of amino acid per 25 grams of protein, the supplements are very expensive sources of protein.

Equivalent of 25 g protein	Arginine/ 25 g protein	Leucine/ 25 g protein	Cost
3 cups skim milk	1,050	2,850	$0.60
2/3 can (4 ounces) tuna	1,800	2,400	$0.80
3 ounces chicken breast	1,600	2,000	$0.65
7 egg whites	2,650	4,200	$0.75
24 pills Twin Labs Amino Fuel	1,020	3,840	$2.80
27 pills Amino Gold	1,050	3,780	$2.60
18 pills Nature's Best	1,320	3,900	$1.80

Jake, a 33-year-old bus driver, took a protein drink after every workout and with every meal. He gained bulk and felt stronger. Were the improvements because of the extra calories in his diet, or the expensive protein drink? Likely, the extra calories.

Bulking up is a matter of dedicating yourself to extra exercise and extra carbohydrates, not to extra supplements. In chapter 16, I address how to gain weight healthfully; this chapter addresses the role of protein in the gaining process. If you are struggling to develop bigger muscles, change your body image, and improve your strength, heed the following tips:

• **Exercise, not extra protein, is the key to developing bigger muscles.** In theory, if you want to gain 1 pound of muscle per week, you need only 14 extra grams of protein per day, the amount in 2 ounces of meat—a mere forkful (Bernadot 1992)!

• **Beware of extra fat.** If you are currently eating large amounts of protein-rich foods, you may be consuming an excessive amount of calories from fat that can easily get stored as body fat, not as bulging biceps.

• **Expensive muscle-building supplements are not the answer.** The amount of protein or amino acids in these formulas is less than that which you might easily get through foods. For example, you would have to eat 5 tablespoons of one popular protein powder at a cost of $1.10 to get the same amount of protein in a much less expensive three-and-a-half-ounce can of tuna that also contains far more nutrients than just protein.

Taking extra amino acids, such as large doses of ornithine or arginine, will not make your muscles bigger or stronger. To date, there's no scientific evidence that individual amino acids have a bodybuilding effect. (For more information, see chapter 12.) Your body needs *all* the essential amino acids to make new muscles. Real food provides the proper balance of all the amino acids, works well, and costs less than amino acid pills. Real food, along with regular exercise, can help you achieve your athletic goals.

9
chapter

Time-Out for a Drink

Basic as it may sound, water is one of the most important nutrients in your sports diet. You can survive for only a few days without water, although you can live for weeks without food. Drinking too little water or losing too much through profuse sweating inhibits your ability to exercise at your maximum potential.

The same athletes who earn an A+ for eating wisely often flunk hydration. Paul, master swimmer, routinely neglected to drink adequate fluids during training and before competitions. Because he was surrounded by lots of water, he falsely assumed that he didn't sweat or need to drink water. He became needlessly fatigued, trained poorly, and did not perform at his best. This oversight cost him attaining his desired personal best performance at several events. For each 1 percent of body weight lost by dehydration, he was forced to slow his pace by 2 percent (Wilmore and Costill 1994). When he began drinking additional fluids on a daily basis, he gained 2 pounds (water weight), felt better, and also swam faster times by simply correcting his chronic state of dehydration.

Water and You

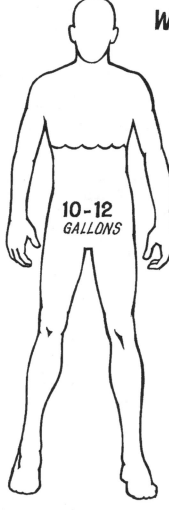

10-12 GALLONS

150 lb. man

Water...

* in blood transports glucose, oxygen, and fats to working muscles and carries away metabolic by-products such as carbon dioxide and lactic acid.

* in urine eliminates metabolic waste products. The darker the urine, the more concentrated the wastes.

* in sweat dissipates heat through the skin. During exercise water absorbs heat from your muscles, dissipates it through sweat, and regulates body temperature. One pound of sweat loss represents about 275 calories of dissipated heat (Wilmore and Costill 1994, p. 248)

* in saliva and gastric secretions helps digest food.

* throughout the body lubricates joints and cushions organs and tissues.

THE DANGERS OF DEHYDRATION

Under extreme conditions, dehydrated athletes suffer severe medical complications. Some individuals have died because misinformed coaches told them never to drink before or during training. Water was once thought to cause stomach cramping, but now we know that athletes should drink as much water as they comfortably can before, during, and after exercise (see table 9.1).

COMMON QUESTIONS ABOUT FLUIDS

To help clarify the confusion about water, fluids, and dehydration, here are the answers to questions commonly asked by thirsty athletes.

Table 9.1   Effects of Dehydration

By weighing yourself before and after you exercise, you can determine how much sweat you lost and the extent to which you dehydrated yourself. Your goal should be to match fluid intake with fluid losses to prevent significant dehydration.

Percent dehydration	Pounds lost for 150-pound person	Effect
1	1.5	Increased body temperature
3	4.5	Impaired performance
5	7.5	Heat cramps, chills, nausea, clammy skin, rapid pulse, 20-30% decrease in endurance capacity
6-10	9-15	Gastrointestinal problems, heat exhaustion, dizziness, headache, dry mouth, fatigue
>10	>15	Heat stroke, hallucinations, no sweat or urine, swollen tongue, high body temperature, unsteady walk

Data from P.G. Cooper (Ed.), and AFAA, 1987, *Aerobics: Theory & practice* (Costa Mesa, CA: HDL Communications).

Sweating It Out

Q. I sweat buckets! After a workout, I'm dripping wet and leave puddles on the floor. Is this healthy?

A. Sweating is good for you! It's the body's way of dissipating heat and maintaining a constant internal temperature (98.6°F). During hard exercise, your muscles can generate 20 times more heat than when you are at rest. You dissipate this heat by sweating. As the sweat evaporates, it cools the skin. This in turn cools the blood, which cools the inner body. If you did not sweat, you could cook yourself to death. A body temperature higher than 106 °F damages the cells. At 107.6°F, cell protein coagulates (like egg whites do when they cook), and the cell dies. This is one serious reason why you shouldn't push yourself beyond your limits in very hot weather.

Men tend to produce more sweat than they need to cool themselves. They sweat large drops of water, which can drip off the skin rather than evaporate, resulting in less cooling effect. In comparison, women tend to sweat more efficiently than men. But both men and women need to be equally diligent with replacing sweat losses.

Replacing Losses

Q. How do I know whether I'm drinking enough fluids to replace sweat losses?

A. The simplest way to tell if you are adequately replacing sweat loss is to check the color and quantity of your urine. If your urine is very dark and scanty, it is concentrated with metabolic wastes, and you need to drink more fluids. When your urine is pale yellow your body has returned to its normal water balance. Your urine may be dark if you are taking vitamin supplements; in that case, volume is a better indicator than color is.

Another way to monitor sweat loss is to weigh yourself before and after you exercise. For every pound you lose, you should drink at least 2 cups of fluid. In hot weather, athletes may easily sweat off 5 to 8 pounds. The weight drop is water loss, not fat loss.

In addition to monitoring urine and weight loss, you should also pay attention to how you feel. If you feel chronically fatigued, headachy, or lethargic, then you may be chronically dehydrated. This is most likely to happen during long hot spells in the summertime. Dehydration is cumulative.

During a very hot week of preseason training, one football player drank like a camel but still couldn't get into water balance. He didn't urinate all day! He dragged through double training sessions and wilted

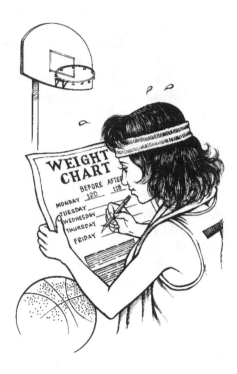

with exhaustion after practice. He sweated so much that he wasn't adequately replacing the fluid loss even overnight; his morning urine was dark and scanty. By the third day into the heat wave, the coach recognized these symptoms of chronic dehydration in many of the players and wisely curtailed practices.

How Much Fluid Is Enough?

Q. Does my thirst tell me if I've had enough to drink?

A. No. You may not feel thirsty, yet you may need more fluids. Your safest bet is to judge by the color and quantity of your urine.

Thirst, as defined by a conscious awareness of the desire for water and other fluids, usually controls water intake. The sensation of thirst is triggered by abnormally highly concentrated body fluids. When you sweat, you lose significant amounts of water from your blood. The remaining blood becomes more concentrated and has, for example, an abnormally high sodium level. This triggers the thirst mechanism and increases your desire to drink. To quench your thirst, you have to replace the water losses and bring the blood back to its normal concentration.

Unfortunately for athletes, this thirst mechanism can be unreliable. Thirst can be blunted by exercise or overridden by the mind. You will voluntarily replace only two-thirds of sweat losses. To be safe, always drink enough to quench your thirst, plus a little more.

Young children, in particular, have a poorly developed thirst mechanism. At the end of a hot day, children often become very irritable, which may be partially due to dehydration. If you are going to spend the day with children at a place where fluids are not readily available, such as at the beach or a baseball game, bring a cooler stocked with lemonade, juice, and water, and schedule frequent fluid breaks to increase everyone's enjoyment of the whole day.

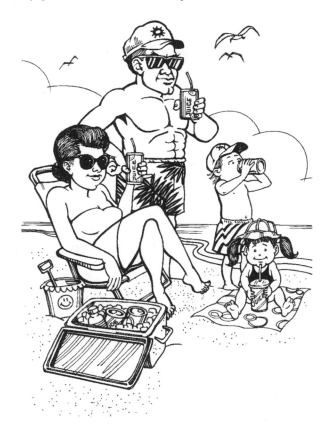

Senior citizens also tend to be less sensitive to thirst sensations than younger adults. Research with active, healthy men aged 67 to 75 years shows that they were less thirsty and voluntarily drank less water when water deprived for 24 hours than similarly deprived younger men aged 20 to 31 years (Phillips et al. 1984). Athletic seniors who participate in any sports should monitor their fluid intake.

Q. How much should I drink before exercise?

A. The exact amount you should drink depends on how large you are (for example, a petite gymnast would drink less than a hulky football player) and how much your stomach can comfortably handle. Assuming that you enter into exercise well hydrated, here are the general guidelines:

• Consume at least 16 ounces of beverages such as water, juice, or a sports drink up to two hours before a competitive event. Because the kidneys require about 60 to 90 minutes to process excess liquid, you'll have the chance to eliminate any excess before competition. For example, if your event is at 10 A.M., drink at least 2 cups of fluids by 8 A.M.

• Drink 4 to 8 ounces or more as tolerated of water or sports drink 5 to 10 minutes before your workout or competition. This fluid in your system will be ready to replace sweat losses. Note that drinking a quart of water before you exercise is less effective than drinking an equal volume while exercising. Researchers aren't quite sure why, but they recommend the optimal approach: Tank up beforehand, plus drink enough to match your sweat losses during long, strenuous exercise (Gisolfi and Copping 1993).

Q. How much should I drink during exercise?

A. During any sporting event, you should start drinking fluids early to prevent dehydration. What you consume at the start will invest in your finish, whether your event is a marathon, a soccer game, or a hike. According to Dr. Larry Armstrong, exercise physiologist at the University of Connecticut, water can travel from stomach to skin in only 9 to 18 minutes after drinking (personal communication, 1996).

In hot weather, drink as much as you can as often as you can. If rapid fluid replacement is important, such as during a football or hockey game, drinking a large volume of fluid initially and maintaining that large volume is preferable to slowly sipping fluids, because the larger volume contributes to faster emptying from the stomach. Of course, this assumes that you can tolerate a large volume of fluid. Be sure to practice high-volume drinking during training. Otherwise, during an event you might end up complaining about stomach sloshing and discomfort from unusually high fluid intakes.

Ideally, you should drink 8 to 10 ounces or as much as you can tolerate every 15 to 20 minutes of strenuous exercise. Under extreme conditions, you might be sweating three times this amount, so that amount of fluid would still leave you with a deficit, but it can significantly reduce the drop in performance that accompanies dehydration.

Always drink before you are thirsty. By the time your brain signals thirst, you may have lost one percent of your body weight, which is the equivalent of 1.5 pounds (3 cups, or 24 ounces) of sweat for a 150-pound person. A 3-percent loss (4.5 pounds) can significantly hurt your performance (Coyle and Montain 1992) and make the difference between winning and losing.

Q. Do I really need to drink eight glasses of water a day?

A. Eight glasses of water might be adequate for a sedentary person, but it is probably too little for many athletes. A general rule of thumb is a liter of water (about one quart) for every 1,000 calories you expend. Hence, the more calories you expend through exercise, the more fluids you'll need.

Rather than count glasses of fluid, you should drink liquids with each meal and monitor your urine output. If you are making trips to the bathroom every two to four hours, you are probably drinking enough.

One sales rep and squash player limited his fluid intake to one cup of coffee in the morning and nothing more until the end of his work day. Because he traveled, he never knew when he'd be able to conveniently find a bathroom. He simply eliminated the "where is a bathroom hassle" by abstaining from fluids. Not only was he chronically dehydrated, which hurt his squash game, but he also had very dark colored, highly concentrated urine that put him at high risk for developing kidney stones.

If you drink more than your body needs, you'll simply urinate the excess. One exercise leader had to go to the bathroom every 30 minutes. She was so concerned about preventing dehydration that she drank a liter every hour, which was needless.

Sodium Replacement

Q. After a sweaty workout, I'm left with a thin layer of salt residue on my skin. Should I eat more salt to replace this loss?

A. Usually, no for the average person who exercises for less than 4 hours at once. Although you may think that you lose a significant amount of salt (more accurately, sodium, a part of salt) when you sweat, you far from deplete your body's supply. In research studies, athletes who lost about six percent of their body weight (the equivalent weight loss of 9 pounds for a 150-pound person) lost only 5 to 7 percent of their body's sodium supply. This is the equivalent of 3,000 to 4,800 milligrams of sodium, or about 1 to 2 teaspoons of salt. (One teaspoon of salt contains 2,300 milligrams of sodium.)

The concentration of sodium in your blood actually increases during exercise because you lose proportionately more water than sodium. Your first need is to replace the fluid; you'll get adequate sodium in the food you eat. For the ordinary athlete, salt depletion is unlikely. Athletes who eat a low-salt diet tend to have low-salt sweat. The less salt they eat, the less they'll lose. The kidneys and sweat glands tend to conserve sodium when it is in short supply.

The amount of sodium that you lose in sweat depends upon how acclimated you are to exercising in the heat. At the beginning of the summer, your sweat is far saltier than at the end of the season. As you adjust to exercising in the heat, you sweat less salt. Training itself also produces changes in sweat gland function, resulting in the production of more dilute sweat. Nature protects you from the potential dangers of becoming salt depleted.

Sodium losses can be easily replaced during your recovery meals after exercise. The average American diet contains 3 to 12 times more sodium than it needs. Sodium occurs naturally in many food items, so you'll get plenty even if you do not add salt to your food. Fruits and juices (popular recovery foods) generally have a low sodium content, but yogurt, pretzels, and spaghetti sauce (equally popular carbohydrates) offer a substantial amount of sodium.

Athletes who exercise hard for more than four hours in extreme heat are at risk of developing medical problems from losing too much salt. If ultraendurance runners, soccer or tennis players in tournament situations, long-distance cyclists, and other people who do extreme amounts of exercise drink too much plain water to replace extreme sweat losses, they may become metabolically imbalanced. They can help prevent hyponatremia (low blood sodium) by eating salty foods during training and, during the event, choosing some foods and sports drinks that contain salt to provide about 250 to 500 milligrams of sodium per hour (the amount in 20 to 40 ounces of Gatorade, for example). During training, they should also practice drinking large volumes of fluids to adapt to the fluid load that will be needed during the event. This will help prevent stomach sloshing.

If you strenuously exercise in the heat for an extended period, such as doing a 100-mile bike ride, an all-day mountain climb with a heavy pack, or repeated days of marathon training in the summer, you might crave salty foods. One hiker commented that after hard summer climbs he seeks out pretzels, popcorn, and other salty snacks. "The salt tastes good to me. I tend to crave it."

Such cravings are your body's way of telling you that you need extra salt. You might want to sprinkle some salt on your recovery meal. The big appetite that likely accompanies this salt craving will help you consume more than enough sodium. See chapter 11 for more information about recovery foods.

Fluid Choices

Q. Do I have to drink water to replace sweat losses?

A. Water isn't the only fluid that will meet your water requirements. Almost any nonalcoholic fluid, such as these, will do:

- Seltzer
- Juice
- Coffee or tea
  (decaffeinated is best)
- Herbal tea
- Lemonade
- Sports drinks
- Soft drinks
- Soups
- Milk
- Smoothies

Even watery foods such as oranges, lettuce, tomatoes, and cucumbers are 85 to 95 percent water by weight and can contribute significant amounts of liquids. Because caffeine has a diuretic effect, opt for herbal tea, decaffeinated iced tea, or decaffeinated coffee for optimal hydration.

Because you will drink more of a beverage if it tastes good to you, be sure to keep pleasing fluids readily available. If your tap water has a disagreeable taste, get a water filter. Or buy bottled water that has a consistently pleasant flavor. Keep your refrigerator stocked with a pitcher of tap water or bottles of spring water. If you get bored with drinking plain ol' water, try seltzer. This sparkling alternative is calorie free, 100-percent pure, and filled with fun bubbles. Add a wedge of lime or a splash of juice for flavor.

Q. Does drinking cold water shock the system or cause stomach cramps?

A. For the average, healthy athlete, drinking cold water does not shock the system or cause stomach cramps. In fact, during hot weather or sweaty exercise, your best bet is to drink a cold fluid because it will cool you off a little faster. You may also find it more palatable and will want to drink more of it.

Drinking cold water in the winter can be a poor choice if you are already chilled. One cross-country skier vividly recalled the time she quenched her thirst from the icy canteen that had been in her backpack for three hours. She was chilled at the time, and the frigid water took its toll. She had to ski very hard for 20 minutes before she warmed herself up again. Hence, if you are skiing, winter hiking, or ice skating in cold weather, you might want to bring along a thermos filled with hot decaffeinated tea with honey, warm soup, hot cocoa, or mulled cider to help warm your body.

Q. Is a soft drink a bad choice for my sports diet?

A. Coke and Pepsi are among the more popular thirst quenchers for sports-active Americans, but they offer zero nutritional value except for 150 calories of refined sugar. Drinking soft drinks is like putting gas in the car but neglecting to put in spark plugs. This sugar does refuel the muscles with carbohydrates, but the natural sugars in juices can do the same trick. Juices also replace the potassium lost in sweat, offer vitamin C (a nutrient that promotes health), and provides numerous other nutrients. Note that commercial sports drinks such as Gatorade, AllSport, or PowerAde are also sugar-filled beverages that offer very little nutritional value.

Rather than judging soft drinks as being good or bad, I look at how many a person is consuming per day:

- A thirsty football player who enjoys a single can of cola can easily fit this 150 calories into his overall wholesome, 5,000-plus calories per day.
- A petite ballet dancer who spends one-third of her 1,400 calories per day training diet on three soft drinks should reevaluate her choices. She could better spend those 450 calories on calcium-rich skim milk to optimize her bone health.

Moderation is the key word. Using the guideline that 10 percent of calories can appropriately come from sugar if you are eating more than 1,700 calories per day, you can determine how many sugary soft drinks (and other sweets) can fit into your sports diet.

Some athletes go to great effort to "de-fizz" a carbonated beverage they want to drink during exercise. They fear the bubbles will hurt their performance or cause an upset stomach. Not the case. Studies show no deleterious effect of carbonation (Zachwieja et al. 1992). Some people actually prefer a carbonated beverage, saying it has a light and refreshing quality.

Q. What about diet soft drinks? Are they bad for my health?

A. If you are on a weight reduction diet, drinking a sugar-free rather than a sugar sweetened soft drink saves about 150 calories (the equivalent of 9 teaspoons of sugar). Diet soft drinks provide a pleasant source of fluid, but otherwise have no positive nutritional content. One or two diet sodas may add enjoyment to a reduction diet, but I advise against drinking liters of diet soft drinks every day (particularly if they are caffeinated); try bottled water or seltzer instead. See table 9.2 for additional information on diet soft drinks.

Table 9.2   Aspartame in Food and Beverages

Many athletes who are cautious about nutrition avoid artificial sweeteners. Nutrasweet (aspartame), in particular, has been controversial because some people report that it gives them headaches or other negative physical reactions. Most researchers, however, believe that aspartame is harmless. It is simply made of two amino acids, aspartic acid and phenylalanine, that naturally occur in protein and exist in high amounts in the diet. For example, one packet of Equal contains 19 milligrams of phenylalanine; this is far less than the 400 milligrams of phenylalanine in a glass of skim milk or the 1,000 milligrams in 4 ounces of hamburger.

If sugar-free soft drinks are an enjoyable part of your diet, the safest advice is to drink them in moderation. Whereas one or two cans can be easily balanced into your diet, the long-term implications from drinking liters day after day, year after year, are yet unknown. If you are that thirsty, drink more water!

The following list compares the aspartame content of commonly eaten foods and beverages. The acceptable daily intake, as established by the FDA, is about 25 milligrams per pound of body weight.

Item	Amount	Aspartame (mg)
Sugar-free gum	1 stick	7
Equal	1 packet	35
Diet hot cocoa	6 ounces	90
Diet gelatin	1/2 cup	80-100
Diet soda	12 ounces	170-195

Data from International Food Information Council, 1992, Intense sweeteners: Effects on appetite and weight management, *IFIC Review* (May); and J. Pennington, 1992, *Bowes & Church's Food Values of Portions Commonly Used*, 16th ed. (Philadelphia: Lippincott).

Sports Drinks

Q. **I'm confused about what to drink, and I want to know if sports drinks are helpful or if water is best.**

A. Water will always be an excellent fluid replacer for most recreational athletes who exercise for less than 60 to 90 minutes. Water is inexpensive, readily available, popular, and what your body needs. It settles comfortably and does a fine job of replacing sweat losses.

If you are at risk of becoming significantly dehydrated during exercise because you are a marathon runner, hockey player, long-distance cross-country skier, or participant in any high-intensity endurance event

ALCOHOLIC BEVERAGES

It is a myth that beer is a good sports drink because it's filled with carbohydrates, potassium, and B vitamins. In fact, it's a very poor sports drink for many reasons:

- **The alcohol in beer has a dehydrating effect.** If you drink beer after exercise, you'll make frequent trips to the bathroom and lose, rather than replace, valuable fluids. Drinking beer before an event increases your chances of dehydration during the event.
- **The alcohol in beer can hurt your sports performance.** If you drink before you exercise, you may end up on the sidelines due to poor performance, if not hypoglycemia. Pre-exercise alcohol can interfere with normal blood sugar control.
- **Beer is a poor source of carbohydrates.** Of the 150 calories in a 12-ounce can of beer, only 50 are from carbohydrates. The rest are from alcohol. Your muscles don't store alcohol calories as glycogen, so with beer you are more likely to get "loaded" than carbo-loaded. Lite beer has even fewer carbohydrates. Here is information comparing carbohydrates in some alcoholic beverages:

Beverage	Amount	Total calories	Carbo calories
86-proof whiskey	1.5 ounces (jigger)	105	—
94-proof whiskey	1.5 ounces (jigger)	115	—
100-proof whiskey	1.5 ounces (jigger)	125	—
Red wine	7 ounces	150	15
Rosé wine	7 ounces	145	15
White wine	7 ounces	140	5

Nutrient data from J. Pennington, 1992, *Bowes & Church's Food Values of Portions Commonly Used*, 16th ed. (Philadelphia: Lippincott).

- **Beer is a poor source of B vitamins.** You'd have to drink 11 cans of beer to get the recommended intake for riboflavin and a lot more to get other vitamins in significant amounts.

I always recommend that athletes get B vitamins from whole-some foods.

If you drink an occasional beer for social reasons, drink plenty of water also. If you are going to drink beer after an event, first quench your thirst with two or three large glasses of water. Then limit yourself to one or two beers, and be sure to eat some carbohydrates such as pretzels or pasta. Don't drink beer or any type of alcoholic beverage on an empty stomach when you are dehydrated; it'll hit you like a ton of bricks!

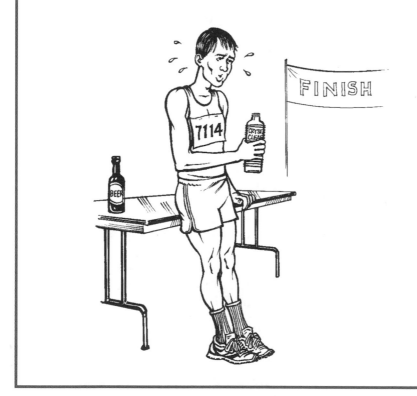

that lasts longer than 60 to 90 minutes, you will have greater stamina if you drink a beverage that contains a small amount of sugar, about 40 to 80 calories per 8 ounces (4%-8% solution). This sugar provides fuel and, in combination with a little sodium, enhances the rate at which your body can absorb the water.

During a moderate to hard endurance workout, carbohydrates supply about 50 percent of the energy. As you deplete carbohydrates from muscle glycogen stores, you increasingly rely on blood sugar for energy.

By consuming carbohydrates during exercise, such as the sugar in sports drinks, your muscles will have an added source of fuel. The sports drinks will also help maintain a normal blood sugar level, so you can exercise longer. Because much of performance depends on mental stamina, maintaining a normal blood sugar level will help you think clearly, concentrate well, and remain focused.

Unlike pre-exercise sugar that in some people results in rebound hypoglycemia, sugar taken during exercise enhances performance. During exercise, the body secretes much less insulin, so a sweetened beverage won't contribute to the "sugar low" that may occur with pre-exercise feedings. (See chapters 4 and 10 for more information about sugar and pre-exercise foods.)

Commercial fluid replacers offer about 50 to 80 calories (12 to 20 grams) of carbohydrates per 8 ounces, a relatively weak solution that quickly empties from your stomach during exercise. If you prefer juices or soft drinks, you should dilute them to this concentration. Otherwise, a highly concentrated drink will likely take longer to empty from the stomach than a commercial fluid replacer will.

Thanks to the power of the media, commercial sports drinks are being perceived as the athlete's edge when it comes to fluid replacements. Although the advertisements may lead you to believe that these special formulations are the ultimate in carbohydration, keep in mind that successful athletes have been drinking homemade sports drinks for years: Cyclists have filled water bottles with tea and honey; marathoners count on friends along the race route to hand them defizzed cola; cross-country skiers have welcomed warm blueberry soup or other sugar solutions at feed stations.

Any fluid replacer, whether commercially prepared or homemade, should achieve the goals of tasting good to stimulate the desire to drink more, replacing lost fluids, providing energy to fuel the muscles, and helping maintain a normal blood sugar level so you can think clearly.

Q. When should I drink a sports drink—before, during, or after exercise?

A. Commercial fluid replacers are diluted beverages designed primarily for highly competitive athletes who need to rapidly replace sweat losses *during* exercise to minimize the risk of becoming dehydrated—football and soccer players, long-distance runners, and racing cyclists. If you choose to drink them 20 to 45 minutes before exercise, note that their sugar content might trigger a hypoglycemic reaction if you are sensitive to swings in blood sugar. If you choose a sports drink after exercise, note that your muscles want carbohydrate-rich fluids to replace the glycogen burned during the event. Most sports drinks have about half the carbohydrates of juices. This means you'll need to drink 16 ounces of Gatorade to get the same amount of carbohydrates as 8 ounces of orange juice or cola. Because of the high price tag on most sports drinks, this can get costly.

If you are, for example, a leisure cyclist who is biking for six hours, you have little physiological need for rapid fluid replacement because you'll have plenty of time to absorb water. You also need not drink a commercial fluid replacer if you are simultaneously snacking on sports bars, bananas, pretzels, and other snacks. These foods negate the purpose of the fluid replacer because their high caloric density delays gastric emptying. According to your taste preferences and budget, you can choose less expensive water along with the food to satisfy your fluid and energy needs, drink lots of nutrient-rich juices, or make your own homemade sports drink (see part IV).

Q. Do sports drinks best replace the sodium lost in sweat?

A. No. Although sports drinks do contain more sodium than you'd get in plain water, they offer relatively low amounts of this electrolyte compared to standard foods (see table 9.3). Don't spend money on a sports drink thinking it will provide needed sodium. The sodium is added primarily to enhance palatability (ACSM 1996). It's a valuable source of sodium only if you exercise for more than 4 to 5 hours..

Q. What about the glucose polymer drinks? Are they best during exercise?

A. Glucose polymers are short chains of glucose molecules. They have become popular with endurance athletes who want carbohydrates that settle comfortably and leave the stomach quickly, but who don't want to drink very sweet liquids or eat solid foods. Polymers are used in some sports drinks such as PowerAde and in many "carbo powders" that provide about 170 calories per 8 ounces.

It is debatable whether a marathoner, triathlete, or other endurance athlete will perform better with a traditional sugared drink (such as defizzed Coke or tea with honey), a polymer drink, or plain water and carbohydrate snacks. What you choose to drink should depend on what works best for your body. Some endurance athletes still feel safest with plain water; it's tried and true. Others prefer a particular brand of sports drink. Some want diluted apple juice or orange sections plus water. Your overall goals are to prevent dehydration and maintain normal blood, and many combinations of water plus carbohydrates can do that job. You have to experiment to determine which combinations you prefer.

Table 9.3   Sodium in Fluid Replacers

The primary purpose of the sodium in sports drinks is to enhance palatability which, in turn, maximizes the rate of fluid absorption. Generally, the gut contains sufficient sodium from the last meal or digestive juices, so there may be little physiological need to add sodium to sports drinks—unless an athlete is exercising for more than 4 hours.

The optimal fluid replacer contains 40 to 80 calories of carbohydrates and 120 to 170 mg sodium per 8 ounces (ACSM 1996).

	Calories	Sodium (mg)
Sports drink (8 ounces)		
Gatorade	50	110
PowerAde	70	70
All Sport	80	55
Exceed	70	50
Soft drink (8 ounces)		
Coke	100	5
Pepsi	105	1
Juice (8 ounces)		
Orange juice	110	2
Apple juice	115	5
Cranberry juice	145	5
Grape juice	155	5
Cranapple juice	175	5
Food		
Orange, large	100	2
Fruit yogurt (8 ounces)	250	250
Potential losses in		
a 2-hour workout:	*1,000*	*1,000*

Nutrient data from food labels and J. Pennington, 1992, *Bowes & Church's Food Values of Portions Commonly Used*, 16th ed. (Philadelphia: Lippincott).

MUSCLE CRAMPS

Muscle cramps are often associated with dehydration. If you have ever experienced the excruciating pain of a severe muscle cramp, you may fearfully wonder if it will strike again. One athlete, who frequently was awakened in the middle of the night by piercing pains in his calf muscles, was eager to find a solution to this disturbing problem. "Perhaps something is wrong with my diet?" he asked, hoping that I'd be able to pinpoint a simple nutritional deficiency.

Because no one totally understands what causes muscle cramps, these unpredictable spasms are somewhat mysterious. They most commonly occur among athletes who work their muscles to the point of exhaustion. They are likely related to overexertion, but fluid loss, inadequate conditioning, and electrolyte imbalance may also be predisposing factors. The solution often can be found with massage, stretching, or, yes, a hard pinch of the upper lip. Other times, nutrition may be involved. Although the following nutritional tips are not guaranteed to resolve this malady, I recommend athletes rule out these possible contributing causes:

• **Lack of water**. Cramps commonly occur when an athlete is dehydrated. To prevent dehydration-induced cramps, drink more than enough fluids before, during, and after you exercise. Always drink enough fluids daily so that your urine is clear, pale yellow, and copious. During a long exercise session, you should drink 8 ounces of fluid every 15 to 20 minutes. After a hard workout, if you are destined to drink alcoholic beverages, be sure to first have plenty of nonalcoholic fluids to replace the sweat losses, because alcohol has a dehydrating effect. One runner eliminated his painful muscle cramps by following the simple advice to first drink water for fluids, then have a beer for social fun.

• **Lack of calcium**. Calcium plays an essential role in muscle contractions. Stories hint that athletes who eliminate calcium-rich dairy products may become plagued by muscle cramps. For example, one ballet dancer found that once she reintroduced

(continued)

yogurt and skim milk into her diet, her cramping disappeared. A mountaineer resolved his muscle cramps by taking Tums, which contain calcium, when hiking. However, some exercise scientists question the accuracy of these anecdotes. A calcium imbalance seems an unlikely cause of muscle cramps because the bones are a huge calcium reservoir. If a dietary deficiency should occur, calcium would be released from the bones to provide what's needed for proper muscle contraction.

Nevertheless, to rule out any possible link between a calcium-poor diet and muscle cramps, athletes plagued by cramps should consume dairy products at least twice each day, for example by eating low-fat milk on cereal and yogurt for a snack. This good nutritional practice certainly won't hurt them, and possibly may help.

• **Lack of potassium**. Electrolyte imbalance, such as lack of potassium, may play a role in muscle cramps. This can also be ruled out by eating potassium-rich foods on a daily basis, focusing on fruits and vegetables. But a potassium deficiency is unlikely to occur as a result of sweat losses, because the body contains much more potassium than even a marathoner might lose during a hot and sweaty race. Nevertheless, a daily potassium-rich diet certainly won't hurt anyone, and in fact is a health-protective choice. See chapters 2 and 11 for more potassium information.

• **Lack of sodium**. Many health-conscious athletes restrict their salt intake, erroneously believing that sodium causes high blood pressure. If they are losing a significant amount of sodium through sweat, they may be putting themselves at risk of developing a sodium imbalance that could contribute to cramps. This is most likely to occur in ultraendurance athletes, such as triathletes or ultrarunners, particularly if they have consumed only water during the event and have eaten no foods or beverages that contain sodium.

I sometimes talk with athletes with low blood pressure who have needlessly imposed a sodium-restricted diet on themselves. They complain to me about cramps, chronic fatigue, and lethargy. They report marked improvement once they reintroduce a little salt into their daily diet.

Although the suggestions for resolving muscle cramps are only suggestions and not proven solutions, you might want to experiment with these dietary improvements if you repeatedly suffer from muscle cramps. Adding extra fluids, low-fat dairy products, potassium-rich fruits and vegetables, and a sprinkling of salt certainly won't harm you, and it may resolve the worrisome problem. I also recommend that you consult with a physical therapist, athletic trainer, or coach regarding proper stretching and training techniques. Nutrition may play no role at all in your cramps.

10

chapter

Nutrition Before and During Exercise

What you eat before you exercise can make or break your workout. Hence, every athlete wants to know what's best to eat before exercising. I only wish I had the winning recipe! The ingredients for the best pretraining or precompetition meal include both physiological and psychological factors. Each person has unique food preferences and aversions, so no one food or "magic meal" will ensure top performance for everyone.

- Herbert, an elite marathon runner, thrives best on two slices of plain bread an hour before his morning run. "It absorbs the stomach juices and settles my stomach." He follows the same routine before he competes.
- Mary Ellen, a rugby player and secretary, avoids any food within four hours of training or competing. Otherwise, she has horrible stomach cramps.
- Tim, a competitive cyclist, claims he must eat cereal. "My magic food is raisin bran with a banana. I've always had my best training rides and races after this breakfast."

- Tracy, a figure skater and seventh-grade student, snacks on a banana before practice sessions but on nothing before a competition. She gets so nervous that she can't keep anything down. "I make sure I eat extra the day before a competition."

Choices of what to eat before exercising vary from person to person and from sport to sport, with no single right or wrong choice. My experience has shown that each athlete has to learn though trial and error during training and competitions what works best for his or her body—and what doesn't work. Some athletes can eat almost anything, others want special foods, and then there are the abstainers who have absolutely no desire to eat anything.

Athletes in running sports, where the body moves up and down, tend to experience more digestive problems than those in sports where the stomach is relatively stable. Jostling seems to be a risk factor for abdominal distress; food eaten too close to exercise time can often "talk back." That's why Walter, a 21-year-old triathlete and college student, eats according to his sport of the day. "When I bike, I enjoy a reasonable meal before the ride and munch on goodies during the workout, or even stop at the dairy for frozen yogurt. When I run, I have to abstain from food for three hours before a workout, or I get diarrhea. That's one reason why I prefer biking to running."

To eat or not to eat . . . that is the question for many active people who wonder about the best way to prevent abdominal discomfort during exercise. Certainly pre-exercise foods that settle comfortably can enhance stamina, endurance, strength, and enjoyment. But with the possibility of pre-exercise food creating intestinal chaos, the threat of diarrhea can turn the thought of pancakes into panic.

Adverse gut reactions occur in 30-50% of endurance athletes. Complaints include

- stomach and upper gastrointestinal (GI) problems (heartburn, vomiting, bloating, "heaviness" of food, and stomach pain) and
- intestinal and lower GI problems (gas, intestinal cramping, urge to defecate, loose stools, and diarrhea).

You should know about some of the predisposing factors for GI problems:

- **Type of sport.** Cyclists, swimmers, cross-country skiers, and others who exercise in a relatively stable position report fewer GI problems than do runners or athletes in running-type sports that jostle the intestines.
- **Training status.** Untrained people who are starting an exercise program report more GI problems than do well-trained athletes who have

gradually built up tolerance to exercise. If you are a novice who is experiencing GI distress, gradually increase your training volume and intensity so your body can adjust to the changes.

• **Age.** GI problems occur more frequently in younger athletes than veterans. This is because the younger athlete may be less trained and possibly have less nutrition knowledge and experience with precompetition eating. Veterans, on the other hand, have had the opportunity to learn from years of nutritional mistakes.

• **Gender.** Women, as compared to men, report more GI problems, particularly at the time of the menstrual period. The hormonal shifts that occur during menstruation can contribute to looser bowel movements.

• **Emotional and mental stress.** Athletes who are tense are more likely to report that food in the stomach lingers longer and settles like a lead balloon.

• **Exercise intensity.** During easy and even moderately hard exercise, the body can both digest food and comfortably exercise. But during intense exercise, the shift of blood flow from the stomach to the working muscles may be responsible for GI complaints.

• **Precompetition food intake.** Eating too much high-protein and high-fat food (such as bacon and eggs or greasy burgers) shortly before exercise can cause GI problems. Tried-and-true low-fat, carbohydrate-rich favorites that are a part of your day-to-day training diet are the safer bet.

• **Food taken during exercise.** Most athletes can tolerate small amounts of familiar foods in their stomachs as long as they don't exercise too hard. If you will be working out at a pace that can last longer than 30-45 minutes, you can both digest food and exercise. But if you do sprint work and all-out efforts, food in your stomach might talk back.

• **Fiber.** High-fiber diets intensify GI complaints. If you are eating large amounts of bran cereal or high-fiber sports bars, try cutting back for a week to see if you feel better.

• **Caffeine and concentrated sugar solutions.** Some athletes seek enhanced performance from drinking a larger-than-usual mug of coffee, but end up with "coffee stomach," diarrhea, and substandard performance. Highly concentrated sugar solutions during exercise are also known to cause stomach distress. Don't confuse the high-carb recovery drinks (about 200 calories per 8 ounces) with low-carb fluid replacers.

• **Level of hydration.** Dehydration enhances the risk of intestinal problems. During training, be sure to practice drinking different fluids on a regular schedule (8 ounces every 15 to 20 minutes of strenuous exercise) to learn how your body reacts to water, sports drinks, diluted juice, and any fluids that you will be drinking during competition.

• **Hormonal changes that occur during exercise.** The digestive process is under hormonal control, and exercise stimulates changes in these hormones. For example, the postmarathon levels of GI hormones in marathon runners tend to be two to five times higher than resting levels. These hormonal changes can result in food traveling faster through the digestive system and explain why some people experience GI problems regardless of what they eat.

PRE-EXERCISE NOURISHMENT

What you eat before you train or compete has four main functions:

1. To help prevent hypoglycemia (low blood sugar), with its symptoms of light-headedness, needless fatigue, blurred vision, and indecisiveness—all of which can interfere with top performance
2. To help settle your stomach, absorb some of the gastric juices, and abate hunger
3. To fuel your muscles, both with food eaten in advance that is stored as glycogen, and with food eaten within an hour
4 To pacify your mind with the knowledge that your body is well fueled

Guidelines for Pre-Exercise Nourishment

To determine the right pretraining or precompetition meal for your body, experiment with the following guidelines. You may find your food preferences vary with the type of exercise, level of intensity, and time of day.

• **Every day, eat adequate high-carbohydrate meals to fuel and refuel your muscles so they'll be ready for action.** Snacks eaten within an hour before exercise primarily keep you from feeling hungry and maintain your blood sugar; they don't significantly replenish muscle glycogen stores. The best refueling occurs within an hour post-exercise.

• **If you will be exercising for more than 60 to 90 minutes, choose carbohydrates with a moderate to low glycemic effect** (see chapter 7 and table 7.3). Yogurt, bananas, oatmeal, bean soup, lentils, and apples are just a few choices. When eaten an hour before exercise, the foods will be digested enough to be burned for fuel, and then will continue to provide sustained energy during the long workout.

- **If you will be exercising for less than an hour, simply snack on any tried-and-true foods that digest easily and settle comfortably.** Bread, English muffins, bagels, crackers, and pasta are a few of the most popular high-carb, low-fat choices.
- **Limit high-fat proteins.** Cheese, steak, hamburgers, and peanut butter take longer to empty from the stomach because fat delays gastric emptying. Cheeseburgers with french fries, large ice cream cones, and pancakes glistening with butter have been known to contribute to sluggishness, if not to nausea. Note that small servings of low-fat protein, however, can settle well and keep you from feeling hungry. One 16-year-old gymnast likes having a scrambled egg for her precompetition breakfast; her brother, also a gymnast, prefers a small slice of cheese pizza. Here are some other appropriate protein choices:

  - Two or three thin slices of turkey or chicken (in a sandwich)
  - One or two slices of low-fat cheese (in pita bread)
  - A spoonful of low-fat cottage cheese (with canned peaches or pineapple)
  - One or two poached eggs (on toast)
  - A glass of skim or low-fat milk (with cereal and banana)

- **Be cautious with sugary foods (such as soft drinks, jelly beans, and even lots of maple syrup or sports drinks) or foods with a high glycemic effect (potatoes, honey, corn flakes, rice; see table 7.3).** Although most athletes perform well after a pre-exercise sugar fix, some athletes who eat these types of carbohydrates within 15 to 120 minutes before hard exercise experience a drop in blood sugar that leaves them feeling tired, light-headed, and needlessly fatigued. By experimenting with eating sugary foods before training sessions, you can learn how your body responds.

  The majority of research currently shows that performance can actually improve with pre-exercise sweets (Ventura et al. 1994). The safest bet, if you simply must have a little bit of something sweet, is to eat it within 5 to 10 minutes of exercise. This short time span is too brief for the body to secrete excess insulin, the hormone that causes low blood sugar. Because the body stops secreting insulin when you start to exercise, you should be able to handle this sugar fix safely if the food settles comfortably.

  Better yet, prevent the need for a quick fix by eating more breakfast and lunch. See chapter 4 for more information about how to resolve sweet cravings.

- **Allow adequate time for food to digest.** Remember that high-calorie meals take longer to leave the stomach than do lighter snacks. The general rule of thumb is to allow at least three to four hours for a

TIMING MEALS BEFORE EVENTS

Time: 8 A.M. event, such as a road race or swim meet

Meals: The night before, eat a high-carbohydrate dinner and drink extra water. The morning of the event, about 6:00 or 6:30, have a light 200- to 400-calorie meal (depending on your tolerance), such as yogurt and a banana, or one or two sports bars, tea or coffee if you like, and extra water. Eat familiar foods. If you want a bigger meal, you might want to get up to eat by 5:00 or 6:00.

Time: 10 A.M. event, such as a bike race or soccer game

Meals: The night before, eat a high-carbohydrate meal and drink extra water. The morning of the event, eat a familiar breakfast by 7:00, to allow three hours for the food to digest. This meal will prevent the fatigue that results from low blood sugar. If your body cannot handle any breakfast, eat a late snack before going to bed the night before. This will help boost liver glycogen stores and prevent low blood sugar the next morning.

Time: 2 P.M. event, such as a football or lacrosse game

Meals: An afternoon game allows time for you to have either a big, high-carbohydrate breakfast and a light lunch, or a substantial brunch by 10:00, allowing four hours for digestion time. As always, eat a high-carbohydrate dinner the night before, and drink extra fluids the day before and up to noontime.

Time: 8 P.M. event, such as a basketball game

Meals: A hefty, high-carbohydrate breakfast and lunch will be thoroughly digested by evening. Plan for dinner, as tolerated, by 5:00 or have a lighter meal between 6:00 and 7:00. Drink extra fluids all day.

Time: All-day event, such as a 100-mile bike ride, triathlon training, or long, hard hike

Meals: Two days before, cut back on your exercise; the day

(continued)

before take a rest day to allow your muscles the chance to replace depleted glycogen stores. Eat carbohydrate-rich meals at breakfast, lunch, and dinner. Drink extra fluids. The day of the event, eat breakfast depending on your tolerance—whatever you normally have before exercising.

Throughout the day, plan to snack at least every one and a half to two hours on wholesome carbohydrates to maintain a normal blood sugar. At lunchtime, eat a comfortable meal. Drink fluids before you get thirsty; you should need to urinate at least three times throughout the day.

large meal to digest, two to three hours for a smaller meal, one to two hours for a blended or liquid meal, and less than an hour for a small snack, according to your own tolerance.

If you are going to participate in a 10:00 road race, you might want to eat only a light 400-calorie breakfast, such as a bowl of cereal with low-fat milk between about 7:00 to 8:00. A hefty 1,000- to 1,200-calorie pancake breakfast might weigh you down. For a noon event, a pancake breakfast at 8:00 could be adequately digested.

• **Allow more digestion time before intense exercise than before low-level activity.** Charlie, a 42-year-old runner and physician, always allows four hours digestion time prior to an intense track workout, but he commonly munches on a bagel 10 minutes before an easy training run. "If I have any food in my stomach before an all-out effort, I feel nauseous. Before an easy training run, however, I can eat almost anything with no stomach problems whatsoever."

Your muscles require more blood during intense exercise than when at rest, so your stomach may get only 20 percent of its normal blood flow during a hard workout. This slows the digestive process. Any food in the stomach jostles along for the ride and may feel uncomfortable or be regurgitated.

During exercise of moderate intensity, blood flow to the stomach is 60 to 70 percent of normal, and you can still digest food. The snacks that recreational skiers, cyclists, and even ultrarunners eat before and during exercise do get digested and contribute to lasting energy during long-term, moderate intensity events.

• **If you have a finicky stomach, experiment with liquified meals to see whether they offer you any advantage** (see table 10.1). Liquid foods tend to leave the stomach faster than solid foods. In one research

Table 10.1   Sample Liquid Meals

Some athletes prefer liquid meals before games because they empty from the stomach more quickly than solid foods do.

Cereal shake

450 calories: 60% carbohydrate, 20% protein, 20% fat

Blend:	2 cups low-fat milk
	1 cup favorite cereal
	Small banana
	4 ice cubes

Optional: 1/4 teaspoon vanilla, dash cinnamon, 1 teaspoon sweetener

Fruit shake

470 calories: 75% carbohydrate, 15% protein, 10% fat

Blend:	1 cup vanilla yogurt
	4-6 peach halves, canned or fresh
	4 graham cracker squares

Optional: dash of nutmeg

study, a 450-calorie meal of steak, peas, and buttered bread remained in the stomach for six hours. A liquified version of the same meal emptied from the stomach two hours earlier (Brouns, Saris, and Rehrer 1987).

Before converting to a liquid pre-event meal, keep in mind that some athletes report that too much liquid "sloshes" in the stomach and contributes to nausea. Always experiment with any new food during training to determine if it offers you any advantage.

• **If you know that you'll be jittery and unable to tolerate any food before an event, make a special effort to eat well the day before.** Have an extra-large bedtime snack in lieu of breakfast. Some athletes can comfortably eat before they exercise, but others prefer to abstain. Both sorts perform well, and both have simply learned how to best fuel their bodies.

• **If you have a "magic food," be sure to pack it along with you when traveling to an event.** Even if it's a standard item such as bananas, pack it so you will be certain to have it on hand.

Even if you have no favorite foods, you still might want to pack a tried-and-true favorite in case of an emergency. If you should encounter delays, such as being stuck in traffic or stranded at an airport, you'll

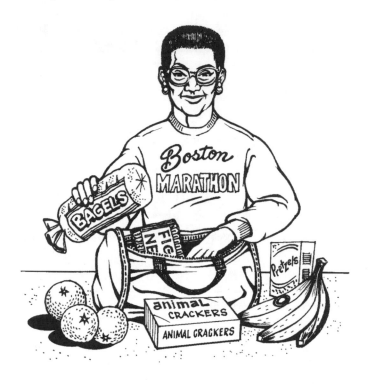

still be able to eat adequately. Emergency foods might include durable carbohydrates that don't easily crumble, such as fig bars, dried fruits, sports bars, or bagels.

• **Always eat familiar foods before a competition.** Don't try anything new!

Pete, a competitive skier, read about a new sports drink that was supposed to be the greatest formula available for nourishment before a race. He drank some for the first time right before a championship event. What a mistake! The liquid gave him a sour stomach; he felt nauseous and performed poorly. He would have been far better off staying with his usual oatmeal. Like many athletes, Pete learned the hard way that he should experiment with new foods only during training.

New foods always carry the risk of settling poorly; causing intestinal discomfort, acid stomach, heartburn, or cramps; or necessitating pit stops. Schedule a few workouts of intensity similar to and at the same time of day as an upcoming competition, and experiment with different foods to determine which (and how much) will be best on race day.

Never, never, never try anything new before a competition, unless you want to risk impairing your performance.

- **Drink plenty of fluids.** You are unlikely to starve to death during an event, but you might dehydrate.
  - Drink an extra four to eight glasses of fluid the day before, so that you overhydrate. You should have to urinate frequently.
  - Drink at least two or three glasses of water up to two hours before the event.
  - Drink another one to three glasses 5 to 10 minutes before the start. For more information about fluids, see chapter 9.

Running on Fuel Rather Than on Fumes

Many athletes take special care to fuel up before they exercise. But some run on fumes because they are afraid that pre-exercise food will result in an upset stomach, diarrhea, and sluggish performance. Without a doubt, too much of the wrong kinds of foods can cause problems but, more often, lack of fuel is the bigger culprit. Morning exercisers, in particular, need to be sure they are appropriately fueled, even if they work out before breakfast.

Skipping breakfast is a common practice among athletes who exercise in the morning. If you roll out of bed and eat nothing before you jump into the swimming pool, teach a step aerobics class, or go for a run, you may be running on fumes. You will probably perform better if you eat a little bit of something before you exercise. During the night, you can deplete your liver glycogen, the source of carbohydrates that maintains normal blood sugar levels. By starting a workout with low blood sugar, you will be likely to fatigue earlier than if you have something to eat.

How much you should eat varies from person to person, ranging from a few crackers to a slice of bread, a glass of juice, a bowl of cereal, or a whole breakfast. If you've had a large snack the night before, you'll be less needy of early morning food. But if you've eaten nothing since a 6:00 dinner the night before, your blood sugar will definitely need a boost. Research has shown good results with 0.5 grams of carbohydrate (2 calories) per pound of body weight one hour before moderately hard exercise, and 2 grams of carbohydrates (8 calories) per pound body weight four hours beforehand. For a 150-pound person, this is the equivalent of 75 to 300 grams (300 to 1,200 calories) of carbohydrate— the equivalent of a small bowl of cereal with banana to a big stack of pancakes (Sherman 1989b).

Researchers can recommend the "best" amount of pre-exercise food, but tolerances vary so greatly from person to person. Some athletes so appreciate the value of pre-exercise food that they get up an hour earlier just to eat. Others have a few bites of a bagel, a banana, or some other easy-to-digest food as they dash out the door, and some habitually run on empty. If you are an abstainer, here are two noteworthy studies that might convince you to experiment with pre-exercise eating.

• Athletes who biked moderately hard for 90 minutes and then performed an intense time trial raced 12.5 percent faster when one hour before the exercise test they ate about 300 calories (0.5 grams of carbohydrate per pound of body weight) as compared to doing the same workout with only water. You might be wondering if they'd have done even better if they'd eaten more. No. Eating twice the amount of carbohydrates, 600 instead of 300 calories, provided no additional benefits (Sherman, Peden, and Wright 1991).

• Cyclists who ate 1,200 calories of carbohydrates (2 grams carb per pound of body weight) four hours before an exercise test were able to bike 15 percent stronger during the last 45 minutes (Sherman et al. 1989). The carbohydrates they ate before they exercised supplied extra fuel for the end of the workout, when their glycogen stores were low.

Although these studies were done with cyclists who tend to report fewer gastrointestinal complaints than athletes in running sports that jostle the stomach, the benefits are worth noting. If you've always exercised on an empty stomach, you may discover you can exercise harder and longer with an energy booster. Experiment during training with eating some carbohydrates within a few minutes to four hours before you exercise: If you swim at 6 A.M., munch on a bagel on the way to the pool. If you work out at lunch, be sure to eat carbs such as cereal for breakfast and perhaps even a banana for a 10 A.M. snack. If you exercise after work, have a carbohydrate-rich lunch and some crackers midafternoon.

Joe, a marathon runner, wondered if his prerun bagel actually provided energy for his workout, or if it simply sat in his stomach. I explained that, despite popular belief, the food that he ate before his moderate exercise did get digested during exercise, but if he were to do extremely intense sprint activity such as a track workout or time trials very little food would get digested. In Sherman's 1991 study, the cyclists absorbed all of the 300 calories (75 grams) of carbohydrates during one hour of moderate/somewhat hard exercise, and 60 percent of the 600-calorie feeding. During intense exercise, however, the stomach does shut down so that more blood can flow to the muscles.

The food you eat before a workout also "tops off" muscle glycogen stores. That is, the cereal you eat at 8 A.M. will fuel your muscles for a midday workout.

Joe also wondered about pre-exercise candy bars. He often felt tempted to raid the vending machine for a quick energy fix. As I mentioned in chapter 4, athletes who eat sugar before they exercise may experience an initial drop in blood sugar during the first 15 minutes of exercise, but the drop is unlikely to result in abnormally low blood sugar that hurts their performance. In fact, most athletes perform better after pre-exercise sugar. Even a candy bar eaten 5 minutes beforehand is unlikely to hurt performance (Neufer et al. 1987). If you know that you are sensitive to sugar swings, you should abstain from sweets, but most active people can handle sugar without a problem.

Feeding Muscles and Mind

For some athletes, food eaten before exercise has more psychological than physiological power. For example, Tim, a cyclist, has to eat cereal before any bike race. No other breakfast is adequate. He carries his cereal and fruit with him whenever he travels to a race, and he feels handicapped unless his appetite is satisfied with muesli topped with a well-ripened banana.

Tim swears that his breakfast contributes not only to strong, successful performances but also to high-quality training and overall well-being. He's confident that the carbohydrates, potassium, calcium, and other nutrients help him win. Undoubtedly they do—if not physiologically, at least psychologically!

Without a doubt, your mind has the power to "convert" any ordinary food into energy-enhancing fuel. Although this attachment to a special food can be helpful, it can also be harmful if the food is unavailable. You may feel handicapped without your magic morsel. For example, one of my clients, a runner, felt crippled when competing in Italy because he couldn't find bran muffins, his favorite food before events.

Carbo-Loading for Endurance Exercise

If you are preparing for an endurance event that lasts for more than 90 minutes—a competitive marathon, triathlon, cross-country ski race, or long-distance bike race—you should saturate your muscles with carbohydrates. But carbo-loading means much more than stuffing yourself with pasta. Here is my nine-step carbohydrate-loading plan to help all endurance athletes fuel optimally for their events.

Carbo-Load Every Day During Training, Not Just Before the Big Event

Your daily diet should be high in carbohydrate, low in fat, and balanced with adequate protein. A daily 60- to 70-percent carbohydrate intake prevents chronic glycogen depletion and allows you not only to train at your best, but also to compete at your best.

The "if some carbohydrates are good, then more will be better" philosophy does not hold true for carbo-loading. If you eat too much, you will likely experience intestinal distress, but your muscles will be no better fueled than if you'd eaten an adequate amount (Rauch et al. 1995). The best target is about 4 grams of carbohydrate per pound of body weight per day. By counting grams of carbohydrates you'll be able to know if your sports diet hits this target (see chapter 7).

Do Your Final Hard Training Three Weeks Before Race Day and Start Tapering Your Training at Least Two Weeks Out

Forget any plans for last-minute training sprees. Put your feet up, rest, and relax for a significant period before the big event. Although hard training builds you up, it also tears you down, and you need time to heal any damage that occurred during training and to completely refuel with carbohydrates. Some exercise scientists suggest you reduce your exercise time down to 30 percent of normal, doing very little exercise in the last 7 to 10 days before the event, other than some short, intense speed intervals to keep you sharp (Houmard et al. 1990).

Tapering properly requires a tremendous amount of mental discipline and control. Most athletes are afraid to taper for such a long time. They are afraid they will get out of shape because they are exercising less. Worry not. The proof will come when you perform better—perhaps 9 percent better! Swimmers, for example, maximized their performance when they tapered for two weeks (Costill et al. 1985). Research suggests a 10- to 13-day taper can be better than a 7-day taper (Zarkadas, Carter, and Banister 1994).

Because you will be exercising less during the pre-event taper, you do not need to eat hundreds of additional calories when carbo-loading. Simply maintain your standard intake. The 600 to 1,000 or so calories that you generally burn during training will be used to give your muscles extra fuel (see table 10.2). If you save the calories that you might have burned during training, you can about double your glycogen stores, and you will be able to exercise harder during the third hour of your event (Rauch et al. 1995).

Table 10.2   Carbo-Loading Guide for Endurance Athletes

Prior to an endurance event that will last for longer than 90 minutes of hard effort, you can give your muscles extra fuel by following this plan that changes your exercise more than your diet:

Number of days before the event	Exercise duration (minutes)	Training diet (% carbohydrates)
21+	120	60-70
5	40	60-70
4	40	60-70
3	20	70
2	20	70
1	Rest day	70
Race	Go for it!	Meal before event, depending on your tolerance

You'll know you have properly loaded if you have gained 2 to 4 pounds (water weight). With each ounce of stored glycogen, you store 3 ounces of water. This water becomes available during exercise and reduces dehydration.

Reprinted, by permission, from W. Sherman et al., 1981, "Effect of exercise-diet manipulation on muscle glycogen storage and its subsequent utilization during performance," *International Journal of Sports Medicine* 2: 115.

Include Adequate Protein Along With the Carbohydrates

Every day, your body needs about 0.6 to 0.9 grams of protein per pound of body weight. Because endurance athletes burn some protein for energy, you should take special care to eat 2 small servings every day of protein-rich foods in addition to getting protein from 2 to 3 dairy servings. See chapters 1 and 8 for more protein guidelines.

Do Not Fat-Load

To achieve the target 20- to 25-percent fat diet, have toast with jam rather than with butter, pancakes moistened with maple syrup rather than with margarine, and pasta with tomato sauce rather than with oil and cheese. A little fat is OK, but don't fat-load.

To achieve a 60- to 70-percent carbohydrate diet, you have to trade in many of the fat calories for more carbohydrates. For example, trade the fat calories in two pats of butter and a dollop of sour cream for a second plain baked potato. When you trade fat for more carbs, you need to eat a larger volume of food to get adequate calories. A one-pound box of spaghetti cooks into a mountain of pasta but is only 1,600 calories. That's a reasonable calorie goal for a hefty premarathon meal, but may be more volume than anticipated. See table 10.3 for a sample carbo-loading diet.

Choose Wholesome, Fiber-Rich Carbohydrates

These promote regular bowel movements and keep your system running smoothly. Bran muffins, whole wheat bread, bran cereal, fruits, and vegetables are some good choices. If you carbo-load on too much white bread, pasta, rice, and other refined products, you're likely to get

Table 10.3   Sample 3,300-Calorie Carbo-Loading Diet

The following diet gets more than 70 percent of the calories from carbohydrates. It would provide 4 grams of carbs per pound of body weight for a 150-pound marathoner. Note that the menu also includes adequate protein (0.8 grams per pound; see chapter 8) to maintain your muscles, yet is still very low in fat and high in carbohydrates.

Breakfast
1 cup orange juice
1/2 cup Grape-Nuts
1 medium banana
1 cup 2% milk
1 English muffin
1 tablespoon jelly   750 calories; 85% carbohydrates

Lunch
2 slices bran bread
3 ounces turkey breast with lettuce, tomato
8 ounces apple juice
1 cup frozen yogurt   750 calories; 65% carbohydrates

Dinner
3 cups spaghetti (6 ounces uncooked)
1 cup tomato sauce (Ragu Hearty)
2 ounces ground turkey
1/4 French bread (4 ounces)   1,300 calories; 70% carbohydrates

Snack
1 cup vanilla yogurt
6 Fig Newtons   500 calories: 80% carbohydrates
Total: *3,300 calories: 75% carb (610 g),*
                                     15% protein (125 g), 10% fat (40 g)

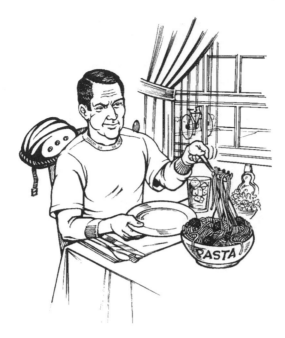

constipated, particularly if you are doing less training. See the section on fiber in chapter 2 for more information. If you are worried about diarrhea, you should avoid fiber-rich foods before an event.

Plan Meal Times Carefully

On the day before the event, you might want to eat your biggest meal at lunchtime so that the food will have more time to digest and pass through your system. Later, enjoy a normal-sized dinner and a bedtime snack. One runner discovered with dismay that the exceptionally hefty dinner she ate the night before a marathon was still sitting heavily in her system on marathon morning.

Drink Extra Fluids to Hydrate Your Body

This reduces your risk of becoming dehydrated.

- Drink about four to eight extra glasses of water and juices during the two days before the event. You should have to urinate frequently.
- Limit dehydrating fluids such as beer, wine, other alcoholic beverages, and beverages containing caffeine.
- On race morning, drink at least three glasses of water up to two hours before the event, one to two cups 5 to 10 minutes before race time. (For more information on fluids, see chapter 9.)

On the Morning of the Event, Eat a Breakfast That You Know Will Settle Well

Food you're familiar with will prevent hunger and help maintain a normal blood sugar level. As a part of your training, you should have practiced eating before races to learn which foods in what amounts work best for you. Don't try any new foods. That festive pancake breakfast may settle like Mississippi mud, and so may the expensive sports bar you've been saving for a special occasion.

Be Sensible

Do not carbo-load on only fruit, or you are likely to get diarrhea. Do not carbo-load on only refined white bread products, or you are likely to become constipated. Do not carbo-load on beer, or you'll get dehydrated. Do not do too much last-minute training, or you'll fatigue your muscles. And do not blow it all by eating unfamiliar foods that upset your system.

EATING DURING ENDURANCE EXERCISE

Ideally, during endurance exercise that lasts for more than 60 to 90 minutes, you should try to keep your body in normal balance by consuming enough fluid to match sweat losses and enough carbohydrate to provide energy and help maintain blood sugar. You can significantly increase your stamina by eating 100 to 300 calories of carbohydrates per hour of endurance exercise (Murray et al. 1991).

More precisely, target about 0.5 grams of carbohydrates per pound of body weight (Coyle et al. 1983). For example, if you weigh 150 pounds, you should target about 75 grams of carbohydrates (300 calories) per hour, which might look like this:

- Six 8-ounce glasses of a sports drink (50 calories per 8 ounces)
- Four cups of a sports drink and a banana
- Two cups of a sports drink plus a sports bar (plus extra water)

Your body doesn't care if you ingest solid or liquid carbohydrates—both are equally effective (Mason, McConell, and Hargreaves 1993). You just have to learn which foods and fluids settle best for your body. I've noticed that runners tend to prefer liquids, whereas cyclists tend to eat both solids and liquids.

Because consuming 100 to 300 calories per hour (after the first 60 to 90 minutes) may be far more than you are used to consuming during exercise, you need to practice eating during training to figure out what foods and fluids do or do not work.

Alex, a novice marathoner, tucked hard candies, gummy bears, and chocolate mints in a waist pack that he wore on his long runs. He also hid two bananas and bottles filled with sports drink on his running loop. Between the snacks and the sports drink, he was able to maintain adequate energy to enjoy his three-hour training runs, and learned what he liked to eat during exercise. Come marathon day, he assigned friends to specific checkpoints along the route; their job was to keep him well supplied with a variety of these carbohydrates. He never "hit the wall," and he was pleased with his time.

Penny, a long-distance swimmer, called me to ask what tastes good with saltwater. She was planning to swim the English Channel. We brainstormed a list of possible ideas, including warm cream of wheat (diluted so she could drink it through a straw), bits of pasta (shells, ziti) that were easy to chew, defizzed cola, animal crackers, and so on. Her favorite turned out to be malted milk balls! It's a good thing she had the foresight to know that her tastes might change during the adventure and that she should have a variety of choices available to her.

Whatever the situation, endurance athletes such as marathon runners, ultradistance cyclists, or Ironman triathletes need to make a nutrition plan far in advance of the event and experiment during training to learn if they prefer grape or lemon sports drinks, solid foods or liquids, sports bars or bananas. By developing a list of several tried-and-true foods, they need not worry about what to eat (and what not to eat) on race day.

Ideally, you should have a defined feeding plan for the event and know your fluid targets, as determined by weighing yourself before and after a workout in different temperatures to determine sweat losses per hour, and your calorie targets. By working with a sports nutritionist or exercise physiologist and the information in table 14.1, you can calculate your calorie needs per hour. You should also figure out how to have these foods and fluids available for you, such as by hiding a bottle of sports drink behind a bush on your training loop, tucking a small bag of raisins into a pocket, putting snacks in a waist pack, or by using a support crew that meets you at designated spots along the route.

During the event, you should try to replace the majority of those calories as tolerated, or target at least 200 to 300 calories of carbohydrates per hour. If you have a support crew, instruct them to feed you on a defined schedule so that you can prevent hypoglycemia and dehydration.

SPORTS BARS

PowerBars, PRBars, GatorBars. You can spend a fortune on these prewrapped bundles of energy. Are they worth it? Some athletes swear yes, others claim no. Here is some information to help you decide on the role of sports bars in your diet.

- **Sports bars are convenient**. In today's eat-and-run society, where meals are a rare occurrence in a busy schedule, a sports bar suits the need for many hungry athletes who seek a hassle-free, somewhat nutritious snack.

- **Sports bars are portable.** Compact and lightweight, these vitamin-enriched bars are very convenient for runners who want to carry a durable snack on a long run, hikers who want a light backpack, or snackers who want to tuck nonperishable food into a pocket. You could also choose low-fat granola bars or breakfast bars from the supermarket as an acceptable alternative at a fraction of the price.

- **Sports bars promote pre-exercise eating—a great way to boost stamina and endurance.** This contrasts to the "don't eat before you exercise" myth that has been perpetuated through generations of athletes and that has perhaps limited their performances. The energy boost associated with eating a pre-exercise sports bar is unlikely to be due to magic ingredients (chromium, amino acids), but rather to eating 200 to 300 calories. These calories (they usually include some form of sugar) clearly fuel you better than the zero calories in no snack. Note that calories from tried-and-true Fig Newtons, graham crackers, bananas, and bagels are also effective pre-exercise energizers.

- **Most sports bars claim to be highly digestible.** One could debate if sports bars are easier to digest than standard food, because digestibility varies greatly from athlete to athlete. I've heard some people comment about how a PowerBar settles heavily in the stomach, while others swear it is the only food they can tolerate during exercise. As with all sports snacks, you have to learn through trial and error during training what foods work for your system and what foods don't. Do not try this pricey treat for the first time before a special event, such as a marathon, bike race, or rugby game only to discover it causes discomfort. (One key to tolerating sports bars is to drink plenty of water along with the bar. Otherwise, the product will settle poorly. Sports bars have a very low water content to make them more compact than fresh fruit, for example, which has a high water content.)

- **Some sports bars tout themselves as fat-free or very low in fat.** They claim that for this reason they digest quickly and empty from the stomach without causing problems.

• **Some sports bars boast about a higher fat content.** This supposedly promotes greater fat burning to help you lose body fat and exercise longer before you "hit the wall." To date, I know of no professional research that suggests that pre-exercise fat enhances weight loss (see chapter 14 for more information about fat burning and weight control). In fact, one study showed no difference in fat burning in athletes who ate a high-carbohydrate or high-fat diet before they exercised (Kavouras et al. 1994).

One possible advantage to including a little fat in the pre-exercise snack may be for sustained energy. By lowering a food's glycemic index, a little fat can provide longer lasting energy for people who will be exercising for more than 90 minutes, such as long-distance bikers, runners, or cross-country skiers. The value of the pre-exercise fat will vary according to individual tolerance. Alternatively, you can enjoy sustained energy by consuming about 0.5 grams of carbohydrate per pound of body weight per hour during endurance exercise, rather than by relying on what you eat before you exercise.

• **Sports bars are expensive.** You'll have to fork over at least one dollar, if not two, to buy most sports bars. The better value is to buy low-fat granola bars or breakfast bars from the supermarket rather than sports bars from the specialty stores or health food centers. A handful of raisins can also do a great job at a very low price! See table 10.4.

Table 10.4   Sports Bars Versus Standard Foods

Although sports bars are a convenient and popular energy source before and during workouts as well as for snacks on the run, standard foods can be just as effective at a fraction of the price.

Sports snack	Calories per ounce	Carbs per ounce	Cost per 100 cal ($)
Banana, 1-1/2" chunk	20	5	.20
Carnation Breakfast bar	119	17	.27
GatorBar	92	21	.81
Growth 1000	128	17	.49
Low-fat granola bar*	110	21	.28
Mr. Big	140	19	.57
PowerBar	100	19	.75
PR* Bar	119	12	1.32
Raisins, 2 tablespoons	91	22	.18

*Nature Valley

Nutrition information from food labels and J. Pennington, 1992, *Bowes & Church's Food Values of Portions Commonly Used*, 16th ed. (Philadelphia: Lippincott).

TOURNAMENTS AND DAY-LONG EVENTS

If you are a competitive swimmer, wrestler, tennis buff, soccer or basketball player, you may frequently be faced with the nutrition
challenges presented by back-to-back events and tournaments that require top performance for hours on end, sometimes days in a row. If
you pay careful attention to what you eat, you'll be able to win with
good nutrition. But as one rugby player commented, "Most players don't
even think about what they will be eating during and between games.
They just eat whatever is around—hot dogs, doughnuts, chips, or nothing." Athletes who give no thought to their nutrition game plan for a
full day of activity can cheat themselves of the ability to perform well
throughout the day.

When you are confronted with extended periods of exercise, your
goals are to maintain proper hydration and a normal blood sugar level.
You have to think constantly about fueling up for the upcoming event,
and then refueling as soon as possible after the first event to prepare for
the next session. As I mentioned earlier, knowing your calorie and fluid
goals can guide your calorie intake and menu planning. Having tried-
and-true sports foods readily available in your gym bag can also make
this an easier task.

Although teaming up with good nutrition can give a team the winning edge, to get a team to dedicate themselves to eating a proper sports
diet can be a challenge. One college coach felt very frustrated by his
team's spirit that inevitably culminated in high-fat pre-event pepperoni
pizza and beer parties that filled the stomach but left the muscles
unfueled and the players dehydrated. No wonder the team was having
a bad season.

The coach took a strong stance.

• He hired a sports nutritionist to educate the players about the importance of pre-event carbohydrates and fluids, and gave the players
lists of foods highest in carbohydrates (see chapter 7 and table 7.4) and
pregame meal suggestions.

• He instructed all coaches and athletic trainers to enforce appropriate between-game eating. With the financial support of the booster's
club, they started to provide bagels, bananas, juices, and other high-
carbohydrate sports snacks and sports drinks for tournament days.

• When traveling to a game, the coach preselected an appropriate
restaurant that could handle the whole team, and he prearranged an
economical buffet with minestrone soup, crackers, spaghetti and tomato sauce, fresh rolls, juice, and frozen yogurt.

• He instructed each player to pack his gym bag with appropriate foods (such as sports drinks, animal crackers, raisins, bananas, bagels) to eat before, during, and between practice sessions and games.

Each player noticed that proper eating helped him perform better, and the team as a whole respected the value of this "win with nutrition" program. And sure enough, they did start to have greater stamina and strength. Although they didn't always win, they no longer got clobbered in the final minutes, and they felt better about their overall efforts.

If you are among the many athletes who give no thought to a sports nutrition game plan during day-long tournaments and repeated events, think again. The right sports diet can indeed enhance your performance. Even varsity athletes and winning teams who are doing well despite poor food choices can do better when they pay attention to their diets. Give food a chance!

TRANSIT PROBLEMS: CONSTIPATION AND DIARRHEA

Problems with constipation or diarrhea are common among athletes. If you've ever been plagued by one or the other during training or at time of competition, you know how worrisome this is and how much it can interfere with top performance. That's why most athletes go to great extremes to promote regular bowel movements.

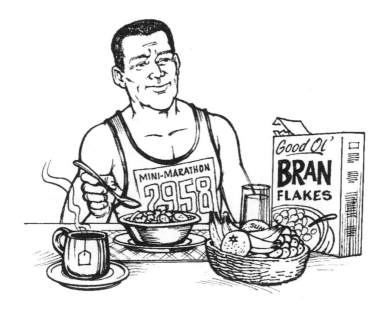

People who fear becoming constipated should faithfully

- eat fiber-rich foods and plenty of fresh fruit and vegetables (see chapter 2) to help prevent constipation,
- drink warm liquids in the morning to encourage regular bowel movements, and
- drink more than enough fluids.

Other athletes struggle with "rapid transit."

Mary complained, "I have to take toilet paper with me whenever I run. I'm plagued by diarrhea and can't figure out why. I feel like a detective and have tried to make dietary changes that might correct the situation. I've tried to determine what triggers the diarrhea by carefully charting for weeks every food and fluid that I've ingested, as well as the times I've exercised and the times I've had diarrhea. I have eliminated suspected problem foods like milk or salads for a week to see if the problem went away, and then looked for changes when I reintroduced these foods into my diet. Nothing. I've allowed at least four hours between eating and exercise. No difference! I've limited broccoli, onions, corn, kidney beans, and other possibly hard-to-digest foods. Not a hint of improvement. I have avoided coffee. Worthless."

Nothing seemed to make any difference. When I looked over Mary's charts, I too was left puzzled. But then I noticed she was chewing gum. That was the culprit! Sugar-free chewing gum contains sorbitol, a type of sugar that can cause gastrointestinal (GI) problems if taken in excess. This lady chewed 20 sticks a day! When she eliminated gum, her GI problems disappeared. What a simple solution to a perplexing problem.

Other athletes aren't quite as lucky and never do find a simple dietary solution. Sometimes they are simply training too much or too fast. Sometimes easy exercise of any type stimulates bowel movements.

Peter, a jogger, was plagued with diarrhea when he started to increase his training mileage. I recommended that he cut back to his baseline mileage for a week, then gradually add on 1 mile per week, rather than 4 to 5. I also advised him to talk with a sports doctor to determine whether he had a medical problem.

For Peter, the solution was to train less intensely. He was trying to run too much, too fast. Like many novice athletes whose bodies have not yet adapted to the stress of intense exercise, he ended up with diarrhea.

If you have persistent problems with diarrhea, intestinal distress, and GI cramping, you should consult your physician. He or she may prescribe some medication to control the problem. You should also consult a sports nutritionist, especially if you are making radical long-term dietary changes. For example, when Larry, a basketball player, discovered he couldn't tolerate milk, he needed help finding alternative, nondairy sources of calcium, riboflavin, and some of the other nutrients in milk. A sports nutritionist who was a registered dietitian helped him find substitutes without sacrificing nutrition.

SPORTS NUTRITION TIPS FOR THE ATHLETE WITH DIABETES

If you have diabetes, your best bet to control your blood sugar is to consistently eat a proper diet (as prescribed by your physician or registered dietitian) and exercise on a regular schedule. Many people with diabetes hesitate to exercise because they are afraid of experiencing hypoglycemia due to abnormally low blood sugar. If you are one of these people, I recommend that you consult with your health care providers to develop a food plan that works for you, read some books about diabetes and exercise (such as the ones listed in appendix B), and practice the following sports nutrition tips.

1. Always exercise after eating, when your blood sugar is on the rise. Do not start to exercise with low blood sugar. Eat a snack first.

2. Always carry sugar in some form with you. (Hard candies and glucose tablets are handy because they aren't messy.) Also carry change with you for a phone call or vending machine.

3. Exercise with someone who knows that you have diabetes and who is aware of the signs of hypoglycemia (confusion, weakness, unconsciousness, convulsions). If your blood sugar plummets, you may stagger and fall; you want your companion to be aware of what's happening. (Some people with diabetes have been misdiagnosed as drunks.) Also make sure your exercise partner knows what to do in an emergency.

4. Most often, you should not change the insulin dose for training but should eat more food. If you repeatedly become hypoglycemic during or after exercise (despite eating more food), you should talk to your doctor about reducing your insulin.

5. To best determine your food and insulin needs, you should monitor your blood glucose during training (for instance, between quarters of a football game or between laps of swimming). You may also need to re-establish these needs when the weather changes from hot to cold.

6. If you are going to be participating in a one-shot bout of high activity (such as an unexpected basketball game), you should eat food before it and you may want to reduce your insulin. Through experience, you'll learn about your body and what strategy works best for you.

7. A person with diabetes has an impaired ability to store and mobilize carbohydrates in the right amounts at the right times, so you should not try to carbo-load. Instead, plan to eat extra calories during exercise.

8. During long-term exercise, replace glucose supplies regularly. When swimming, you may want to pop out of the pool after 50 laps to drink a small can of orange juice; during a marathon, you'll need to eat sugar or snacks along the route.

9. On a long day trip of, say, hiking or cycling, eat six small meals containing both carbohydrate and protein. Be overprepared with extra emergency food in case you get unexpectedly delayed. Explain to your friends beforehand that you are unwilling to share the food with them, or bring more than enough for everyone.

10. Drink plenty of fluids before and during exercise to prevent yourself from becoming dehydrated. You need more fluid if your urine is dark and there is little of it.

11. Because exercise has a lingering effect, you should eat more than usual after exercising. Otherwise, you may become hypoglycemic that night or even the next day.

DIGESTING NUTRITION ADVICE

Advice about what to eat before and during exercise must be taken with a grain of salt, so to speak, because each person's digestive tract is metabolically unique. By experimenting with a variety of fluids, foods, and eating patterns before, during, and after practice you'll gradually discover the best choices for your body. In contrast to the wrong foods that can destroy your performance, the right foods in the right amounts can optimize your chances for success. Eat wisely and win!

11
chapter

Nutrition for Recovery

Billy, a 47-year-old runner, noticed that he wasn't recovering from the Boston Marathon as quickly as his peers; he wondered if a poor diet was making the difference. "Preparing for Boston, I ate a blue-ribbon diet. I chose bagels instead of doughnuts, apples instead of potato chips, pasta rather than burgers. I really wanted to run well, and I ran my best time ever—2:32. Afterward, I rewarded myself with my standard high-fat junk food diet. I felt tired and abnormally achy for more than a week. If I'd eaten better, would I have recovered faster?"

Other competitive athletes have expressed similar concerns. Football players want to know what they should eat after morning practice to prepare for the afternoon session. Bodybuilders wonder if they should eat extra protein after workouts to repair muscles. Tennis champs seek out foods that will prepare them for the next day's match. Swimmers search for the proper foods that will get them through a heavy season of training and competing without letting them deteriorate and experience chronic fatigue.

PREVENTING CHRONIC FATIGUE

Athletes can become chronically fatigued for a variety of reasons, including excessive training, inadequate rest, and improper nutrition. If you have a strenuous and prolonged training schedule in addition to other commitments and responsibilities, you may find yourself with too little time for proper eating and sleeping.

Listed here are some symptoms of chronic fatigue syndrome. If you are experiencing two or more of these symptoms, take heed!

- Unusually poor performances in training and competition
- Failure to improve performance despite diligent training
- Inability to perform better in competition than during practice
- Loss of appetite and body weight
- Insomnia
- Joint and muscle pains that have no apparent cause
- Frequent colds or respiratory infections
- Irritability and anxiety that may be accompanied by depression

Rather than getting to the point of chronic fatigue, you should take steps to prevent it:

- Eat a proper sports diet that provides adequate carbohydrates and protein.
- Allow recovery time between bouts of intense exercise.
- Plan your schedule so you can get enough sleep at night.
- Try to minimize stress in your life and curtail disruptive activities that might drain your physical and mental energy reserves.

Data from W. Sherman and E. Maglischo, 1991, "Minimizing chronic fatigue among swimmers: Special emphasis on nutrition," *Sports Science Exchange* 4 (35). Gatorade Sports Science Institute.

Proper nutrition enhances performance. When you are confronted with the rigors of a tough training schedule, remember that what you eat after a hard workout or competition does affect your recovery. For the serious athlete, foods eaten after exercise require the same careful selections as the meal before exercise. By wisely choosing your foods and fluids, you will recover more quickly for the next workout.

If you are a recreational exerciser who works out three or four times per week, you need not worry about your recovery diet because you have enough time to refuel your muscle glycogen stores before your next workout. But you should be concerned about your recovery diet if you are a competitive athlete who does two or more workouts per day, such as a football player at training camp who practices morning and afternoon, a competitive swimmer who competes in multiple events per meet, a triathlete who trains twice per day, an aerobics instructor who teaches several classes daily, or a basketball player who needs to endure the entire season of intense training and competing. In order to recover and refuel for the next bout, you should pay particular attention to what you eat after the first session.

Athletes commonly have reasons to eat inadequately after exercise, including that they don't feel hungry and don't have time. This chapter addresses the consequences of giving in to these excuses and outlines important considerations for optimal recovery from either exhaustive daily training, one hard competition, or multiple events in the same day or weekend. For more information, refer to chapter 10.

RECOVERY FLUIDS

After you finish a hard workout, your top dietary priority should be to replace the fluids you lost by sweating so that your body can get back into water balance (see chapter 9). The best choices for replacing sweat losses include one or more of the following:

- Juices, which supply water, carbohydrates, vitamins, and minerals (electrolytes)
- Watery foods such as watermelon, grapes, and soups that supply fluid, carbohydrates, vitamins, and minerals
- High-carbohydrate sports drinks or soft drinks, which supply fluids and carbohydrates (but minimal, if any, vitamins or minerals)
- Commercial fluid replacers, which supply fluids, some carbohydrates and electrolytes, and a few vitamins if fortified with them
- Water, which tends to be convenient, well tolerated, and least expensive

To determine how much fluid to replace, you need to know how much water you lose during a strenuous event. You can estimate this by weighing yourself before and after a hard training workout. Your goal is to lose no more than 2 percent of your body weight (for example, 3 pounds for a 150-pound person). By drinking on a schedule (8 ounces every 15 to 20 minutes of hard exercise), you can prevent dehydration.

One football player was shocked to discover that on a relatively cool day, he'd lost 8 pounds during the morning football practice—5 percent of his body weight and the equivalent of a gallon of sweat! (One pound of sweat loss represents 16 ounces of fluid.) He became aware of the importance of drinking more. He started bringing a water jug to practice so he wouldn't feel guilty for taking more than his share from the limited water supply on the playing field. He drank at every opportunity during practice, and then made sure that he finished the whole gallon, plus more on very hot days, between the morning and afternoon practices. These steps to prevent dehydration helped him recover easily.

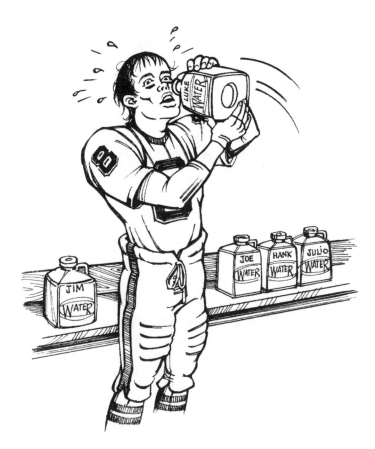

If you become dehydrated during an unusually long and strenuous bout of exercise, you should drink frequently for the next day or two. Your body may need 24 to 48 hours to replace the sweat losses. You'll know that you are adequately rehydrated when your urine is clear, pale yellow and you have to urinate frequently. A small amount of dark urine is still concentrated with metabolic wastes. (If you take vitamin supplements, your urine may be a dark color; you'll need to judge your hydration status by the volume of urine.) See chapter 9 for additional information on fluids and rehydration.

RECOVERY CARBOHYDRATES

Your muscles can replace glycogen at the average rate of about 5 percent per hour. Thus, it takes at least 20 hours to fully replenish depleted muscles. Ideally, you should consume carbohydrate-rich foods and beverages within 15 minutes after your workout; that is, when the enzymes responsible for making glycogen are most active and will most rapidly replace the depleted glycogen stores at the rate of 7 to 8 percent per hour (Ivy et al. 1988).

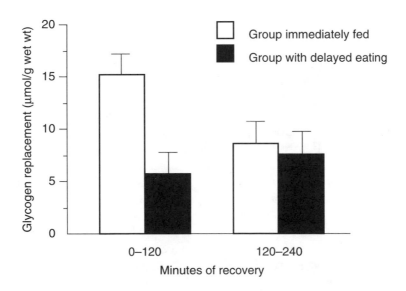

The two test groups show that eating within 15 minutes after exercising replenishes glycogen stores faster than delaying eating for two hours.

Adapted, by permission, from J. Ivy et al., 1988, "Muscle glycogen synthesis after exercise: Effect of time carbohydrate ingestion," *Journal of Applied Physiology* 64: 1481.

More precisely, your target intake is 0.5 grams of carbohydrate per pound of body weight every two hours for six to eight hours (Ivy et al. 1988). Let's assume that you weigh 150 pounds:

150 lb × 0.5 g carbs/lb = 75 g carb = 300 calories carb

Thus, you'll need about 75 grams (300 calories) of carbohydrates within the first two hours. (One gram of carbohydrate contains 4 calories, so this converts to 300 calories.) Two hours later, you should eat another 300 calories of high-carbohydrate foods.

Your body will naturally want this amount, if not more. If you've been exercising so hard that you have concerns about replacing depleted glycogen stores, the chances are good that you are very hungry for lots more calories! You can eat more than the calculated amount, but extra carbohydrates will not hasten the recovery process.

Liquids and solid foods will refuel your muscles equally well, and foods with a moderate-to-high glycemic effect will provide the quickest replenishment (see chapter 7). Some popular 300-calorie, carbohydrate-rich food suggestions are listed here:

- 8 ounces of orange juice and a medium bagel
- 16 ounces of cranberry juice
- one 12-ounce can of soft drink (not diet) and an 8-ounce fruit yogurt
- one bowl of corn flakes with milk and a banana

Commercial high-carbohydrate sports drinks and carbohydrate powders can also refuel your muscles. But be aware that these carbo drinks lack most of the vitamins and minerals that accompany wholesome natural foods (unless they are fortified with them). They also tend to be more expensive than standard foods.

As I mentioned before, most fitness enthusiasts can recover at their own pace because they don't deplete themselves of carbohydrates in their typical 30- to 45-minute workout. In contrast, endurance athletes and others involved in exhaustive daily training or repeated and closely scheduled competitions should pay careful attention to quickly refueling.

Elaine, a cyclist and physical therapist, knew that she should eat recovery carbohydrates after racing, but she was tired of yet another plate of pasta; she wanted meat. Like many endurance athletes, she'd eaten primarily carbs for the three days prior to her event, and now she wanted something else. She satisfied this craving and properly refueled by eating a hamburger supplemented with lots of carbohydrates: a thick kaiser roll, minestrone soup with crackers, lemonade, and frozen yogurt. The hamburger became an accompaniment to the other carbohydrate-rich choices, and she ended up with a high-carbohydrate diet after all.

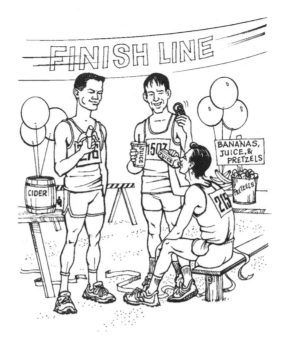

PROTEIN

Don't avoid protein in your recovery diet. In fact, some protein can actually enhance glycogen replacement in the initial hours after hard exercise. Protein, like carbohydrate, stimulates the action of insulin, a hormone that transports glucose from the blood into the muscles. Protein eaten along with carbohydrates (such as protein-rich milk with cereal, a slice or two of turkey on a bagel, or a little lean meat in spaghetti sauce) provides a winning combination! A good ratio is 1 gram of protein for every 3 grams of carbohydrates (Zawadski, Yaspelkis, and Ivy 1992). See table 11.1.

Although lots of extra protein is unnecessary after exercise to repair muscles and enhance the recovery process (Brouns 1993), you do need the recommended amount of protein (see chapter 8). In some cases, carbohydrate-conscious athletes shun protein, forgetting that adequate amounts are essential for a well-balanced diet that sustains overall good health. They should specifically plan in some protein to balance out their diet.

RECOVERY ELECTROLYTES

When you sweat, you lose not only water but also some minerals (electrolytes) such as potassium and sodium that help your body function

Table 11.1   Recovery Foods: Balancing Carbohydrates and Protein

Protein, in addition to carbohydrates, helps to optimize glycogen recovery. This study shows how the right balance of carbohydrate and protein enhanced the recovery of nine male cyclists who exercised hard, depleted their glycogen stores, and then ate either only protein, only carbohydrates, or a combination of carbohydrates and protein. The results indicate that protein stimulates the activity of insulin, a hormone that enhances glycogen replacement (Zawadski et al., 1992).

Feeding	Carb (g)	Protein (g)	Glycogen stores 4 hours after exercise (micromoles glycogen/g protein)
1	0	40	+30
2	112	0	+103
3	112	40	+142

Note: 112 g carb = 448 calories; 40 g protein = 160 calories

normally. You can easily replace these losses with the foods and fluids you consume after the event. Based on the assumption that the harder you exercise, the hungrier you'll get and the more you'll eat, you'll consume more than enough electrolytes from standard postexercise foods. You won't need salt tablets or special potassium supplements. For example, Pete guzzled a whole quart of orange juice after his 2:32 marathon. This replaced three times the potassium he might have lost. A third of a quart, which contains 600 milligrams of potassium, would have done the job! He also munched on a bag of pretzels that more than replaced sodium losses.

Potassium

Potassium is a mineral involved in maintaining normal water balance in your body. Although potassium-rich orange juice is a particularly good choice for a recovery fluid, many athletes find that orange juice is too acidic and settles uncomfortably. Alternatives include almost any natural juices, particularly pineapple or apricot nectar. Another alternative is to drink plain water for fluid and eat a banana for potassium. See table 11.2 for the potassium content of some popular recovery foods, noting that some are surprisingly low in potassium.

Table 11.2   Potassium in Some Popular Recovery Foods

A pound of sweat contains about 80 to 100 milligrams potassium. During 2 to 3 hours of hard exercise (expending 1,200 to 1,800+ calories), you might lose 300 to 800 milligrams of potassium. The following chart rank-orders some fluids and foods for potassium content. In general, natural foods are preferable to commercial products. See tables 1.3, 1.4, and chapter 2, "Increasing Your Potassium Intake," for a complete potassium list.

Food	Mg potassium/ serving	Mg potassium/ 100 calories (amount)
Potato	840 1 large (7 ounces)	380 1/2 large potato
Yogurt	530 8 ounces, low-fat	370 2/3 cup
Orange juice	475 8 ounces	420 7 ounces
Banana	450 medium	450 1 medium
Pineapple juice	330 8 ounces	230 6 ounces
Raisins	300 1/4 cup	230 3 tablespoons
Beer	90 12 ounces	60 8 ounces
AllSport	55 8 ounces	70 10 ounces
PowerAde	30 8 ounces	45 11.5 ounces
Cranapple juice	40 8 ounces	30 6 ounces
Gatorade	30 8 ounces	60 16 ounces
Coke	0 12-ounce can	0 8 ounces

Nutrition information from food labels and J. Pennington, 1992, *Bowes & Church's Food Values of Portions Commonly Used,* 16th ed. (Philadelphia: Lippincott).

If you are tempted to replace potassium losses with commercially prepared fluid replacement beverages, look closely at table 11.2 and note that most of these special sports drinks are potassium poor.

Commercial fluid replacement drinks are designed to be taken during intense exercise. They are very diluted, which helps them empty faster from the stomach. They are not the best recovery foods in terms of electrolyte content, carbohydrates, and overall nutritional value unless you drink large volumes.

Sodium

Another electrolyte that you lose when you sweat is sodium (a part of salt). Although you lose a little sodium under ordinary exercise conditions, you do not come close to depleting your body's stores. For the average fitness participant, replacing salt losses either after or during exercise is of no major concern (see chapters 2 and 9).

In most cases, the typical American diet more than adequately replaces sodium losses. Popular recovery foods such as yogurt, muffins, pizza, and spaghetti have more sodium than you may realize! If you need extra salt, you will crave it. Sprinkle a little salt on your food or choose some salty items such as pretzels, crackers, or soup (see table 11.3).

In extreme circumstances, such as an ultraendurance event that lasts for more than 4 hours in the heat, you have a higher risk of becoming sodium depleted. To prevent this, be sure to consume salted fluids or foods during the event.

Table 11.3   Sodium in Some Popular Recovery Foods

A pound of sweat contains about 400 to 700 milligrams of sodium. During two to three hours of very hard exercise, you might lose 1,800 to 5,600 milligrams of sodium. The more you have adapted to exercising in the heat, the less sodium you'll lose. If you need salt, you'll crave it. Notice that it's easy to get sodium through unsalty foods such as bread and bagels.

Recovery food	Sodium (mg)
Pizza, 1/2 of 12" cheese	1,300
Macaroni and Cheese, 1 cup Franco-American	1,060
Spaghettios, 1 cup	990
Chicken Noodle Soup, 1 cup Campbell's	830
Spaghetti sauce, 1/2 cup Ragu	820
Salt, 1 small packet	500
Bagel, 1 small Lender's	320
Cheerios, 1 cup	290
American cheese, 1 slice (2/3 ounce)	260
Pretzels, 1 Dutch	220
Saltines, 5	180
Bread, 1 slice Pepperidge Farm Hearty Slices	180
Potato chips, 20	140
Gatorade, 8 ounces	110
Frozen yogurt, 1 cup	100
Beer, 12 ounces	15
Coke, 12 ounces	10
Orange juice, 8 ounces	5

Data from food labels and J. Pennington, 1992, *Bowes & Church's Food Values of Portions Commonly Used,* 16th ed. (Philadelphia: Lippincott).

REST

As I discussed in chapter 7, rest is a very important part of your training program.

> The day after his marathon, Dave felt compelled to hop back on his feet and start training for the next event two months away. "I feel guilty if I don't run every day. I'm afraid I'll become unfit, fat, and lazy if I miss a day of training."

Like many compulsive exercisers, Dave allowed no recovery time in his exercise program. He neglected the important physiological fact that rest is essential for top performances. I told him that rest would enhance his recovery process, reduce his risk of injury, and invest in his future performance.

I recommended that Dave not attempt a training run on the day after a major marathon. If he insisted on exercising, I instead suggested that Dave try an alternative form of exercise that would limber up his tight muscles but not pound his joints. He took a gentle bike ride to the swimming pool and slowly swam laps for 15 minutes, easing his guilty conscience and loosening his muscles.

Time is necessary for the recovery process of healing and refueling. To completely replace depleted glycogen stores, the muscles may need up to two days of rest with no exercise and a high-carbohydrate diet. There's no way Dave could have done quality training with his battered muscles. He admitted that he was being compulsive and not wise. (See chapter 15 for more discussion about how to handle compulsive behaviors.)

Dave's muscles were sorer by the second day after the marathon, but his achiness was normal. You can expect to experience worse soreness on the second day after strenuous exercise that damages your muscles (such as downhill running). If the pain persists, you should consult a sports medicine specialist for some professional help. And, of course, you should keep eating a variety of wholesome foods with all the vitamins, minerals, and protein needed to enhance the healing process.

The same athletes who avoid rest after an event also tend to overtrain while preparing for an event. Many athletes train for two or three hours per day, thinking this will enhance their performance. Unlikely. Research has shown that swimmers performed just as well on one 90-minute training session per day as they did with double workouts of two 90-minute sessions (Costill et al. 1991). Quality training is better than quantity training; do not underestimate the power of rest.

12
chapter

Supplemental Strategies

You've undoubtedly heard the message time and again that you can get the vitamins you need from the foods you eat. To date, neither the American Dietetic Association (American Dietetic Association 1996) nor one government health organization recommends that you include supplements as a part of your daily diet. Yet surveys repeatedly show that many Americans fail to eat adequate fruits, vegetables, whole grains, and low-fat dairy foods. Should public health officials recommend that we take supplements to compensate for our poor eating habits? Or should they put more emphasis on teaching Americans how to eat healthfully despite a hectic lifestyle?

VITAMINS VERSUS FOOD

Vitamin supplements are very popular among today's athletes. Surveys suggest that about 75 percent of all athletes take some type of supplement, ranging from a simple multivitamin pill to a complex assortment of wonder pills. Supplementation practices differ among sports. About 6 percent of male basketball players take supplements, in comparison to 100 percent of bodybuilders (Burke and Deakin 1994).

Confusion stems from the $4 billion vitamin industry's advertisements that have convinced millions of people of a need to supplement their diets. One working mother who didn't have time to eat right was swayed by advertisements to believe that supplements would compensate for her poor eating habits. So was a banker, who reported taking vitamins as health insurance to help protect him from the stress of hard squash games and the negative effects of drinking a few beers afterward. A construction worker in training for a triathlon expressed this concern: "I'm so active, I must need more vitamins than my diet can provide." A personal trainer with a busy schedule was convinced that taking supplements could help her have enough energy to get through her active day.

Like many active people who are constantly feeling stressed, grabbing hit-or-miss meals, juggling work with workouts, fighting fatigue, and exercising intensely, you may have turned to vitamin supplements as a panacea to guard your health, compensate for a diet filled with processed foods, enhance your athletic abilities, boost your energy, and promote future "super health." But take note: The same ads and salespeople that entice you to take supplements generally downplay the importance of food. You still need to eat well, regardless of the number of pills you pop. A supplement, if you chose to take one, should be part of a larger plan for an optimal sports diet. Your first priority should be to choose the fundamental foods that supply the vitamins and other nutrients you need.

Too many people take a vitamin pill breakfast in preparation for their chocolate chip cookie lunch. They naively believe that a vitamin supplement satisfies 100 percent of their nutritional needs. They are wrong. Yes, they may get 100 percent of their vitamin needs with the pill. But we also need protein, minerals, energy, fiber, and phytochemicals— nonvitamin compounds in foods that protect our health (see table 2.6). No vitamin provides energy (calories) nor does it compensate for a meal of sugars and fats. Pill poppers are naive to think that a pill of any type can magically make up for an erosive lifestyle. It's also unlikely that any of the commonly occurring diseases of aging, such as diabetes or heart disease, is caused by the deficiency of a single nutrient.

VITAMIN SUPPLEMENTS: WHAT THEY ARE AND WHAT THEY AREN'T

The purpose of this chapter is to take a look at some of what is and is not known about nutritional supplements. Then you can decide if you should spend more money on fruits and vegetables than on

THE FUNDAMENTAL FORTY NUTRIENTS

Carbohydrates

Protein (9 essential amino acids)

- histidine
- isoleucine
- leucine
- lysine
- methionine
- phenylalanine
- threonine
- tryptophan
- valine

Fat

- linoleic acid

Vitamins

Fat soluble (4)

- A
- D
- E
- K

Water soluble (9)

- B-1 (thiamin)
- B-2 (riboflavin)
- B-6 (pyridoxine)
- niacin
- B-12
- folacin
- biotin
- pantothenic acid
- C (ascorbic acid)

Minerals

Major (3)

- calcium
- phosphorous
- magnesium

Trace (9)

- iron
- zinc
- iodine
- copper
- manganese
- fluoride
- chromium
- selenium
- molybdenum

Electrolytes

- sodium
- potassium
- chloride

Water

The following substances are being studied to determine possible human requirements:

- aluminum
- arsenic
- boron
- cadmium
- choline
- cobalt
- nickel
- silicon
- strontium
- titanium
- tin
- vanadium

By eating a variety of foods from the Food Guide Pyramid, you will get the fundamental 40 nutrients required to maintain good health. Plus, you'll get even more fiber, phytochemicals, and food substances that protect your health.

Data from National Academy Press, 1989, Recommended dietary allowances, 10th rev. ed. (Washington, DC: National Academy Press).

supplements and more time on living a healthier lifestyle by exercising regularly, reducing stress, and laughing. Because researchers have yet to determine the entire role of vitamins in the diet, stay tuned and be sure to take care of your whole health. Vitamin supplements are only one part of the picture.

What Are Vitamins?

Vitamins are metabolic catalysts that regulate biochemical reactions within your body. Your body cannot manufacture vitamins, which is why you must obtain them through your diet. To date, 13 vitamins have been discovered, each with a specific function. For example, thiamin helps convert glucose into energy, vitamin D controls the way your body uses calcium, and vitamin A is part of an eye pigment that helps you see in the dim light. The trick is to get enough of a vitamin to invest in optimal health, without getting too much and experiencing harmful reactions.

Historically, vitamins have been studied in terms of short-term nutritional deficiencies based on the minimal amount of a nutrient required to prevent diseases such as beriberi and scurvy and as coenzymes that regulate body processes. The Recommended Dietary Allowances (RDAs) were developed to define that need. They are not minimal requirements, but rather provide at least a 30 percent margin of safety to cover the nutritional needs of 97 percent of healthy Americans and account for human variability. For example, the amount of vitamin C that prevents the deficiency disease scurvy is 10 milligrams per day; the recommended intake is 60 milligrams, or 6 times the minimum amount. You can meet these recommended intakes even if you are eating on the run, by choosing a variety of wholesome foods from the five food groups (refer to chapter 1).

What Vitamins Are Not

You need adequate vitamins to function optimally, but no scientific evidence to date proves that extra vitamins offer a competitive edge. Despite claims to the contrary, supplements will *not* enhance performance, increase strength or endurance, provide energy, or build muscles.

If you have a vitamin deficiency that is impairing your performance, a supplement can correct that problem. However, vitamin deficiencies usually are related to a larger medical problem that needs attention, such as anorexia, unhealthful weight reduction, malabsorption problems, or years of extremely poor eating habits.

Some people claim they feel better and have more energy when they take vitamins. These anecdotal claims raise questions about individual

Vitamin Breakdown

VITAMIN	RECOMMENDED INTAKE	FUNCTIONS
(retinol) A	5,000 IU	Necessary for healthy eyes, skin, and linings of the digestive and urinary tracts and the nose
B₁ (thiamin)	1.5 mg	Helps transform carbohydrates into energy
B₂ (riboflavin)	1.7 mg	Necessary for energy release and for healthy skin, mucous membranes, and nervous system
B₃ (niacin)	20 mg	Helps transform food into energy; necessary for growth and for production of hormones
B₆ (pyridoxin, pyridoxamine)	2.0 mg	Necessary for synthesis and breakdown of amino acids; aids in metabolism
Folic acid (folate)	0.4 mg	Necessary for production of blood cells and healthy nervous system

Vitamin		Amount	Function
	BIOTIN	0.3 mg	Needed for metabolism of carbohydrates, fats, and protein
	Pantothenic acid	10 mg	Needed for metabolism of carbohydrates, fats, and protein
	B₁₂	6.0 mcg	Needed for synthesis of red and white blood cells and for metabolism of food
	C (ascorbic acid)	60 mg	Necessary for healthy connective tissue, bones, teeth, and cartilage; enhances immune system
	D (cholecalciferol)	400 IU	Needed for calcium and phosphorus metabolism and for healthy bones and teeth
	E (tocopherol)	30 IU	Necessary for nourishing and strengthening cells
	K	70 to 140 mcg	Necessary for blood clotting

responses to vitamins and point out that each person is metabolically unique. Or perhaps the pill taker experiences a placebo effect—the positive response that accompanies a belief that a pill will help them feel better. Maybe the vitamins are being taken as part of a "health kick" that includes eating better, exercising regularly, and taking supplements. These lifestyle changes, rather than the supplement itself, perhaps deserve credit for increasing the feelings of well-being.

Vitamins and Athletes

Many active people wonder if exercise increases their vitamin needs. For the most part, no. Exercising doesn't burn vitamins, just as cars don't burn spark plugs. Vitamins are catalysts that are needed for metabolic processes to occur. There is no evidence to date that vitamin supplementation improves performance in people who are adequately nourished. Also keep in mind that the more you exercise the more you eat and the more vitamins you consume. Most athletes consume more calories, and therein more vitamins, than inactive people with smaller appetites. Deficiencies are more likely to occur in a sedentary person who eats very little, such as an elderly grandparent, as compared to the sports-active person who eats lumberjack portions.

Studies suggest that the established RDAs for a few vitamins might be low for active people. For instance, the current recommended intake for riboflavin (vitamin B-2, important for converting food into energy) is 0.6 milligrams per 1,000 calories. A more appropriate intake for active people is 1.1 milligrams per 1,000 calories (Belko 1987). Yet a higher need doesn't mean you should rush out to buy riboflavin. You can easily get adequate riboflavin in a breakfast of cereal with milk!

If in your busy training schedule you occasionally eat poorly, you may wonder if a supplement could compensate for the grease and goo.

> Pat, a 46-year-old office manager, was a tournament golfer. She consumed a well-balanced diet six out of seven days a week. Fridays were her downfall because of fatigue and work stress. She'd inevitably "go off the deep end" and comfort herself with doughnuts, ice cream, and cookies, and then she'd take megadoses of vitamin supplements to protect herself from nutritional deficiencies.

I assured Pat that a nutritional deficiency would not develop overnight. She could survive on less than 100 percent of every vitamin every day because she stores vitamins in her body, some in stockpiles (A, D, E, K—the fat-soluble vitamins) and others in smaller amounts (B,

C—the water-soluble vitamins). Like most healthy people, she probably had enough vitamin C stored in her liver to last six weeks. One day of suboptimal eating would not have resulted in a nutritionally depleted body. Nutritional deficiencies develop over the course of months or years, such as can happen with the person who is anorexic or who eats an inadequate vegetarian diet.

Supplements for Special Situations

Although I always advise athletes to first try to get their vitamins through wholesome foods, I do recommend a simple multivitamin supplement for individuals at risk of nutritional deficiencies. Supplements are appropriate for people who are facing these issues:

• **Restricting calories.** Dieters who eat less than 1,200 to 1,500 calories daily may miss out on some important nutrients.

• **Allergic to certain foods.** People who can't eat certain types of foods, such as fruits or wheat, need to compensate with alternative vitamin sources to avoid deficiencies in some nutrients.

• **Lactose intolerant.** The inability to digest the milk sugar found in dairy products is a common occurrence among African-American and Hispanic people. Avoiding dairy foods can result in a diet deficient in riboflavin and the mineral calcium.

• **Pregnant.** Expectant mothers require additional vitamins, but they should consult with their physicians before taking a supplement.

• **Contemplating pregnancy.** Women who are thinking about becoming pregnant should be sure to have a diet rich in folic acid. They should also take a multivitamin with 400 micrograms of folacin. This B vitamin helps to prevent brain damage in the fetus at the time of conception and can help reduce the risk of some types of birth defects. See table 12.1 for foods rich in folic acid.

Needless to say, mothers-to-be should eat well every day to fortify their bodies with the nutrients needed for not only today's health but also future health during pregnancy. For example, if you enter pregnancy with low iron stores, a situation common to female athletes, you may likely end up anemic. Pregnancy is already tiring enough. Why add more fatigue to the picture? Rather than call upon good nutrition during pregnancy as one calls upon a fire truck in an emergency, start eating a blue-ribbon diet today that focuses on folic acid, iron, and calcium.

• **Total vegetarians.** People who abstain from eating any animal foods may become deficient in vitamins B-12, D, and riboflavin. Those who eat a poorly balanced vegetarian diet can also become deficient in protein, iron, and zinc.

Table 12.1   Foods Rich in Folic Acid

Folic acid is found primarily in dried beans, colorful vegetables, and a few fruits. The RDI is 400 micrograms per day.

Food	Amount	Folic acid (micrograms)
Spinach	1 cup cooked	260
Lentils	1/2 cup cooked	180
Avocado	1/2 medium	110
Asparagus	5 spears	100
Broccoli	1 cup cooked	80
Romaine lettuce	1 cup shredded	80
Lima beans	1/2 cup cooked	80
Chick-peas	1/2 cup canned	80
Kidney beans	1/2 cup canned	65
Orange	1 large	60
Peas, green	1/2 cup	50
Bread, whole wheat	2 slices	30
Peanut butter	2 tablespoons	25
Egg	1 large	25
Chicken liver	4 ounces cooked	880

Data from J. Pennington, 1992, *Bowes & Church's Food Values of Portions Commonly Used*, 16th ed. (Philadelphia: Lippincott).

Vitamins as Health Insurance

When it comes to nourishing your body, the American Dietetic Association recommends you should always plan to get the vitamins you need from the food you eat—food first. If you do this, you'll likely have no need to take a supplement to prevent deficiencies. (People who care enough to take supplements usually are the ones least likely to need them). Then, if you wish to take a supplement for "health insurance," take a single one-a-day standard multivitamin. It is unlikely to harm you and it may have positive long-term benefits, as I will explain in the upcoming paragraphs. (American Dietetic Association 1996)

Many athletes who prescribe a wide array of supplements for themselves have little knowledge of how vitamins work or what doses are appropriate. They figure that if a little bit is good, then a lot must be better. They may also think that "natural" means "harmless." Not the case. Athletes who take megadoses of supplements do an excellent job not only of supporting the vitamin industry, but also of setting themselves up for toxic reactions. For example, high doses of vitamin B-6 (greater than 1.0 gram per day over a period of months) may cause numbness, loss of muscle coordination, and paralysis; too much nicotinic acid (taken to reduce blood cholesterol) may lead to liver damage. In general, any dose greater than 10 times the Daily Values (listed as "1000% of the DV" on the supplement's nutrition label) is considered a megadose and should be taken under a physician's guidance (see table 12.2).

If you are currently taking supplements and are not knowledgeable about vitamins, I recommend that you get a nutrition checkup with a registered dietitian (RD). The RD will be able to evaluate your diet and tell you not only what nutrients you are getting but also the best food sources for those you are missing. To find an RD, call the American Dietetic Association's referral network at 1-800-366-1655. You can also call the nutrition department at your local hospital or sports medicine clinic, or look in the Yellow Pages under dietitian and select a name followed by RD.

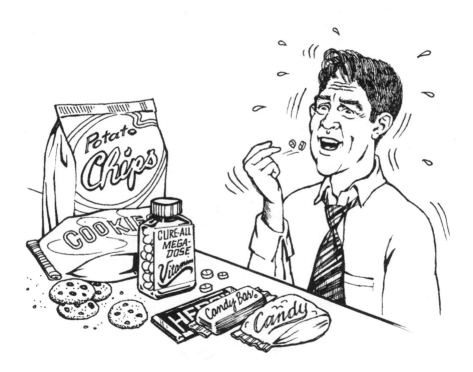

Table 12.2   Guidelines for Dietary Supplements

Because so many athletes are taking vitamins in a hit-or-miss fashion, the U.S. Olympic Sports Medicine Committee established guidelines for dietary supplements. They emphasize that supplements are just that—supplements. They are not replacements pills for a good diet.

Nutrient	Supplement range	Other considerations
Beta carotene	3-20 mg 5,000-33,000 IU	No data on individuals under 18 years
Vitamin C	250-1,000 mg	No data on individuals under 18 years
Vitamin E	100-400 IU	No data on individuals under 18 years
Iron (males)	Because of the risk of iron overload, iron supplements are recommended for males only if a medical workup (which includes a nutrition checkup and blood tests) indicates a problem with iron deficiency.	
Iron (females)	Because women are at high risk for iron-deficiency anemia, a medical checkup is recommended yearly. This should include a nutrition checkup and blood tests. If the tests suggest a need for extra iron, supplement at 100% RDA.	
Multivitamin or mineral	100% of the RDA or the Estimated Safe and Adequate Daily Dietary Intake (ESADDI)	
B-complex	100% RDA	
B-6	Less than 500 mg/day, to reduce risk of toxic reaction	
Niacin	Large doses may impair performance. Individuals using high doses to reduce blood cholesterol levels should do so only under medical supervision.	
Calcium	500-1,000 mg (A 2:1 calcium to magnesium ratio is recommended.)	
Chromium	50-200 mg; research does not support above this amount.	
Zinc	14-20 µg, the amount found in most multivitamin or mineral pills. Amounts exceeding this may be toxic.	

Beyond Dietary Deficiencies

As we age and look to the future, many athletes consider taking vitamins for health protection and injury prevention. Supplements are viewed as therapeutic agents that might enhance longevity. Because many of the diseases of aging are affected by diet, many older athletes are not only eating wisely but also taking supplements to complement their total health program. To date, the verdict is unclear whether health benefits can be attributed to supplements of the antioxidant nutrients A, C, and E, or to the other known and yet unknown compounds in the fruits, vegetables, and other wholesome foods rich in these vitamins.

Regarding heart disease, high levels of antioxidants, particularly vitamin E, along with other antioxidants such as vitamin C, beta carotene (a precursor to vitamin A found in plants), and selenium, may play a vital preventive role. According to one hypothesis, the so-called "bad" LDL cholesterol only becomes bad when it is oxidized and then damages the blood vessels in the heart. When vitamin E travels with LDL and vitamin C travels in the blood plasma, these vitamins can inhibit oxidation and thereby reduce oxidative damage and heart disease. Two large studies on men and women have shown that those who took about 100 international units (IU) of vitamin E for at least two years had a 40 percent lower risk of heart disease (Stampfer et al. 1993; Rimm et al. 1993).

The antioxidants may also reduce the formation of cancerous tumors. They seem to work by blocking the destructive, but natural, process known as oxidation. Antioxidant vitamins apparently help your body's defenses limit this damage.

Some people hypothesize that active people need to take additional vitamin E to counteract the free radicals that are formed during exercise, which could increase the risk of heart disease and cancer. According to Dr. William Evans, PhD, exercise physiologist at Pennsylvania State University, "We've looked for evidence of free-radical damage in response in endurance athletes, and we just don't see it." Although the general recommendation to take an antioxidant supplement may be sound, Evans believes that exercise is unlikely to cause the type of free-radical damage that will be detrimental to your health. As you train, you enhance your ability to counteract the free radicals with free-radical fighting enzymes that double, triple, and quadruple in their activity. This enhancement is all part of the training response (Evans 1994).

The question also arises: Can supplemental vitamin E reduce the risk of injuries? One study with cyclists who were training and competing very strenuously suggests that 330 mg of vitamin E for five months reduced signs of oxidative damage to the cells (Rokitzki et al. 1994).

HOW TO CHOOSE A SUPPLEMENT

If you choose to take a vitamin supplement, you may feel overwhelmed by the myriad choices: name brands, store brands, stress formulas, all-natural products, and so on. The following guidelines can help you sort through the hype and zero in on the best bets. Above all, think "food first." Taking a multivitamin and mineral supplement does not compensate for a high-fat, low-fiber, unbalanced diet.

• Choose a supplement with the vitamins and minerals close to 100% of the Daily Values (DV). Don't expect to find 100% of the DV for calcium and magnesium listed on a label, because these minerals are too bulky to put in one pill.

• Don't buy supplements that contain excessive doses of vitamins and minerals, particularly minerals. High doses of one mineral can offset the benefits of another. For example, too much zinc can interfere with the absorption of copper.

• Choose a supplement with beta carotene, not vitamin A. Beta carotene, the precursor to vitamin A, acts as the antioxidant. Opt for a supplement that contains chromium, a nutrient that may be lacking in American diets.

• Buy a supplement before its expiration date, and store it in a cool, dry place.

• Ignore claims about "natural" vitamins; they tend to be blends of natural and synthetic vitamins and offer no benefits. The exception is vitamin E, which is more potent in its natural form, but the difference is inconsequential.

• Chelated supplements offer no advantages, nor do those made without sugar or starch, nor those with the highest price tag.

• Take a vitamin with a label that states it has passed the 45-minute dissolution test. A supplement is of little value unless it is absorbed by the body.

• To optimize absorption, take a supplement with or after a meal.

Data from *Environmental Nutrition Newsletter*, 52 Riverside Drive, New York, NY 10024. (August, 1993)

But the importance of this is not yet fully understood. Will reducing oxidative damage help reduce injuries? Stay tuned!

To date, nutrition researchers have not determined the optimal level of the antioxidant vitamins for protection from heart disease, cancer, and injuries. As I noted in chapter 2, getting adequate vitamin C and A is easy to do by eating lots of fruits and vegetables. (Table 12.3 has additional food suggestions.) But getting even the RDI for vitamin E (30 IU) is difficult. Most food sources high in vitamin E are also high in fat. To get 100 IU, a protective amount of vitamin E, from natural foods highest in E, you'd have to eat 2 cups of almonds, 7 cups of peanuts, or 2 cups of olive or corn oil. Eating this would displace the carbohydrates you need to fuel your muscles! Or, you could chow down on 6 cups of kale, 4 cups of sweet potatoes, or 19 cups of spinach. Most athletes on the run lack the time or interest for this.

MINERALS

Minerals are present in all living cells. They occur freely in nature in the soil and water, and travel through the food chain by being absorbed into the plants that grow in the soil and then into the animals that consume the plants and water. Vegetables of the same species can differ in mineral content, depending on the soil in which they were grown.

Each mineral has a unique role in the body. For instance, calcium maintains the rigid structure of the bones, potassium and sodium control water balance in the body, iron assists with oxygen transport, magnesium activates enzymes and is required for muscular contraction, zinc is involved in growth and healing.

As with vitamins, you can get the minerals you need if you eat a wide variety of wholesome foods, especially whole grains, fruits, and vegetables. Iron and zinc can be exceptions to that general rule, particularly for those who abstain from red meat; the same is true for calcium for those who abstain from dairy products. But people who eat foods rich in iron and calcium generally get ample amounts of other minerals at the same time.

Iron

Iron is a necessary component of hemoglobin, the protein that transports oxygen from the lungs to the working muscles. If you are iron deficient, you are likely to fatigue easily upon exertion. These athletes are at highest risk of suffering from iron deficiency anemia:

Table 12.3   Antioxidants in Foods

Some of the best sources of the antioxidant vitamins C and A (made from carotenoids) are listed in tables 1.3 and 1.4. When you eat these foods, eat piles of them! The best sources of vitamin E are in plant oils, and it's harder to eat piles of those because the foods have more calories. Nevertheless, be sure to include some of these healthier high-fat foods when balancing your day's fat budget.

Food	Portion	Vitamin E(mg)
Almonds	1/4 cup	14
Peanuts	1/4 cup	4
Sunflower seeds	1/4 cup	28
Olive oil	1 tablespoon	2
Oil, canola	1 tablespoon	3
Oil, safflower	1 tablespoon	6
Spinach, cooked	1 cup	2
Wheat germ	1/4 cup	5
RDA		8-10

Data from J. Pennington, 1998, *Bowes & Church's Food Values of Portions Commonly Used*, 17th ed. (Philadelphia: Lippincott).

- Female athletes who lose iron through menstrual bleeding
- Athletes who eat no red meat (the best dietary source of iron)
- Marathon runners, who may damage red blood cells by pounding their feet on the ground during training
- Endurance athletes, who may lose significant amounts of iron through heavy sweat losses
- Teenage athletes, particularly girls, who are growing quickly and may consume inadequate iron to meet their expanded requirements

Getting Enough Iron

Follow these tips to help you boost your iron intake.

- Eat lean cuts of beef, lamb, pork, and the dark meat of skinless chicken or turkey three to four times per week.
- Select breads and cereals with the words *iron-enriched* or *fortified* on the label. This added iron supplements the small amount that naturally occurs in grains. Eat these foods with a source of vitamin C (for example, orange juice with cereal, tomato on a sandwich) to possibly enhance iron absorption.

- Use cast-iron skillets for cooking. They offer more nutritional value than stainless steel cookware! The iron content of spaghetti sauce simmered in a cast iron skillet for three hours may increase from 3 to 88 milligrams for each half-cup of sauce.
- Don't drink coffee or tea with every meal, particularly if you are prone to being anemic. Substances in these beverages can interfere with iron absorption. (Drinking them an hour before a meal is better than afterward.)
- Combine poorly absorbed vegetable sources of iron (nonheme iron, 10-percent absorption rate) with animal sources (heme iron, 40-percent absorption rate). For example, eat broccoli with beef, spinach with chicken, chili with lean hamburger, and lentil soup with turkey.

For a list of foods highest in iron, refer to table 12.4. For more information about the importance of iron-rich meats, refer to chapters 1, 8, and 15.

Too Much of a Good Thing

Maintaining adequate iron balance is important for top sports performance. But having iron levels too high, or iron overload, is cause for concern. It can be a risk factor for heart disease and heart attacks, particularly if you also have high LDL cholesterol. Iron may promote production of free radicals that oxidize the LDL and cause damage to blood vessels and heart tissue.

Iron overload is a genetic condition that happens in about 1 in every 250 people. It can also be associated with arthritis and diabetes. Men and postmenopausal women are most susceptible because they have relatively low iron requirements; they should not take iron supplements unless recommended by their physicians. The best way to identify iron overload is by having your blood tested for serum ferritin to measure the amount of iron stored in the body. A level of 200 micrograms or higher signals danger.

Zinc

The mineral zinc is a part of more than 100 enzymes that make your body function properly. For example, it helps remove carbon dioxide from your muscles when you exercise. Zinc also enhances the healing process.

Because the zinc from animal protein is absorbed better than zinc from plants, vegetarian athletes are at risk of eating a zinc-deficient diet. For a list of foods rich in zinc, refer to table 12.4.

Table 12.4   Iron and Zinc in Foods

The Daily Value for iron on food labels is based on 18 milligrams; the recommended amount for most men is 10 milligrams, for women 15-18. This target iron intake is set high because only a small percentage is absorbed. The best iron sources are from animal products and fish.

The recommended intake for zinc is 15 milligrams. This is also set high, and may be hard to consume. Athletes who sweat heavily and incur zinc losses through sweat should make 15 milligrams their target, however.

	Iron (mg)	Zinc (mg)
Animal sources[1]		
Liver, chicken, 4 ounces cooked	9	5
Beef, 4 ounces	3	6
Turkey, 4 ounces dark meat	2	5
Pork, 4 ounces	1	3
Oysters, 6 medium raw	6	75
Shrimp, 12 large	2	1
Chicken breast, 4 ounces	1	1
Fish, 4 ounces haddock	1	1
Tuna, 3 ounces light	1	1
Egg, 1 large	1	0.5
Fruit and juice		
Prune juice, 8 ounces	3	0.5
Apricots, 5 halves dried	0.8	0.3
Dates, 10 dried	1	0.2
Raisins, 1/3 cup	1	0.1
Vegetables and Legumes[2]		
Refried beans, 1 cup	4.5	3.5
Spinach, 1/2 cup cooked	3	1
Tofu, 1/4 cake	2	1
Peas, 1/2 cup	1	1
Broccoli, 1/2 cup	1	0.3
Dairy		
Skim milk, 1 cup	0.1	1.0
Cheddar cheese, 1 ounce	0.2	1.0
Grain		
Cereal, Total, 1 cup	18	0.7
Raisin Bran, Kellogg's, 3/4 cup	18	4
Cream of wheat, 1 cup	9	0.3

	Iron (mg)	Zinc (mg)
Pasta, 1 cup cooked, enriched	2	1
Bread, 1 slice enriched	1	0.2
Brown rice, 1 cup cooked	1	1.2
Other		
Brewer's yeast, 1 ounce	5	
Molasses, 1 tablespoon blackstrap	3.5	0.2
Wheat germ, 1/4 cup	2	3.5

[1]Animal sources of iron and zinc are absorbed best (except for iron from eggs).
[2]Vegetable sources of iron and zinc are poorly absorbed.
Nutrient data from J. Pennington, 1992, *Bowes & Church's Food Values of Portions Commonly Used*, 16th ed. (Philadelphia: Lippincott).

Chromium

The rumor has spread throughout gyms and health clubs that chromium supplements can help athletes lose fat, build muscle, and boost their metabolisms. This sounds too good to be true. In fact, it isn't true. But let's look at some of what is known about chromium.

Chromium is a mineral that helps insulin transport glucose out of the blood and into the muscle cells. Because chromium is associated with insulin, it is involved in transporting amino acids into muscles, burning fat, and storing glycogen. Although true chromium deficiency is rare and has yet to be documented among athletes, some scientists believe that borderline chromium deficiencies are common, and may indeed have something to do with the high incidence of diabetes in older people. If you eat a diet based on refined foods such as white flour products and sugary treats, you may be eating inadequate chromium. Choosing more foods from table 12.5 would likely be to your health advantage.

Well-controlled scientific studies have yet to suggest that chromium offers an advantage for athletes who are not chromium deficient. In one study, football players who received chromium supplements showed no greater increases in muscle mass or strength, or decreases in body fat, than football players who trained without supplements did (Clancy et al. 1994). In another study (Hallmark 1996) with untrained 24-year-old men who followed a 12-week strength training program, those who took 200 micrograms of chromium per day increased their strength by 23%—this was less than the 33% increase in those who took no chromium. Body fat stayed the same in both groups. The researchers saw no benefits to taking chromium supplements.

Table 12.5   Foods Rich in Chromium

The RDI for chromium is 120 micrograms for adults. Chromium is often sold in the form of chromium picolinate. Picolinate is a natural derivative of the amino acid tryptophan; it forms a stable complex with chromium and enhances the absorption of chromium into the body.

The following lists some of the best food sources of chromium. Note that very little chromium is found in highly processed and refined foods such as sugar and white flour.

Food	Chromium (μg/serving)
Prunes, 3	60
Peas, 1 cup cooked	60
Brewer's yeast, 2 tablespoons	60
Corn, 1 cup canned	55
American cheese, 1 ounce	50
Chicken breast, 4 ounces	50
Cucumber, 1	50
Peanut butter, 1 tablespoon	40
Mushrooms, 1/2 cup cooked	30
Shredded wheat, 2 ounces	30
Potato, 1 medium baked	30
Beer, 12 ounces	30-60
Oysters, 6 medium raw	22
Apple, 1 medium with skin	19
Whole wheat bread, 1 slice	12
Wheat germ, 1/4 cup	6

ENERGY ENHANCERS AND MAGIC POTIONS

If running faster, jumping higher, and getting stronger could be achieved by taking a magic pill, wouldn't athletes be happy! No more hours of endless training and carefully planned eating. You could simply pop a pill or drink a potion to achieve your goals. Offering such items for sale is certainly unethical, and in some cases illegal, but eager athletes yearning for success will pay a high price for improved performance.

If you have taken special pills and potions that you think have improved your performance in any way, the improvements may simply be because you felt more confident or believed the supplement would help. Your mind is very powerful and can elicit from you performances that may be far beyond your expectations. This is called the *placebo effect*. You can get this same benefit by believing that eating the world's best sports diet will help you win with good nutrition!

Scientific research continues to support the proven way to improve performance: hard training and proper eating. No scientific data, to date, supports any of the following effects from these intriguing products:

- Protein supplements do not build megamuscles.
- Bee pollen has no energy-enhancing effect.
- Ginseng will not make you faster.
- Spirulina is not the final cure for aches and injuries.
- MCT oil is not a magic energizer.

Common Questions About Energy-Enhancing Food Substances

Research does suggest that some food substances might have an ergogenic effect. The following questions address some probing questions that today's athletes are asking about certain supposed ergogenic aids.

Q. Can extra branch-chain amino acids (valine, leucine, and isoleucine) prevent the mental fatigue that is associated with exhaustion?

A. Fatigue is associated with biochemical changes that occur in your brain as well as in your muscles. Athletes who are exhausted have a high level of brain serotonin, a substance that has been associated with drowsiness. Tryptophan is the precursor of serotonin. Branch-chain amino acids (BCAAs) inhibit the uptake of tryptophan, reducing the level of brain serotonin and, theoretically, the feeling of fatigue.

Although the research offers mixed opinions, today's consensus is that taking supplemental BCAAs such as valine, leucine and isoleucine will be unlikely to correct this problem (Burke and Deakin 1994; Davis 1995). Low doses of BCAA supplements tend to have little effect upon brain serotonin, and large doses not only are unpalatable but also can contribute to dehydration, and they may create a toxic reaction. The better way for you to reduce mental fatigue is to consume adequate carbohydrates during endurance exercise. Adequate carbohydrates from sports drinks or solid foods reduce the use of BCAAs for fuel, reduce the amount of tryptophan in the blood, and consequently reduce brain serotonin levels and fight fatigue (Brouns 1993). Chapter 10 provides more information about eating during exercise.

Q. Do extra branch-chain amino acids enhance recovery from exhaustive endurance exercise?

A. Possibly, but more research is needed. The BCAAs are quickly available for use during periods of recovery. The branch-chain amino acid glutamine is needed for a strong immune system. It is also good for making protein during recovery (Brouns 1993).

Q. Will creatine enhance performance in athletes, such as oarsmen, hockey players, 100-meter sprinters, and wrestlers, who do short bursts of high-intensity exercise?

A. Possibly. Creatine is a naturally occurring compound found in meat and fish. (Vegetarians tend to have lower creatine levels than meat eaters.) Creatine is also available in powder and pills. Creatine phosphate is used by the muscles to generate energy for 1 to 10 seconds of intense work. Prior to exercise, 5 grams of creatine monohydrate dissolved in 8 ounces of water and taken in the morning, at noon, in the afternoon, and in the evening for five days increases muscle creatine. This may allow muscles to perform better during brief, all-out exercise bouts (Greenhaff 1995).

Creatine is not a drug, so it is unlikely to become a substance banned by the International Olympic Committee. The use of creatine raises a lot of political questions: Is taking creatine supplements any different than taking extra carbohydrates? Do creatine supplements contradict the spirit of fair play in sports?

Q. Can athletes like sprinters, speed skaters, and rowers who do short-term, intense exercise enhance endurance by buffering lactic acid?

A. Perhaps. When you exercise at a very high intensity, your muscles generate metabolic acids that hinder muscular function. Taking bicarbonate (as in baking soda) in a dose of 0.15 grams per pound of body weight one to two hours before the exercise task can buffer the acids and thereby enhance performance during an event that lasts 1 to 7 minutes, such as 1,500-meter running, 400-meter swimming, and rowing events. Be aware, however, that athletes who "soda load" commonly experience intestinal distress (Horswill 1995). If you are tempted to use buffers, you not only should weigh the ethics of this practice, but also should determine during training if you can tolerate the buffer without side effects that hurt performance. Also note that some athletes respond better than others.

Q. Is "fat-loading" a valid dietary recommendation to enhance stamina?

TOO GOOD
TO BE TRUE?

Today's magazines are filled with claims that sound too good to be true:

>   Burn fat faster!
>   Reduce fat thighs in 30 days!
>   Run faster and longer!

Whether you are concerned about body fat, fatigue, energy, speed, muscle mass, or dehydration, you can easily find a solution with a high price tag. Clearly, the sports supplement industry is a multimillion dollar booming business that thrives on our hopes and aspirations.

How can you tell if a claim is true? It's hard. Even the most knowledgeable sports scientists can have trouble telling if

- the "research" is cited from professionally respected journals,
- the claims are based on research done on athletes, not on rats or sick people, or on false research,
- the claims are valid but taken out of context,
- the claims are based only on anecdotes or phony testimonials, or
- the endorsement from the prestigious university or medical center is unauthorized.

The safest bet is to remember that if the claim *sounds* too good to be true, it probably *is* too good to be true!

A. No. Although the fat loading hypothesis is intriguing, there is insufficient evidence to support the notion that eating extra dietary fat will improve endurance performance by increasing the use of fat for fuel and decreasing the reliance upon the limited carbohydrate (glycogen) stores. Yes, hard training helps your muscles adapt to greater fat burning. But eating excess dietary fat does not enhance endurance. At best, trained muscles can utilize only 8 to 12 percent of the fats that pass through the muscle (Sherman and Leenders 1995). Despite what ads for fat burning foods and pills suggest, scientific evidence still says that exhaustion correlates with carbohydrate depletion.

The Best Energy Enhancers

Without a doubt, a proper sports diet with adequate fluids and carbohydrates is the best investment in top performance. Your dietary goals are to prevent dehydration and maintain normal blood sugar. This means you should follow these guidelines:

- Be well fueled every day so you can train at your best. Target intake: 3 to 5 grams of carbohydrate per pound of body weight per day (see chapter 7).
- Be well hydrated every day, and drink extra fluids before and after exercise to prevent dehydration. Goal: to urinate every two to four hours a clear, pale yellow urine (see chapter 9).
- Consume adequate carbohydrates and fluids during exercise that lasts longer than 60 to 90 minutes. Target intake: 0.5 grams of carbohydrate per pound of body weight (about 300 calories if you weigh 150 pounds) per hour of exercise, as tolerated, after the first 60 to 90 minutes and 8 ounces of fluid every 15 to 20 minutes.
- After exhaustive exercise, recover with adequate carbohydrates. Target intake: about 75 grams (300 calories) of carbohydrates every two hours for six to eight hours.
- Allow adequate rest days for your muscles to refuel and recover. Target: at least one week's taper before competition, and during training at least one day with no exercise and another easy day or a day off per week.

For additional information about energy enhancers, refer to the recommended readings in appendix A. The basic thing to remember is that although food is not magical or mystical, in combination with an appropriate training program, food does work, and it is legal and safe. You will always win with good nutrition!

Caffeine: A Stimulating Topic

Because caffeinated beverages are popular around the world, athletes in all cultures wonder if caffeine can help enhance exercise performance. Some athletes swear yes, while others disagree.

Pat, a 27-year-old swimmer, always drinks a cup of coffee before he races. "Maybe the effect is psychological, but I think that caffeine enhances my performance. My muscles seem to work more easily."

Jean, a soccer player, avoids the stuff. "A cup of coffee before a game would put me over the edge. I'm already jittery, and a caffeine jag is the last thing I need!"

Henry, a runner, prefers his coffee after he exercises. "Drinking coffee on an empty stomach nauseates me. I prefer my brew after I run, as I relax with a nice meal and the morning paper."

For some folks, coffee is a priceless "perk-me-up" before exercise. For others, it's a worthless beverage that makes them jittery and gives them "coffee stomach." Some researchers have suggested that caffeine can significantly enhance an athlete's endurance. In a 1978 study (Costill, Dalsky, and Fink 1978), runners who had the caffeine equivalent of 2 cups of coffee (330 milligrams of caffeine) one hour prior to exhaustive running ran 15 minutes longer than when they exercised to exhaustion without the caffeine. In a more recent study (Trice and Haymes 1995), bicyclists who took 2.5 grams of caffeine per pound of body weight (about 175 grams of caffeine for a 150-pound person, the amount in 1 cup of coffee) exercised for 29 percent longer during high intensity cycling.

Because caffeine stimulates the release of fats into the blood, researchers originally thought that the working muscles would burn more of these fats for energy and spare the limited muscle glycogen stores. With no evidence to support this hypothesis of enhanced fat metabolism (Clarkson 1993), it now seems less likely, particularly among competitive athletes who are already wired on adrenaline with similar fat-releasing effects.

Caffeine's energy-enhancing effect is more likely related to its ability to make exercise seem easier. Through its stimulant effect upon the brain, caffeine may reduce the fatigue associated with long bouts of exercise. In one study, subjects pedaled as hard as they could for two hours on special bicycles that recorded the amount of energy they expended. They worked 7 percent harder after taking caffeine than when they cycled without it, despite perceiving the effort as equal (Ivy et al. 1979).

If you are chronically tired from the rigors of your training program, you may be particularly attracted to caffeine for this reduction in perceived exertion. But if you are hyper with precompetition adrenaline, you are unlikely to need the additional stimulation of caffeine. In fact, caffeine may even put you over the edge if you have a low tolerance for it.

Also note that caffeine taken before exercise has a diuretic effect, particularly if you are unaccustomed to drinking coffee. In hot weather, every drop of fluid can count, and you should seriously consider the risks and benefits of pre-exercise coffee. One basketball player I counseled avoided coffee before games; otherwise, he'd be running too often to the bathroom.

Recent research suggests that caffeine taken *during* exercise, as opposed to before exercise, does not promote greater urine loss (Wemple, Lamb, and Blostein 1994). Maybe this helps explain why so many

Table 12.6   Caffeine in Beverages and Nonprescription Drugs

Apart from being a drug of everyday life, caffeine is 1 of more than 50 drugs banned by the International Olympic Committee. The irony is that small doses of caffeine (such as taken socially) may enhance performance, whereas high doses (such as are banned) are counter-productive to performance.

Olympians with more than 12 micrograms of caffeine per milliliter of urine can be disqualified from competition. To get this level, one would have to deliberately consume in two or three hours the equivalent of one of the following:

- 4 10-ounce mugs of coffee
- 16 colas
- 24 Anacin
- 4 Vivarin

This is clearly an abnormally high amount.

	Average caffeine (mg)
Beverage	
Coffee (10 ounces)	
Brewed, drip method	230
Instant	130
Decaffeinated	5
Tea, 10 ounces brewed	80-120
Iced tea, 12 ounces	70
Hot cocoa, 8 ounces	5
Soft drink, 12 ounces*	
Pepsi Light	35
Dr. Pepper	40
Pepsi Cola	40
Coca Cola	45
Diet Coke	45
Tab	45
Mountain Dew	55
Drug	
Anacin, 2 tablets	32
Excedrin, 1 tablet	65
No Doz, 1 tablet	100
Dexatrim, 1 tablet	100

*Children who drink a can of cola can receive the equivalent in caffeine to the adult who drinks a cup of coffee. Root beer and other caffeine-free beverages are better alternatives for parents to offer their children.

Caffeine data from International Food Information Council, 1993, *Caffeine and Health: Clarifying the Controversies* (Washington, DC: Author); and J. Pennington, 1992, *Bowes & Church's Food Values of Portions Commonly Used*, 16th ed. (Philadelphia: Lippincott).

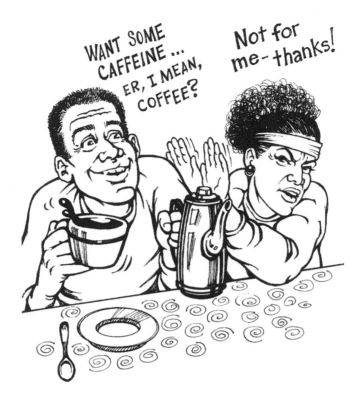

endurance athletes talk about performing better when they take swigs of defizzed cola.

Whereas a cup or two of coffee before exercise may be helpful, more may be of little value. A 1995 study (Pasman et al. 1995) showed that well-trained cyclists performed equally well with about 350 milligrams of caffeine as with 850 milligrams. So if you're tempted to jazz yourself up with a second mugful, think again. You may find that the second mug will do you in with the caffeine jitters. Plus, too much caffeine is illegal according to the International Olympic Committee. Table 12.6 on page 224 lists the caffeine amounts in some common perk-me-ups.

Many folks drink a warm mug of coffee not for an energy boost but because a warm liquid promotes regular bowel movements and helps clean them out before they exercise. This may be the most justifiable reason for some athletes to include this brew in their sports diet. After all, if you are so tired that you choose coffee for its stimulant effect, you should probably be resting and not dragging yourself through a workout. Be sure no trouble is brewing in your desire for caffeine!

For more information on caffeine as a part of your daily diet, see chapter 2.

part

Weight Management

13
chapter

As a Matter of Fat

Most athletes appreciate the beauty of their strong muscles and healthy bodies, but some hate their body fat with a vengeance.

> One of my clients, a dance instructor, grabbed her inner thigh and exclaimed with disgust, "See this? I hate it. I can't seem to lose this handful of flab no matter how hard I train or how many leg lifts I do." A basketball player yanked a handful of flesh around his hips and cringed. "This spare tire drives me crazy. I hate the way it bulges over my uniform shorts. I always feel so fat compared to my teammates."

Mind you, neither of these athletes was overweight or overfat. Compared to the average American, they were trim and well below normal fat levels. The dancer was 19 percent fat; the Reference 24-year-old woman is about 27 percent fat. The basketball player was 10 percent fat; the Reference 24-year-old man is about 15 percent fat.

However, when they compared themselves to their colleagues, they perceived themselves as blimps. Like most scantily clad athletes, they somehow always seemed to be too fat and were never able to get perfectly thin. Even among the nation's top women runners—a very lean group of women—body fatness is an issue. When surveyed about their desired weight, more than half wanted to lose about 2 to 4 pounds (Clark, Nelson, and Evans 1988).

WHY DO WE HAVE IT?

Although excess body fat is excess baggage that slows us down, we do need a certain amount of fat for our bodies to function normally. Fat, or *adipose tissue*, is an essential part of our nerves, spinal cord, brain, and cell membranes. Internal fat pads the kidneys and other organs; external fat offers a layer of protection against cold weather. For the Reference man, essential fat comprises about 4 percent of body weight (that is, 6 fat pounds for a 150-pound man). In comparison, the Reference woman has about 12 percent essential fat (15 fat pounds for a 125-pound woman). Table 13.1 further describes the various levels of body fatness.

Women store essential fat in their hips, thighs, and breasts. This is readily available to nourish a healthy baby if a woman becomes pregnant. The handful of fat that the dance teacher grabbed on her inner thigh included essential fat that nature wanted her to have. No wonder she had trouble losing that small bulge; it was supposed to be there.

If you are a woman fighting the battle of the bulging thighs, you may be fighting a losing battle. The activity of the enzymes that store fat in women's thighs and hips is very high compared to other fat storage areas in women and to fat storage in the hips and thighs of men. Plus, the activity of the enzymes that release the fat is low, making it difficult to lose fat in these areas. The easiest time for women to lose fat in this area is during the last trimester of pregnancy and breastfeeding. At those

Table 13.1 Defining Body Fatness

| Classification | Image | Percent fat | |
		Males	Females
Very low fat	Skinny	7-10	14-17
Low fat	Trim	10-13	17-20
Average fat	Normal	13-17	20-27
Above normal fat	Plump	17-25	27-31
Very high fat	Fat	25+	31+
Essential fat		3-5	11-13

Adapted from B. Getchell and W. Anderson, 1982, *Being fit: A personal guide* (New York: John Wiley and Sons).

times, the activity of the fat-storing enzymes drop, and that of the fat-releasing enzymes increases. Nature, again, is protective of a woman's ability to care for her offspring.

BODY FAT FACTS

We are all familiar with the "fats of life"—the fat thighs, tummy bulges, and spare tires. Here is a short trivia quiz to test your fat knowledge.

1. **True or False? To reduce the fat around the stomach and hips, you should incorporate sit-ups into your exercise program.**

False. Spot reducing sounds like a great idea. Entrepreneurs have made fortunes by designing exotic exercise machines that "melt away" fat spots, if not overnight then at least within a week. According to exercise physiologist Frank Katch at the University of Massachusetts in Amherst, the concept of spot reducing is silly (Katch et al. 1984). That is, you can't reduce through vigorous exercise only the fat cells in one localized area of your body. The fat burned during prolonged exercise comes from all areas of your body, not just the part being worked most vigorously; and it is the burning of fat in combination with a calorie deficit for the entire day that reduces body fat. It's not the muscle movement itself.

Katch commandeered 19 college students to do 5,004 sit-ups over the course of 27 days. He compared fat measurements from the exercised and unexercised parts of their bodies and found them to be equivalent at the beginning and end of the study. Both abdominal and shoulder blade fat experienced similar changes. Granted, the stomach muscles got stronger, but the stomach fat changed at the same rate as the other body fat. Efforts to spot reduce just didn't work!

Some people spend hours exercycling or stair stepping, trying to burn off the fat in their thighs to no avail. As Wendy complained, "My thighs have gotten bigger instead of smaller." She had built thigh muscle from the rigorous exercise but had not lost body fat. When you lose fat, you lose it from everywhere, not just in one place. And the rigorous exercise might contribute to additional bulk that you dislike.

2. **True or False? To lose body fat, you have to do low-intensity, fat burning exercise.**

False. To lose fat, you have to create a calorie deficit for the day. You can do this by adding on exercise of any type, eating less, or combining the two. Just be sure that by the end of the day you have eaten fewer calories than you needed! That way, you'll dip into the stored body fat and burn it for energy.

Some people think the key to body fat loss is doing fat burning exercise, or low-intensity exercise that uses more fat than muscle glycogen for fuel. Wrong. No studies have shown that burning fat during exercise impacts upon loss of body fat (Zelasko 1995). But because you can sustain low-intensity exercise for longer than high-intensity workouts, you can easily burn off more calories, let's say, in one hour of slow jogging (600 calories) than in 10 minutes of fast running (150 calories).

3. True or False? If you add on exercise, you'll lose body fat.

False. To lose body fat you have to create a calorie deficit for the entire day. That is, you have to burn off more calories than you consume. Exercise can help contribute to the calorie deficit, but exercise is often overrated as a way to reduce body fat. Exercise is better used as a tool to help maintain weight loss, because it helps relieve stress (which can reduce stress eating), helps you feel good about yourself, boosts your metabolism, and increases the desire to feed yourself healthfully.

Many people do successfully lose weight by adding on exercise. That's because they start a total health campaign that includes not only adding on activity but also subtracting some calories. After they work out, they tend to feel great, they've relieved stress, and they have less of a desire to unwind after a hectic day by munching through a bag of chips as they had done prior to starting the exercise program.

But some of my clients come to me complaining that they have lost no weight, despite hours of working out. That's often because they are rewarding themselves afterward with generous amounts of calories that replace all they burned off. Despite popular belief, appetite tends to keep up with your exercise load (except in extreme conditions); the more you exercise, the hungrier you will eventually get and the more likely you will be to eat enough to replace the calories you burned off (assuming you take the time to do so). Nature does a wonderful job of protecting your body from wasting away, particularly if you are already lean with little excess fat to lose! Another factor that influences the effectiveness of exercise as a means to lose weight relates to the toll of exercise on your total daily activity. That is, some avid exercisers put all their effort into exercising hard for one or two hours per day but then do little spontaneous activity the rest of the day (Thompson et al. 1995). This pattern is common among athletes who claim to maintain weight despite increased activity and restricted calories.

If you do want to use exercise to promote weight loss, perhaps the most effective type of exercise is exercise that builds muscle. Unlike aerobic exercise that burns calories primarily during the exercise session but very few thereafter, strength training boosts your metabolism throughout the entire day and night. Muscle tissue actively burns calories. The more muscle mass you have, the more calories you burn. In a study with men and women ages 50 to 70 who strength trained three days per week for 12 weeks, metabolic rate increased 15 percent and they lost 4 pounds of fat without actively dieting (Nelson et al. 1994).

4. True or False? If you become injured and are unable to exercise for a week, your muscles will turn into fat.

False. Muscle does not turn into fat, nor does fat turn into muscle. They are two separate entities and are not interchangeable. Perhaps you've noticed a fat layer on roast beef or pork chops. A similar fat layer occurs with humans. The fat tissue is a layer of fat-filled cells that covers the muscles. Muscle is the protein-rich tissue that performs exercise. When you exercise, you build up muscle tissue. When you consume fewer calories than you expend, you reduce the fat layer.

If, due to injury or illness, you are unable to exercise, your muscles may lose their tone, but they won't turn into fat. Unexercised muscle tissue actually shrinks in size. For example, Joe, a skier, broke his leg and was shocked to see how scrawny his calf looked when the cast was removed five weeks later. Once Joe started exercising again, he rebuilt the muscle to its original size.

If you overeat (as often happens with inactive athletes who are also bored, depressed, and hopeful that chocolate chip cookies will cure all ailments), you will become fatter. I often counsel wounded football players who gain 10 to 20 pounds after an injury. They continue to eat lumberjack portions although they need fewer calories. The extra fat takes up more space than the muscle, and the players feel and look flabby.

5. True or False? Cellulite is a special kind of fat that appears after a person has repeatedly gained and lost weight.

False. Cellulite is a fad description of the bulging orange peel appearance of fat that sometimes appears on the hips, thighs, and buttocks. Although much is written about cellulite, little is actually understood about it. Some medical professionals believe that the bumpy, dimpled appearance of cellulite may result from restrictions of connective tissue separating fat cells into compartments. If you overeat and fill the fat cells, the compartmental restrictions may cause the fat to bulge.

Women are afflicted by cellulite more than men because their skin is thinner and their fat compartments are larger and more rounded. Also, women tend to deposit fat in their hips, thighs, and buttocks, areas in which cellulite appears easily, but men tend to deposit fat around their waists.

Some medical specialists suspect a genetic predisposition toward cellulite may exist. If a mother has cellulite, the daughter is likely to acquire it as well. Cellulite generally appears as a person ages, because the skin loses its elasticity and becomes thinner.

BODY IMAGE:
WAITING FOR THE RIGHT BODY

> Helen, a tall and stocky rugby player, was sensitive about her bulky body. Her brothers had teasingly referred to her as a gorilla. As I measured her body fat, Helen anxiously awaited the moment of truth.

"Your weight is fine, Helen," I said. "You simply have a lot of muscle and a big bone structure. You have very little excess fat." Although Helen perceived herself as being overweight, she was actually quite lean and not overfat.

Visual appearance and body weight are deceptive for athletes who tend to compare themselves to their teammates. We all come in different sizes and shapes, most of which are genetically determined. Although you can change your body to a certain extent by losing fat or building muscle, you can't do a complete makeover. Even if you lose the excess baggage, sometimes you still won't end up with the body you want.

> Janice, one of my clients, complained, "I just hate my megalegs. Can't I do anything to slim them down?"

I questioned Janice about her mother's, sisters', aunts', and grandmothers' legs. She acknowledged, "We all have thunder thighs. They are the trademark of our family." I invited Janice to reevaluate her body shape goals and become a bit more realistic in her expectations given this genetic predisposition. "You may not like your legs, Janice, but they are yours forever. You can trim them a bit by losing some fat, but you are unlikely to transform them into toothpicks. I recommend that you let go of your dissatisfaction with your body, accept yourself for the sincere and caring person you are, and focus on the things in life that really matter. You are wasting a lot of mental energy worrying about your thighs. Enjoy your life instead of putting life on hold as you wait for the right body."

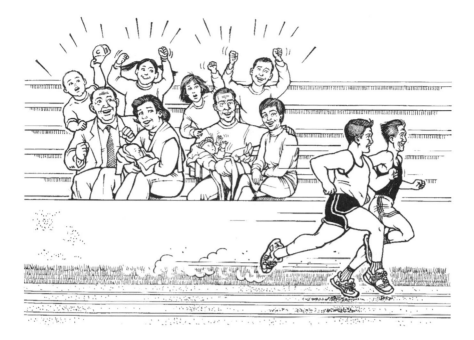

Janice is just one of many of my clients who express deep frustrations about their body images. Unfortunately, the media strongly promote the idea that everyone is supposed to possess a bean stalk body and that the pears and apples among us are slothful gluttons. Far from the truth!

We all come in different sizes and shapes unique to our genetic makeup (Bouchard 1991). Just as some of us have thick hair, others have thin hair; some have blue eyes, others have brown eyes. No one seems to care about hair thickness or eye color, but the media have made us all care about body fatness. As a result, too many self-conscious people feel inadequate because of repeated failures at transforming themselves into a shape they aren't meant to be. For example, one husky high school soccer player wanted to transform herself into a petite ballerina, an unrealistic vision. She thought she could diet away the excess pounds and become lean and lanky. She failed to recognize that she had little fat to lose. Most of her weight was solid muscle, not flabby fat.

Body Types

Like it or not, you are born with a specific body shape that is yours for life. The three standard body type classifications are:

- Ectomorph—Relatively long legs and arms, narrow fingers and toes, and a delicate bone structure
- Mesomorph—Heavy bone and muscle development, broad hands, and a muscular chest
- Endomorph—Round and soft, often with slender wrists and ankles and relatively small facial features

Body shapes can also be classified into four categories:

- The Pear—Normally has narrow shoulders, a small chest, and an average waist; fat concentration is usually in the hips and thighs
- The Apple—Usually has a round tummy, with no visible waistline; fat concentration is in the waist; limbs are thin
- The Inverted Triangle—Usually has broad shoulders and narrow hips; fat concentration is generally in the chest
- The Hourglass—Broad hips and chest and a small waist; fat concentration normally in the chest and hips

APPLE   PEAR   INVERTED   HOURGLASS
TRIANGLE

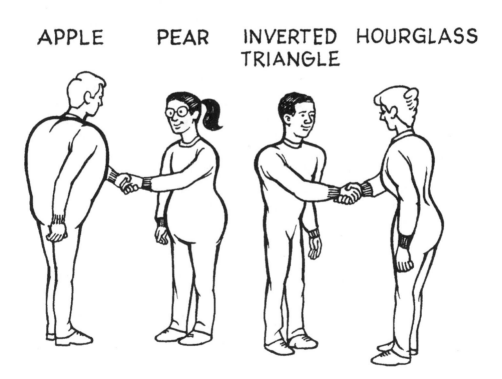

Are You Imagining the Wrong Body?

Because of today's appearance consciousness, you undoubtedly hold an image of what you are supposed to look like. If a woman, you are supposed to be sleek, slender, and slim; if a man, bulky, muscular, and trim. Yet few people naturally possess their desired physique. Most of us are ordinary mortals, complete with bumps, bulges, fat, and fleshiness. Women, in particular, are designed with a natural roundness and softness that tends to get rounder and softer with aging.

In general, about one-third of all Americans are truly dissatisfied with their appearance, women more than men. A woman will most commonly complain about her thighs, abdomen, breasts, and buttocks. A man expresses dissatisfaction with his abdomen, upper body, and balding scalp. Sometimes the problem is imaginary (such as when the anorexic skater complains about her fat thighs); sometimes it is real, and ranges from a mild complaint about love handles that hang over the running shorts to a major preoccupation with thunder thighs that results in relentless dieting and exercise.

Even lean athletes, particularly women, are not immune from the epidemic of body dissatisfaction despite their fitness. Many perceive themselves as having unacceptable bodies, and they go on to develop eating disorders out of desperation. In fact, the best predictor of who will develop an eating disorder relates to who struggles most with body image.

What you look like on the outside should have little to do with how you feel on the inside. But in reality, the thinking goes like this:

1. I have a defect (fat thighs) that makes me different from others.
2. Other people notice this difference.
3. My looks affect how these people see me—repulsive, ugly.
4. I'm bad, unlovable, inadequate.

This type of thinking is common among young dancers experiencing body changes as they blossom from girls into women and develop hips and thighs, runners feeling pressure to be thinner, exercise leaders who think every student scrutinizes their bulges, and numerous other people who think they have an imperfect body.

Learn to Love Your Body

If you are dissatisfied with your body, you might think the solution is to lose weight, pump iron, or do thousands of sit-ups. This "outside" approach to correcting body dissatisfaction tends to be inadequate. Concern about what you look like is really a mask for how you feel

MAKING PEACE WITH YOUR BODY

"Your body is your house, and you might as well make it your home," suggests Marcia Hutchinson, body image specialist. But chances are you are discontent with at least one body part. Rather than judging yourself from the outside in, your better bet is to make peace with your body and to love yourself from the inside out. Here are some tips for developing a healthy body image and boosting your self-esteem.

- **Honor your personal history.** Your perception of your body has been shaped by past experiences. By acknowledging your personal story, you will become more conscious of your past destructive thoughts and dieting programs and become more receptive to choosing healthier behaviors.

- **Accept yourself the way you are and live in the now.** If you accept yourself as you are, you will be able to channel your energy into positive changes that will boost your healthy eating and exercise program. Enjoy life today, rather than living in the past or being afraid of the future.

- **Create a positive mental outlook and positive self-talk messages.** By creating, nurturing, and sustaining a positive mental outlook, you'll be able to feel good about who you are. Give yourself positive messages that reinforce all your good qualities and skills. You'll start to view yourself differently.

- **Steer away from comparisons.** Rather than trying to live up to picture-perfect images, recognize that attractiveness is a multidimensional combination of a variety of aspects, including the inner attractiveness that makes you unique.

- **Give yourself praise and rewards.** Acknowledge the positive steps you make in taking care of yourself, and create rewards that recognize the effort you are putting into your body image wellness program.

Data from *Reshaping your body, rethinking your mind: A practical guide to enhancing body image & improving self esteem* by Lauve Metcalfe, 450 West Valle del Oro, Tucson, AZ 85737.

about yourself— your self-esteem. Given that about 25 percent of your self-esteem is tied to how you look, you can't feel good about yourself unless you like your body and feel confident with how you look. Weight issues are often self-esteem issues.

The best approach to resolving your body shape issues is to learn to love the body you have. As I mentioned before, so much of what you look like, your size and shape, is genetically determined. You can slightly redesign the house that nature gave you, but you can't totally remodel it, at least without paying a high price.

If you are struggling with your body image, you need to think back to identify when you first got the message that something is wrong with your body. Perhaps it was a parent who lovingly remarked that you looked good, but that if only you'd lose a few pounds you'd look even better, the siblings who teased you about your thunder thighs, or the relative who molested you. (Sexual abuse is a common cause of body hate.) Then, you need to take the following steps to be at peace with your body and to like yourself:

- Rename your disliked body part (that is, rename "ugly jelly belly" a more loving "round tummy").
- Identify the parts of your body that you do like.
- Give yourself credit for your attractive body parts with positive talk.

Don't dwell on the negative, but instead love all the good things your body does for you. It rides bikes, runs races, and lets you have fun. How could you enjoy sports without your body? A healthy body can come in all types of sizes and shapes; you can even be fat and fit.

With practice, you'll come to learn that appearance is only skin deep and that your real worth is the loving, caring, and concern you offer to your family and friends. You'll be able to muster the courage to face scary situations. You can even put on that bathing suit and feel at peace!

AT WAR WITH THE SCALE

Some people give too much power to this metal monster.

> Paul, a marathoner, clearly remembers, "One morning I got so mad at the scale. It told me I'd gained 3 pounds, and I'd been starving myself for half a week. I angrily jumped up and down on it until it broke. That's the last time I've weighed myself!"

Paul can laugh now when he recalls that story, but he wasn't laughing at that time.

If you are caught up in worrying about your weight, I advise against weighing yourself daily. You'll likely refer to yourself as being "good" when the pounds drop, and "bad" when they go up. Nonsense. You are the same lovable person, regardless of a pound up or down.

A scale measures not only fat but also muscle gain, water, food, intestinal contents, the coffee you drank just prior to being weighed, and so on. It tells you information that may be irrelevant. For example, if you increase your exercise program, decrease your food intake, build up muscle, and lose fat, the scale may indicate that your weight has remained the same. You will feel thinner, look thinner, and your clothes will be looser, but you will not get the psychological rewards if the scale has dampened your spirits. Scales can also be inaccurate.

Some athletes play games with the scales and fool only themselves. For example, runners, racquetball players, and other athletes who perspire heavily often prefer to weigh themselves after a hard workout. During exercise, they may have lost 5 pounds. That's 5 pounds of sweat, not fat.

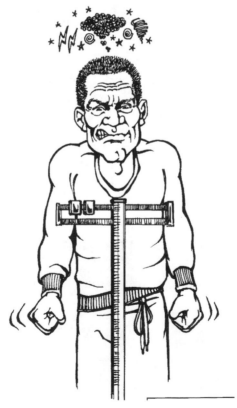

The only time to weigh yourself (if you insist) is the first thing in the morning. Get up, empty your bladder, and then step on the scale before you eat or drink anything. You'll be weighing your body, pure and simple. If you weigh yourself at the end of the day, you'll also be weighing your dinner, beverages, and other foods that are in your intestines.

Also remember that weight is more than a matter of willpower. Weight, like height, is largely under genetic control. When it comes to height, you have likely accepted the fact that you can't force yourself to grow six inches. But when it comes to weight, you may demand your body to lose an inappropriate number of pounds.

Certainly, if you are overfat, you can reduce to an appropriate level of body fatness. Weighing yourself weekly on the scale can be a positive reinforcer. But if you are an already lean athlete who is struggling to drop those final 5 pounds below an appropriate weight, you may

HOW MUCH SHOULD I WEIGH?

Although only nature knows the best weight for your body, the following guidelines offer a method to estimate the midpoint of a healthy weight range (plus or minus 10 percent, depending on whether you have large or small bones).

Women: 100 pounds for the first five feet of height, 5 pounds per inch thereafter.

Men: 106 pounds for the first five feet of height, 6 pounds per inch thereafter.

For example, a woman who is five feet, six inches could appropriately weigh 100 + 30 = 130 pounds. (Range: 117-143.)

A man who is five feet, ten inches could appropriately weigh 106 + 60 = 166 pounds. (Range: 149-183.)

Although athletes commonly want to be leaner than the average person, heed this message: If you are striving to weigh *significantly* less than the weight estimated by this guideline, think again. Pay attention to the genetic design for your body, and don't struggle to get too light. The best weight goal is to be fit and healthy rather than sleek and skinny.

feel like a failure and question your own self-worth: "Why can't I do something as simple as lose 5 pounds?"

Some athletes are between a rock and a hard place when it comes to meeting the weight demands of their sport. For example, wrestlers, rowers, ballet dancers, and figure skaters participate in a sports system that does not accommodate athletes as designed by nature. This raises ethical concerns. Should genetically stocky people be discouraged from ballet, figure skating, gymnastics, and other sports that favor thinness? Should wrestlers be encouraged to drop 15 pounds to a lower weight class? The sports' governing bodies need to be reminded that weight is more than a matter of willpower and that health and fitness are more important than weight.

BODY FAT MEASUREMENTS: FACT OR FICTION?

When I counsel athletes who have a poor concept of an appropriate weight, I measure their body fat rather than rely on a scale and height–weight charts. The fat measurement helps put into perspective the proportion of an athlete's body that is muscle, bone, essential fat, and excess fat. The scale provides a meaningless number because it doesn't indicate the composition of the pounds. Whereas some pounds are desirable muscle weight, others are less desirable fat weight. Obviously, the muscle weight contributes to top athletic performance in most sports. The fat weight is the bigger concern, because excess fat can slow you down.

Believe me, judging from the tension that radiates from a weight-conscious athlete's body, I believe that getting your body fat measured ranks high on the list of anxiety-provoking life experiences! This number unveils the real truth. Hulky football players are often humbled to learn that 20 percent of their brawn is flab. It's excess fat they lug around, not solid, steely muscle. Weight-conscious gymnasts are often thrilled to learn that they are leaner than they thought.

If you want to have your body fat measured, you'll certainly want to have it done correctly by a qualified health professional to eliminate any possibility of being told that you are fatter than you really are. Inaccurate readings send people into a tizzy! If you later want to get remeasured, always try to have it done by the same person using the same technique to ensure greater consistency.

These are four common methods to estimate percent body fat:

- Underwater weighing, which sounds intriguing and traditionally has been considered the most accurate method

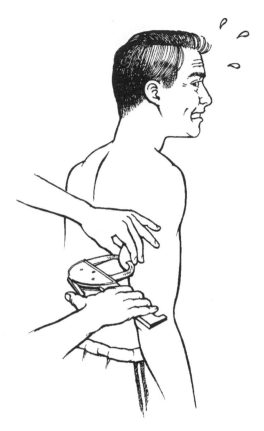

- Skinfold calipers, which are more convenient, less sensational, and relatively accurate
- Bioelectrical impedance analysis (BIA), which is a snazzy, computerized method with increasing accuracy
- Near infrared reactance (NIR), which measures the thickness of the skin at only one site, which may poorly represent overall body fat

When it comes to measuring body fat, there is no simple, inexpensive method to date that's 100 percent accurate. Underwater weighing, calipers, electrical impedance, and near infrared reactance all have potential inaccuracies. The following information evaluates these options to help you decide the best way to estimate your ideal weight, should you want to quantify the fats of life.

Keep in mind that body fat measurements should be included as part of a conversation about an appropriate weight for your body. That is, if you are far leaner than other members of your genetic family but have a higher percent fat than you desire, you may already be lean for your body. For example, a five-foot, six-inch walker lost 50 pounds, from 200 to 150, and wanted to reach a seemingly appropriate weight goal of 130 pounds. Because she couldn't seem to lose beyond 150 without severely restricting her intake, I measured her body fat. She was 28 percent fat—the higher end of "average" but far leaner than anyone else in her family. I suggested that she be at peace with this healthier weight and remember that she was already very thin for her body.

Underwater Weighing

With underwater weighing, the subject exhales all the air in his or her lungs and then is weighed while submerged in a tank of water. Despite popular belief, this technique does not measure body fat. It measures body density. Body density translates mathematically into percent fat. During the translation, however, significant error can creep into the picture. The equations for translating density into fat are most appropriate for the "standard" male. This excludes a lot of very thin runners and very muscular body builders. The same equations can be inappropriately used for girls on the high school swim team, 50-year-old marathoners, and professional football players.

Body density differs among all types of athletes and is affected by age, gender, and race. Children and senior citizens differ from each other in body densities. The anorexic ballerina with osteoporotic, low-density bones is far different from the standard male and may receive an inaccurate percent fat estimate unless the difference in density is accounted for using a population-specific equation.

Errors with underwater weighing also stem from the inexperience of the victim being weighed. If you've never been submerged into a weighing tank, you are likely to be nervous and may not completely exhale all the air in your lungs before going under the water. This will affect the density reading. Exercise physiologists have estimated that as little as 2 cups of air can affect body fat measurements by as much as 3 to 5 percent. Intestinal gas can also disrupt the accuracy, as can poorly calibrated equipment. Many portable underwater weighing systems (the kinds that show up at road races, health fairs, and runners' expos) may lack the precision of a weighing system used in a research laboratory.

Needless to say, if you are looking for a perfect measurement tool, underwater weighing has sources of error. But so do the other methods.

Skinfold Calipers

Skinfold calipers are large "pinchers" that measure the thickness of the fat layer on specific body sites. They are best used by health professionals who have been well trained in the technique. Active people often are measured by students or novice technicians who may be using imprecise or poorly calibrated calipers at crowded health fairs or fitness events. A hasty measurement an inch above or below the established pinch point can add 5 to 15 millimeters of fat to the measurement. Those little millimeters can translate inaccurately into a high body fat reading.

I often get phone calls from frenzied athletes who were measured at a health fair and are told that they are overfat when they suspect that they're really not. When I carefully remeasure them in my unrushed, uncrowded office, I can get a much better reading. I can also use my professional judgment to determine if the number I get seems to be reasonable for that person. The eyeball method is fairly reliable!

Individual fat patterns also contribute to inaccurate calculations. For example, one female skier had inherited abnormally fat arms. An arm measurement is used in many conversion formulas. According to one calculation that used this arm measurement, the skier's body was 28 percent fat, but according to another method that adjusted for the fat arms, she was 19 percent fat. That's quite a variation.

Even accurate measurements commonly translate into erroneous information because of inappropriate conversion equations. In order to be most accurate, the measurements from a runner, wrestler, body builder, or gymnast should be plugged into sport-specific conversion equations. This seldom happens for the average athlete. In harried situations, such as at some health fairs, the technicians are unlikely to take the time to switch formulas. They can even forget to convert from male to female equations. One rushed technician incorrectly used a man's formula on a woman. The poor lady ended up with a measurement of 8 percent more fat than she really had and a depressed state of mind. She had frustrations about her weight until she decided to get her fat remeasured under more peaceful conditions.

As you can see, the accuracy of body fat measurements using calipers depends on the precision of the technician, the accuracy of the caliper, and the appropriateness of the conversion equations. Repeated measurements by different technicians using different calipers and different equations can yield widely different results.

Skinfold caliper measurements are often used to measure *changes* in body fatness. I often record on a monthly basis the measurements of people losing a significant amount of weight through regular exercise. By comparing the numbers (either as measurements in millimeters or converted into percent fat), the dieters can monitor changes. People recovering from anorexia also appreciate repeat skinfold measurements as a way to see they are rebuilding muscle, not just gaining fat. This use of calipers may not give a 100% accurate picture but shows trends, particularly when the same technician measures the dieter each time, using the same calipers and same conversion equations.

Bioelectrical Impedance

Body composition is commonly measured by using bioelectrical impedance analysis, a computerized system that sends an imperceptible electrical current through the body via an electrode attached to the wrists and ankles. The flow of the current is affected by the amount of water in the body. Because water is in only fat-free tissue, the current flow can be translated into percent body fat.

Measuring body composition by bioelectrical impedance is a simple procedure that takes just 5 minutes to perform. The machine is portable, easy to use and popular at road races and health fairs. Although popular, this method also can be problematic, particularly among athletes. Due to the nature of the conversion equations, the body fatness of lean athletes is sometimes overestimated, and the fatness of overweight people is sometimes underestimated. With new sport-specific equations being developed, you can anticipate improved accuracy.

You will get an inaccurate reading if you are dehydrated, so don't bother to get measured after hard exercise or after you've had any alcoholic beverages. Both of these factors affect the water level in your body and will alter the reading. Other factors that may affect the accuracy of the measurement include premenstrual bloat, food in the stomach, and carbo-loaded muscles (water gets stored along with the carbohydrates). If you are improperly positioned during the test (say, with part of your arms touching your body), you will also get an inaccurate reading. This error can easily happen in crowded exhibitions.

Even if you are in water balance and accurately positioned, you still might receive an incorrect measurement. The calculations are based on the assumption that the standard person is 73-percent water. Research has shown that young people tend to be 77-percent water, older folks 71 percent. Exercise scientists are developing new prediction equations to resolve this problem. Be sure the person measuring you uses up-to-date equations.

Near Infrared Reactance

Commonly known as the Futrex 5000 method to measure body composition, near infrared reactance measures fat thickness based on principals of light absorption and reflection. An instrument that emits an infrared light beam is placed over the arm muscle. It measures the light that is absorbed by the muscle and fat and is reflected off the bone. This measurement is commonly taken at the biceps only. The accuracy of the translation into percent body fat varies, depending on the population being measured. If you are very lean, be forewarned that NIR might overestimate your percent fat, and if you are overweight, NIR might underestimate your percent fat. More research is needed to validate this method among athletes. And the measurement of only one site limits accuracy, particularly for people with genetically fat arms.

What's the Use?

Until researchers find the definitive method to measure body fat, here's my advice: Consider body fat measurement as a comparative measurement to reflect changes in your body as you lose fat, gain muscle, shape up, and slim down. Don't expect more accuracy than is possible (see table 13.2). The standard error is plus or minus 3 percent. Hence, if you are measured at 15 percent, you might be 12 percent or 18 percent. That doesn't take into account another 3 percent biological error due to individual variations in body fatness.

Your best bet is to see how the measurements change over time. Have the same person measure you at bimonthly intervals over the course of a year. Calipers and electrical impedance are generally the most available and least expensive methods. Although not 100% accurate, they provide enough information to help you assess trends in your body fat changes.

Table 13.2   Variability in Body Fat Measurement

Just as getting weighed on different scales results in different pound values, getting body fat measured by different people using different methods results in different body fat numbers. This study done on 57 white males (average age 22 years) demonstrates the significant variability that occurs even under scientific conditions (Stout et al. 1994).

Measurement method	Average reading (percent fat)	Range (percent fat)
Underwater weighing	15	4.4-34.5
Calipers	12.5	4.5-26.5
Futrex 5000	14	4.5-32.5
Futrex 1000	18.5	10.0-37.0
BIA	18	9.0-31.0

Data from J. Stout, J. Eckerson, T. Housh, G. Johnson, and N. Betts, 1994, "Validity of body fat estimations in males," *Med Sci Sports Exerc* 26(5): 262.

WORDS OF WISDOM

Even better than entrusting your fate to a random number, I strongly recommend that you listen to your body. Each person has a set point weight at which the body tends to hover. You may slightly overeat one day, slightly undereat the next, but your weight will stay more or less the same. If you drop below this natural weight, your body will start to talk to you. You may fight a nagging hunger, become obsessed with food, and feel chronically fatigued. On the other hand, if you are above your set point, you will feel fat and flabby.

My experiences counseling athletes of all ages and weights indicate that you likely do know your comfortable weight zone. As Tricia, a five-foot, two-inch masters swimmer, acknowledged, "I can diet down to 110 pounds, an appropriate weight for the average person of my height. But I don't stay there. My body is most comfortable at 117 to 120. That's heavier than most people my height, but that's what's normal for me and where I fit in with the rest of my family. Everyone is heavyset."

She had learned through years of unsuccessful dieting that she'd never be able to fit her ideal image of perfectly thin. She has now accepted her build and recognizes that she can healthfully participate in sports regardless of the few extra pounds. Weight, after all, is more than a matter of willpower, and happiness is not based on thinness.

14
chapter

Lose the Weight, Keep the Energy

Many athletes maintain a trim appearance without effort. They exercise regularly and eat what they want. But others battle with weight and believe they will always be too fat, never too thin. They have been influenced by advertisements, the media, and their peers to think that thin is good and thinner is better.

Some competitive athletes in weight-oriented sports such as wrestlers, dancers, gymnasts, figure skaters, and distance runners, strive to be lighter and leaner even though they have no excess fat according to nature's standards. Other recreational exercisers know they have excess flab and want to improve their self-images. All of these sports-active dieters should learn how to lose weight while maintaining enough energy to train.

High-energy, low-calorie reducing programs are possible. You can lose weight while enjoying a balanced sports diet. The trick is to wisely choose what and when you eat. And before attempting a weight loss program, you might want to get your body fat measured (see chapter 13). By knowing what percentage of your weight is excess body fat, you'll have a valid perspective for what an appropriate weight goal should be. All too often I counsel active people who weigh more than they desire, but their weight is primarily muscle with little excess fat.

No wonder they struggle with trying to reduce. They have no excess weight to lose!

THE BALANCING ACT

Like many athletes, Jan, a high school runner and dieter, felt totally confused about how to lose weight during training. "I know that for running I'm supposed to eat carbohydrates for muscle fuel, for dieting I'm supposed to avoid fats, and for building and protecting my muscles I need some protein. But how can I eat a balanced diet and still lose weight?"

Jan needed a game plan for good nutrition (see chapter 1). I reviewed with her the Food Guide Pyramid as well as calorie information. Because it's important to understand calories (or more correctly, kilocalories or kcals, the amount of heat needed to raise one liter of water by one degree Centigrade), I repeat here that calories come from

- carbohydrates (16 calories per teaspoon),
- proteins (16 calories per teaspoon),
- alcohol (28 calories per teaspoon), and
- fats (36 calories per teaspoon).

Excess calories from fats are the main dietary demons. Your body can very easily store excess dietary fat as body fat, whereas you are more likely to burn off excess calories of carbohydrates. Butter, margarine, oil, mayonnaise, salad dressing, and grease are obvious fats; fats are also hidden in meats, cheeses, peanut butter, nuts, and other protein foods. Excess calories from alcohol also quickly add up and can easily inflate your body fat stores, as can the calories from the high-fat munchies that commonly accompany the alcohol.

Eat Fat, Get Fat?

In this day and age of low-fat, no-fat, reduced-fat, and fake-fat foods, Jan had heard clear messages that if she eats fat she will get fat and will raise her risk for developing heart disease and cancer. So, she restricted her fat intake, assuming that less fat would contribute to leanness and health, but she didn't lose weight.

Another athlete, Paula, a lean yet avid fat avoider, came to me determined to lose just 3 more pounds. Paula was running 5 miles every day after work, swimming or lifting weights before work, and biking 40 to 50 miles on Saturdays. "I'm doing lots of exercise. I don't eat any fatty foods; I haven't had junk like cookies or ice cream for two years. I just can't understand why I haven't lost weight." Like many health-conscious athletes, Paula had taken the popular advice to stay away from fatty foods, but to no avail. What was wrong?

Weight reduction is more complex than adding on exercise and eliminating dietary fat. And confusion abounds among athletes like Jan and Paula, as well as among obesity researchers, about the best way to lose body fat. These factors contribute to the confusion:

• **The body has a complex and highly sophisticated system for regulating its fat stores.** The "one diet fits all" approach to losing weight is not appropriate; different people have different types of fatness. Some overweight people are apple shaped with fat tummies, others are pear shaped with big hips; some have beer bellies, others have fat distributed equally everywhere; some are genetically heavy people, others are genetically lean; some are men, others are women. And all these people likely differ in their ability to easily lose body fat (Bouchard, 1991).

• **Weight loss research tends to be done in controlled situations with limited availability of food.** The reality of real life eating is much different! Research subjects have no opportunities to cheat, nor do they participate in birthday parties and social eating feasts that can contribute extra calories.

• **Short-term reducing diets don't show the whole picture.** Do the results hold true for the long run? Long-term dieting and denial of favorite foods, including ones that contain fats, commonly lead to binge eating and regaining weight.

CALORIES DO COUNT

Weight control is based on a calorie budget, not only on a fat gram budget. Fat loss occurs when you burn off more calories than you eat. That is, if you require 2,400 calories per day to maintain your weight but eat only 2,000 calories, you will lose fat. The kind of calories that you eat may be of less consequence. That is, if you choose to spend 300

WHAT YOU MUST KNOW TO LOSE WEIGHT

As the debate continues regarding the best way to lose weight, here's what I think you need to know and account for in your weight loss plans.

• **Diets don't work.** Dieting and denial lead to overeating, if not binge eating.

• **Your body has a *set point*.** A predetermined weight that is appropriate for your body. You may not like this number, but you can't easily change it (Leibel, Rosenbaum, and Hirsch 1995).

• **Calories count.** But the mathematics of weight loss is not consistent. Just as your body can rev up its engines to burn off a few excess calories if you overeat, it can also lower the throttle when energy is scarce. This is how the body tries to maintain a set weight (Leibel, Rosenbaum, and Hirsch 1995).

of your 2,000 calories on high-fat peanut butter instead of fat-free bagels, you can still lose body fat. Fatty foods that fit into your calorie budget are not inherently fattening (Alford, Blankenship, and Hagen 1990). Take a look at your friends. I'll bet that you know of several people who eat fat but are not. You can appropriately eat 25 to 30 percent of your calories from fat (see chapter 1).

Some people eat thinking that fat-free means calorie-free, and they eat lots of fat-free foods. Bad idea! Excess calories, regardless of the source, will ultimately be stored as fat (Hill et al. 1992). Dieters who try to fool the dieting system by eating only fat-free foods fool only themselves. For example, Sharon, a personal trainer, reported she'd been known to eat a whole box of fat-free pretzels for a snack. Paul, a bodybuilder, routinely polished off a half gallon of fat-free frozen yogurt, and Nancy, a swimmer, used to eat at least six fat-free bagels per day. No wonder they all complained they hadn't lost weight even though they hadn't eaten foods containing fat. They were eating too many calories; they needed to create a calorie deficit to lose body fat.

The "eat no fat, lose body fat" advice tends to work best for overweight people who eliminate fatty foods and lose weight because they eat fewer calories. For example, instead of having 700 calories of bacon, eggs, and buttered toast for breakfast, Elliott switched to 400 calories of cereal and banana as part of a conscious effort to lose 50 pounds, and he successfully dropped weight due to the continued calorie deficit.

In contrast, when already lean people eat a low-fat diet, they commonly feel driven to eat more calories of carbohydrates to compensate for the reduced fat calories. Weight reduction becomes increasingly hard if you strive to be lighter than nature designed (Leibel et al. 1995). For example, Paula, who wanted to lose 3 pounds but was already at her set point weight, reported she felt driven to eat lots of rice cakes, pretzels, and other low-fat foods.

I recommended that Paula include some fat in her diet so that she could

- eat a wider variety of food and enjoy better dietary balance (her extremely low-fat diet was lacking in protein, iron, and zinc),
- feel more satisfied (foods with fat provide a pleasant feeling of fullness), and
- be more at peace with food.

Her fat-free food plan created guilt feelings whenever she succumbed to eating a food with fat. For example, she declined a piece of birthday cake because it contained fat. She said she would have felt too guilty if she had eaten some. I reminded Paula that other thin people enjoyed the cake and didn't get fat from eating it. Clearly, she was confusing appropriate dieting with her desire to be in control. This desire to control fat had little to do with weight and more to do with rigidity. See chapter 15.

Because only excess fat calories are fattening, you can eat fat as a part of your calorie budget. Note that many lean athletes eat fat and are thin. You can, too, as long as you don't overeat total calories. Just as fat-free does not mean calorie-free, fat-filled does not mean off limits. Within nutritional reason, you should spend your calories on the foods you want to eat and enjoy eating. That includes cheese, chips, and ice cream—all of which can fit into a balanced diet and your fat and calorie budget in "diet portions." If you deny yourself your favorite foods, you will be more likely to end up bingeing on these items.

MEAL TIMING: DOES IT MATTER WHEN YOU EAT?

If you tend to eat most of your calories at night because of your hectic work or training schedule, you may have wondered if the huge evening intake makes you fat.

Patrick, a 25-year-old triathlete and office helper, certainly had no success with dieting by day and eating by night. "I eat only an orange for breakfast because I'm not hungry after my morning run. I don't want to eat much lunch because food in my stomach can interfere with my afternoon workout. Come evening, I try to diet but generally devour whatever food I can find in my kitchen because I'm absolutely ravenous. Despite all my training and attempts to diet, I haven't lost weight. It seems as though I should have wasted away to nothing by now but I haven't, and I feel very discouraged. Is that because of all the nighttime eating?"

Maybe yes, maybe no. One survey of 1,800 women found no connection between weight and big evening meals (Kant et al. 1995). But the night eaters did consume more fat, protein, and alcohol, and less carbohydrate, vitamin C, B-6, and folic acid—indicative of a fast food diet. In comparison, a smaller research study (Halberg 1983) suggests otherwise. When subjects were allowed to eat as much as they wanted but only in one meal per day, when they ate their one meal at night, they tended to eat 600 calories more than when they had their one meal as

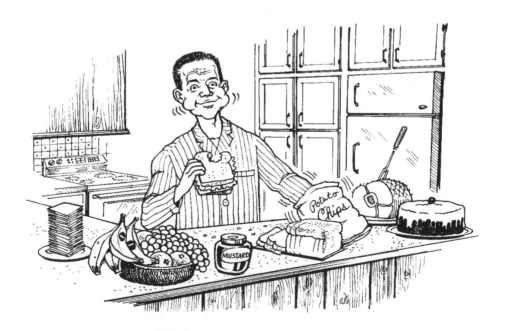

breakfast. It seems that if you don't eat much food before evening, you cultivate an enormous appetite that is hard to satisfy; you'll likely overeat and gain weight. As Patrick rationalized, "I feel as though I deserve to eat whatever I want. I've starved myself all day, I've worked hard, I'm tired, and I need a reward."

The bottom line for dieters is that you should eat appropriately during the day and then eat less at night. You'll not only have more energy for training, but you'll also prevent yourself from getting too hungry and overeating. Remember that when you get too hungry, you may no longer have the energy to care about how much you eat. You simply want to eat and eat.

WEIGHT LOSS WITHOUT MARTYRDOM

To lose weight healthfully and successfully keep it off, you should pay attention to these guidelines:

- How much you eat. There is a "diet" portion of any food.
- When you eat. Eat big breakfasts, rather than big dinners.
- Why you eat. Are you bored, stressed, lonely, or actually hungry?

These three keys can help you to implement a successful weight reduction program without dieting. Diets don't work.

If you are thinking about going on a diet, think again. *Diet* is a four-letter word, of which the first three letters spell *die*. Dieting conjures up visions of cottage cheese, grapefruit, rice cakes, and shredded wheat with skim milk. The typical dieter has very few fun memories associated with dieting. Diets teach denial and willpower. They also set the stage for going off the diet, binge eating, and developing disordered eating patterns (see chapter 15).

Because I'm a dietitian, most people assume that I put people on diets. I don't. People who go on a diet simply go off a diet. Not only do they have a 95-percent chance of regaining all the lost weight, but they're also in danger of regaining proportionately more fat than muscle. That represents a lot of wasted (or is that waisted?) effort.

> In her search for success with weight reduction, Amy, a 39-year-old bank teller, came to me for her "last hope" diet. "I've been on every diet in the book. You name it, I've done it. I've eaten grapefruit for breakfast, lunch, and dinner. I've avoided fats like the plague. I've consumed more salads than I care to think about. I have lost at least 500 pounds, but have regained 520. Maybe *you* can put me on a successful diet?"

WEIGHT LOSS
AFTER PREGNANCY

Q. "My baby was born four months ago and I still haven't lost all the weight. Will I lose weight naturally, or should I start to diet?"

A. Be patient! New mothers need to remember that life has seasons. The first year after pregnancy may not be the season to be as lean or as athletic as desired. Pregnancy lasts for 9 months, and many women need 9 to 12 months to return to their prepregnant physiques (see page 54). Don't try to crash diet now.

Your better bet is to focus on eating healthfully and to trust that healthy eating will contribute to the return of your appropriate weight. But this process often gets confounded because motherhood brings its own set of nutritional challenges and frustrations. When your baby cries, your life stops, and so do many healthful eating habits! Fatigue, stressful life changes, family adjustments, and lack of energy to shop and cook can also take their toll on the quality of your diet. You may also lack the mental energy you need to reduce your weight.

The stresses and frustrations that accompany motherhood can interfere with your desired weight loss plans and may even contribute to weight gain. If you are now home all day with readily available food, you may comfort yourself with soothing "drugs" such as candy, cookies, and other special treats. Your intentions to exercise may get confounded by physical exhaustion or lack of time and childcare. If this is the case, you might want to pay a baby-sitter so you can have some time to exercise. This may help you feel better—and feel better about yourself.

If you fear that you'll end up overweight for the rest of your life, take note of a survey of new moms. The women, who were all runners, reported that most returned to running 5 weeks after delivery, and were at their prepregnancy weight in five months (Lutter and Cushman 1982). Yes, there can be a lean life after pregnancy, as verified by the many mothers you see in the world around you who are lean. For now, love yourself from the inside out, enjoy your baby, and be gentle on yourself.

I explained to Amy that I wouldn't put her on a diet because diets don't work. Instead, I offered to teach her how to eat healthfully. By eating healthfully, she would lose weight. More importantly, she'd be able to exercise energetically, become and stay healthier, and learn how to keep the weight off for the rest of her life.

A PERSONALIZED FOOD PLAN

During her first meeting with me, Amy expressed her embarrassment about her inability to eat less. "I feel childish that I can't do something as simple as lose weight. I know what I should do to lose weight, and I just don't do it." I assured Amy that I have helped many knowledgeable dieters who have been humbled by their lack of control over food. Successful weight reduction isn't as easy as it sounds. That's why professional advice, individually tailored to a person's lifestyle and food preferences, is far more successful than packaged programs or self-inflicted diets.

If you, like Amy, want to lose weight once and for all, I recommend that you get personalized, professional guidance from a registered dietitian (RD). This health professional has fulfilled specific educational requirements, has passed a registration exam, and is a recognized member of the nation's largest organization of nutrition professionals, the American Dietetic Association. Because some states lack specific standards defining who can rightfully call themselves a dietitian or nutritionist, you'll best protect yourself from frauds and nutrition gurus if you seek guidance from RDs.

Here are some ways to locate your local registered dietitian:

- Call the American Dietetic Association's referral hot line (1-800-366-1655). They will give you a list of registered dietitians in your ZIP code. Request a dietitian who specializes in your specific concern: weight control, eating disorders, sports nutrition, cholesterol reduction, or whatever.
- Look in the Yellow Pages under dietitian and select a name followed by RD.
- Call the outpatient nutrition clinic at your community hospital.
- Ask your physician for a recommendation, or inquire at a local sports medicine clinic or health club.
- Call your state's dietetic association (see your phone book).

THIRTEEN TIPS
FOR SUCCESSFUL WEIGHT REDUCTION

The following tips helped Amy lose weight. They may help you develop your own winning way with food, especially if you work with a registered dietitian. These tips can also be appropriate for people who want a healthy food plan for maintaining weight.

Tip #1. Write Down What and When You Eat or Drink in a Day and Why

Keep accurate food records of every morsel and drop for three days. Also record why you eat. Are you stressed, hungry, or bored? Include the time and amount you exercise as well. Evaluate your patterns for potentially fattening habits such as skimping at breakfast, nibbling all day, overeating at night because you've gotten too hungry, entertaining yourself with food when you're bored, or rewarding yourself with chocolate when you're stressed.

Pay careful attention to your mood when eating. Amy discovered there were times when a hug and human comforting could have better

RESTING
METABOLIC RATE

Some people think they deserve to eat only if they exercise, but that's not the case. You need hundreds of calories every day simply to live. Here's how a 150-pound man burns calories while only resting in bed all day.

Organ	Calories per day	Percent of resting metabolic rate
Brain	365	21
Heart	180	10
Kidney	120	7
Liver	560	32
Lung	160	9
Other tissues	370	21

nourished her than food. She acknowledged that eating a tub of pop-corn certainly diverted her loneliness or anxieties, but it did nothing to resolve the problem that triggered the eating.

If you eat for reasons other than for fuel, you need to recognize that food is *fuel* and should not be abused like a drug. Food becomes dangerously fattening when it is eaten for entertainment, comfort, or stress reduction. And no amount of any food will solve any problem.

Tip #2. Become Aware of Meal Timing

If you eat lightly during the day and excessively at night, experiment with having a bigger breakfast and lunch and a lighter dinner. See chapters 3 and 4 to review how eating earlier in the day prevents you from getting too hungry, losing control, and overeating in the evening.

Amy was surprised that I thought her diet breakfast of cereal with skim milk was too skimpy and contributed to her overeating later in the day. She thought that diets were supposed to start at breakfast. I told her to start her diet at dinner; she needed more energy to get through the day.

Tip #3. Learn Your Calorie Budget

Know how much you can eat and still lose weight so you can be sure you are eating adequately at breakfast and lunch. Most people are surprised to learn how many calories they deserve to eat. They try to eat far too little, end up too hungry, and then blow their diets.

Tip #4. Subtract 20 Percent of Your Total Calorie Needs

Amy deserved to eat about 2,200 calories per day to maintain her weight. She subtracted 400 calories (20% × 2,000 = 400) from 2,200, leaving her 1,800 for her reducing diet. In the past, she had tried to reduce on 1,000 to 1,200 calories per day. She was skeptical about the proposed reducing plan of 1,800 calories. "If I can't lose weight on 1,000 calories, why should I lose on 1,800?" she questioned.

I reminded her that when she cut back too much, she got too hungry and blew her diet. She also lost muscle, slowed her metabolism, consumed too few of the nutrients she needed to protect her health and invest in top performance. Slow and steady weight loss stays off; quick weight loss is quickly regained.

Theoretically, if you eat 500 fewer calories per day than you normally do, you should lose one pound per week, because one pound of fat is the equivalent of about 3,500 calories:

260 Nancy Clark's Sports Nutrition Guidebook

$$500 \text{ calories} \times 7 \text{ days/week} = 3{,}500 \text{ calories/week} = 1 \text{ pound body fat}$$

This equation does not always hold true; nature makes weight loss harder for people who try to get below their set point weight (Leibel, Rosenbaum, and Hirsch 1995).

Tip #5. Divide Your Calorie Budget Into Three Parts of the Day

For Amy, her 1,800-calorie reducing diet worked out to 600 calories per section of the day:

Breakfast/snack	600 calories
Lunch/snack	600 calories
Dinner/snack	600 calories

Amy was initially hesitant with this plan and complained, "I'm afraid I'll get fat from eating so much breakfast and lunch." I reminded her of these points:

- She wouldn't gain weight from eating more at breakfast or lunch. Even if she ate too much, she could compensate by eating less at night. She'd have more energy to exercise and burn calories.
- If she skimped on those meals, she'd be likely to overeat at night.
- She was simply trading in the evening diet-blowing calories for wholesome foods earlier in the day.
- She'd be eating fewer calories than before, even though it seemed like more. And she'd be burning more with her increased exercise.
- If she wasn't hungry at night, she could eat less dinner.

Tip #6. Read Food Labels

Become familiar with the calorie content of the foods you commonly eat and then balance your calorie budget according to the rules for a well-balanced diet. That is, include at least three of the five food groups at each meal (see chapter 1). Too many dieters eat the same food(s) all the time, such as apples, apples, apples; this limits their intake of natural vitamins and minerals.

Amy was an expert calorie counter, and she commented that she tended to get neurotic about counting calories. I reminded her to count calories loosely and to consider them a general guideline and helpful tool to determine the appropriate amount of food to eat. By listening to her body and learning what 600 calories felt like, she could then use that feeling for future reference. For example, when at a restaurant she

To estimate your daily calorie requirement:

1) Determine your resting metabolic rate (RMR), the number of calories you need simply to breathe, pump blood, grow hair, and be alive, **120 lb.** by taking your body weight x 10.

Healthy Body Weight (lb.) x 10 Calories = 1200 Calories (RMR)

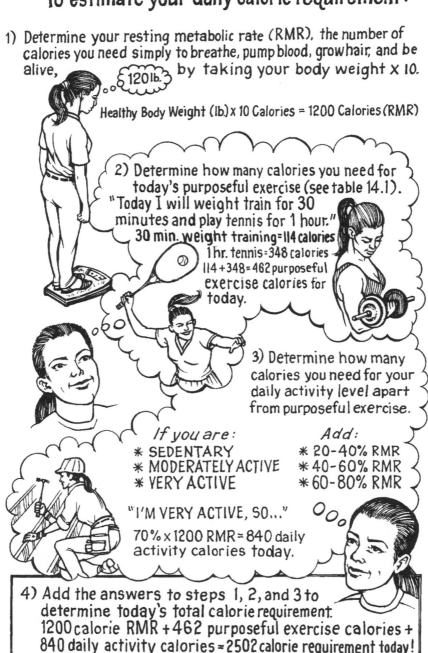

2) Determine how many calories you need for today's purposeful exercise (see table 14.1).
"Today I will weight train for 30 minutes and play tennis for 1 hour."
30 min. weight training = 114 calories
1 hr. tennis = 348 calories
114 + 348 = 462 purposeful exercise calories for today.

3) Determine how many calories you need for your daily activity level apart from purposeful exercise.

If you are: Add:
* SEDENTARY   * 20-40% RMR
* MODERATELY ACTIVE * 40-60% RMR
* VERY ACTIVE   * 60-80% RMR

"I'M VERY ACTIVE, SO..."
70% x 1200 RMR = 840 daily activity calories today.

4) Add the answers to steps 1, 2, and 3 to determine today's total calorie requirement.
1200 calorie RMR + 462 purposeful exercise calories + 840 daily activity calories = 2502 calorie requirement today!

Table 14.1   Calories Burned During Exercise

You can use this information to determine a reasonable estimate of the amount of calories you burn when exercising at a comfortable pace. If you are pushing yourself hard, add more calories.

Activity	Calories per hour per pound body weight
Badminton	2.6
Bicycling, 10 mph	2.7
Chopping wood, ax	2.3
Dancing, ballroom	1.6
Dancing, modern	2.6
Farming, light	2.3
Farming, heavy	3.2
Gardening, hoe, dig	3.2
Golf, walking	2.3
Horse grooming	3.5
House cleaning	1.6
Hiking, hilly	3.6
Horseback riding, trot	2.8
Jogging, 6 mph	4.2
Jumping rope	3.8
Mopping	1.7
Painting, outside	2.1
Racquetball	4.1
Rowing machine	3.1
Sawing, by hand	3.3
Scrubbing floors	2.9
Scuba diving	3.8
Skating, ice	2.6
Snow shoveling, light	2.9
Skiing, cross-country	3.7
Skiing, downhill	2.6
Snowshoe walking	4.5
Squash	4.3
Swimming, slow crawl	3.5
Soccer	3.7
Table tennis	1.9
Tennis, singles	2.9
Tennis, doubles	1.8
Volleyball	2.2
Walking, 3.5 mph	2.4
Waterskiing	3.0
Weight training	1.9

Adapted from B. Stamford and P. Shimer, 1990, *Fitness without exercise* (New York, NY: Warner Books).

could tell the right amount to eat by matching the at-home dinner's 600-calorie feeling of fullness with the same fullness from a restaurant's meal with an unknown calorie content.

Tip #7. Eat Slowly

Overweight people tend to eat faster than their normal weight counterparts. The brain needs about 20 minutes to receive the signal that you've eaten your fill. No matter how much you consume during those 20 minutes, the satiety signal doesn't move any faster. This explains why soup is an excellent first course for dieters. It takes time to eat, and it decreases the appetite for the main entrée. Try to pace your eating time so that you eat less and avoid the discomfort that often occurs after rapid eating.

Amy had the bad habit of inhaling her meals in a matter of minutes. She'd eat nonstop, without enjoying the pleasures of the meal. I encouraged her to put her fork down frequently—she didn't have to eat nonstop—and to *taste* the food. After all, the best part about food is its taste. She wasn't taking the time to enjoy that, and she was missing one of life's pleasures.

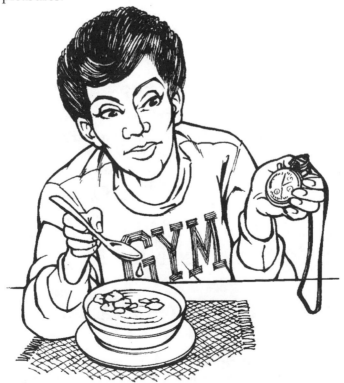

Because Amy had eaten quickly for most of her life, I suggested that she practice eating slowly at least one meal per day, and then build that up to two, then three meals. She discovered that lunchtime became more enjoyable once she gave herself permission to relax and enjoy the meal as well as the mealtime. She also felt less tempted to eat dessert, because the slowly savored lunch satisfied her appetite.

Tip #8. Eat Your Favorite Foods Regularly

If you deny yourself permission to eat what you want to eat, you are likely to binge. However, if you give yourself permission to eat these foods in diet portions, you will be less likely to blow your reducing plan. That is, if chocolate glazed donuts are among your favorites, have one once or twice a week. When eating this treat, do remember to chew it slowly, savor the taste, and fully enjoy it. You'll free yourself from the temptation to devour a dozen donuts in one sitting.

Amy's downfall was ice cream. "I can go for four days without an ice cream fix, but then I inevitably end up eating a whole pint." I encouraged her to eat ice cream for lunch at least twice per week to prevent those unnecessary binges. She discovered that she had little desire for ice cream once she knew that she could have some, and she stopped craving ice cream because of her better eating patterns. By preventing herself from getting too hungry, she lost interest in rich treats!

Tip #9. Keep Away From Food Sources That Tempt You

Out of sight, out of mind, and out of mouth! If you spend a lot of free time in the kitchen, you might want to relax in the den, where food is less likely to be readily available. At parties, socialize in the living room, away from the buffet table, and away from the snacks. At the market, skip the aisle with the cookies.

Amy used to walk home from work by way of the ice cream shop. No wonder she'd succumb to temptation! I suggested that she walk down another street. This became the simple solution to what had been a major problem.

Tip #10. Post a List of Ten Pleasurable Activities That Require No Food

When you are bored, lonely, tired, or nervous, you need to have some strategies in mind other than eating. For example, you might want to call a friend, write a letter, take a bath, water the plants, listen to music by candlelight, go for a walk, take a nap, or meditate. Food is designed to be fuel, not entertainment.

Amy overate when she felt stressed. I encouraged her to ask herself prior to indulging, "Am I hungry, or am I stressed?" If the answer was "stressed," she learned to recognize that no amount of food would resolve the stress so she shouldn't even start to eat. A phone call to her best friend became the slimming alternative.

Tip #11. Each Week, Plan a Day Off From Dieting

You don't have to lose weight every day. If you are confronted with a hectic schedule and wonder how you will survive the day's stresses, give yourself permission to fully fuel yourself. You'll need the energy to cope. If you are going to a fancy wedding and want to enjoy the full dinner, go right ahead! Remember that every day you can choose to lose, maintain, or even gain weight.

Amy had always attempted a diet as a nonstop event that lasted until she reached her goal weight. She liked my recommendation to plan in a treat once a week. "Knowing that I will enjoy going out to eat on Friday night helps me stay with my reducing program the rest of the week."

Tip #12. Exercise Consistently

Exercise regularly, but do not overexercise. If you do too much, you will likely end up injured, tired, and irritable. Exercise should be for fun and fitness, not simply for burning off calories. Be sure that you enjoy yourself.

Amy would sometimes punish herself with double workouts, longer runs, and harder bike rides to burn more calories. Although she did expend 500 to 600 calories per session, she'd end up too hungry by day's end and would inevitably replace that calorie deficit, plus more. I encouraged her to stop using exercise as punishment. She should be training to improve her performance, not pounding herself to burn calories. I reminded her that the "E" in exercise stands for enjoyment.

Tip #13. Think "Fit and Healthy"

Every morning before you get out of bed, visualize yourself as being fitter and leaner. This will help you start the day with a positive attitude. If you tell yourself that you are eating more healthfully and are successfully losing weight, you will do so more easily. Positive self-talk is important for your well-being.

Amy constantly reminded herself that she'd rather be healthier and leaner than to overeat. She took smaller portions. She made a daily eating plan and stuck to it. On her way home after work, she visualized herself eating a pleasant (but smaller) dinner, chewing the food slowly, savoring the taste, relaxing after dinner with a book rather than cookies, and successfully following her food plan. By practicing this scene before she arrived home, she discovered that she was better able to carry through with her good intentions.

Amy also reminded herself that when she ate well, she felt better and trained better. She also felt better about herself. After years of unsuccessful dieting, she liked feeling successful, perhaps even more than feeling thinner.

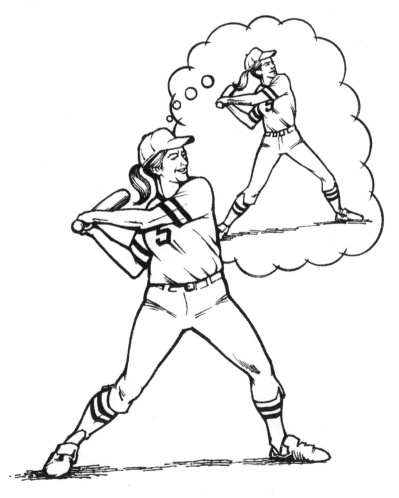

WRESTLING WITH WEIGHT: DIETING TIPS FOR ATHLETES WITH WEIGHT LIMITS

If you are a wrestler, boxer, jockey, or rower, you are probably not overweight. But you may have to cut weight to achieve a lower weight standard for your sport or else be denied permission to compete. Use the following tips as well as the information in this chapter to help you lose weight healthfully.

• First of all, get a realistic picture of how much weight you have to lose by getting your body fat measured (see chapter 13). The absolute minimal weight includes 5 percent fat for men and 12 percent fat for women. The minimum weight recommended for wrestlers commonly includes about 7-percent body fat. Trying to achieve a weight that will result in your having to starve yourself to lose muscle or to dehydrate yourself to lose water weight is difficult and can hurt rather than enhance your performance.

If you don't have access to calipers or another means to measure your percent body fat, give yourself the less professional "pinch test." If you can pinch more than half an inch of thickness over your shoulder blade or hips, you can safely lose a little more weight.

• Start to lose weight early in the season or, better yet, before the start of the season. That way, you'll have the time to lose weight slowly (1 to 2 pounds per week) and more enjoyably. Your goal is to achieve and stay at your lowest healthy body-fat level.

• Remember that it is counterproductive to lose weight rapidly before an event. If you do, depleted muscle glycogen and dehydration will take their tolls. In a study with wrestlers who quickly lost about 8 pounds (4.5 percent of their body weight), the wrestlers performed 3.5 percent worse on a six-

(continued)

minute arm crank test designed to be similar to a wrestling competition. These results suggest that rapid weight loss in athletes prior to competition may serve as a detriment rather than offer a competitive advantage (Hickner et al. 1991).

Athletes who struggle and starve to get to a low weight tend to fool only themselves. Remember, the odds are against the starved wrestler who crash diets to make weight as compared to the well-fueled wrestler who routinely maintains or stays within a few pounds of his fighting weight during training.

• To lose weight, follow the calorie guidelines outlined on p.260. No matter how much weight you have to lose, be sure to eat at least 1,500 calories of a variety of wholesome foods every day to prevent vitamin, mineral, and protein deficiencies. Do not eliminate any food group.

• Water is not extra weight. Your body stores the precious water in a delicate balance. If you disrupt this balance, you will decrease your ability to exercise at your best. Using diuretics, rubber suits, saunas, whirlpools, or steamrooms to dehydrate yourself is dangerous.

• When replacing sweat loss after workouts, note that juices, sports drinks, and soft drinks all have calories. Ration them wisely! The lowest-calorie fluid replacer is water.

• If you are worried that strict dieting as a teenager will stunt your growth, note that you will catch up after the competitive season. Many wrestlers are short in stature not because of malnutrition but rather because of genetics. They tend to have short parents. Small people often select a low-weight sport because they are more suited for that than for football or basketball.

15
chapter

Overcoming Eating Disorders

Food and exercise go hand in hand. Most athletes love to eat and welcome the fact that the more they exercise, the more they can eat. But some athletes are overwhelmed by food obsessions and eating disorders. They worry constantly about what they'll eat, when and where they will eat, how much weight they will gain if they eat a normal meal with their friends, how many hours they will have to exercise to burn off those calories, how many meals they should skip if they overeat by a few morsels, and so on. They are consumed by the endless frets revolving around food, weight, exercise, and dieting.

Betsy, a 16-year-old runner, says that her obsessions with food began when her high school track coach advised her to lose 5 pounds, 5 pounds she didn't have in excess. She ended up losing muscle and strength.

Peter, a 40-year-old lawyer, started having cookie fixations during his struggle to attain a lower than ever racing weight for the Boston Marathon. His diet of 1,500 calories per day consisted of nothing for breakfast or lunch, then 30 Oreos after his run. He was just too hungry to cook a healthy dinner, so he madly devoured cookies until he panicked that he might gain weight.

Sally, a 31-year-old compulsive swimmer, reported constant food thoughts after she had lost 20 pounds. She wanted to weigh 99 pounds, even though 110 pounds was a good weight that she could comfortably maintain. She'd finish one meal and then immediately start thinking about the next because she was still hungry. She lived in fear of overeating.

EATING DISORDERS AMONG ATHLETES

Eating disorders among sports-active people seem to be on the rise. Coaches commonly express concerns about some of their athletes, especially those in sports that emphasize weight such as running, gymnastics, wrestling, and lightweight crew. Research indicates that eating disorders are widespread among all college athletes.

• About one-third of collegiate female athletes have some type of disordered eating pattern, be it anorexia (self-induced starvation), bulimia (binge eating, followed by self-induced vomiting), laxative abuse, excessive exercise, crash diets, or other unhealthy weight loss practices. (Rosen et al. 1986)

• Three percent of 695 athletes in midwestern colleges met the diagnostic criteria for anorexia, and 21.5 percent met the criteria for bulimia (Burkes-Miller and Black 1988). (See the next section for these diagnostic criteria.)

• The majority of people with eating disorders exercise compulsively. The athlete with anorexic tendencies exercises as a means to create a calorie deficit and be thinner; the athlete with bulimic tendencies exercises to burn off the calories consumed during a binge (Yates 1991).

Approximately half of all dieters report abnormal eating binges; many of these dieters abuse exercise as a means to help control their weight. Some call themselves "athletes," when in reality they can be better named "compulsive exercisers." Many live in fear of getting fat, and they constantly restrict their food in hopes of losing weight. They live with chaotic eating patterns and body hatred.

If you are among the lucky few who effortlessly maintain their desired weight, you probably think that all this talk about food and weight is ridiculous. However, if you are a runner, dancer, gymnast, wrestler, or other weight-conscious athlete who constantly strives to be thinner, you may experience some degree of an obsession with food. If you believe that you spend more time thinking about food than the average person does, keep reading.

I estimate that at least 30 to 40 percent of my clients at SportsMedicine Brookline are obsessed with food, and they represent only a minority

WHAT IS ANOREXIA?

People with anorexia nervosa tend to either consistently restrict food or restrict and then binge and purge. The following definition is used by the American Psychiatric Association (1994):

- Intense fear of gaining weight or becoming fat, even though underweight
- Disturbance in the way a person experiences his or her body (i.e., claiming to "feel fat" even when emaciated), with an undue influence of body weight or shape on self-perception
- Weight loss to less than 85 percent of normal body weight or, if during a period of growth, failure to make expected weight gain leading to 85 percent of that expected
- Refusal to maintain body weight over a minimal normal weight for age and height
- Denial of the seriousness of the current weight loss
- Absence of at least three consecutive menstrual cycles

Data from the *Diagnostic and Statistical Manual of Mental Disorders*, 1994, 4th ed., revised. Copyright 1994 American Psychiatric Association.

of athletes who seek professional nutrition guidance. Most athletes who are obsessed with food struggle on their own for years before asking for help. They are embarrassed that they can't seem to resolve their food imbalances. One 45-year-old woman confided that I was the first person in 30 years to whom she had talked about her bulimia.

Food, for these athletes, is not fuel. It is "The Fattening Enemy" that thwarts their desire to be perfectly thin. Their goal is thinness at any price—and that price is often mental anguish, physical fatigue, injuries that fail to heal, and impaired athletic performance. These athletes perform suboptimally because they eat poorly. One high school runner failed to connect her inability to finish track workouts with her one

WHAT IS BULIMIA?

The person with bulimia nervosa may purge via self-induced vomiting or the misuse of laxatives, diuretics, or enemas (purging type) or use other inappropriate compensatory mechanisms to prevent weight gain, such as fasting or exercising excessively (nonpurging type). The definition used by the American Psychiatric Association (1994) includes

- Recurrent episodes of binge eating, characterized by both of the following:
  1. Eating an unusually large amount of food in a discrete period of time (the amount eaten is larger than most people would eat during a similar time period and under similar circumstances)
  2. Feeling out of control during the eating episode and unable to stop eating or control what and how much is eaten

- Compensating for the food binge to prevent weight gain, such as inducing vomiting; misusing laxatives, enemas, or other medications; fasting; or exercising excessively
- Binge eating and purging, on average, at least twice a week for three months
- Evaluating self-worth according to body shape and weight

Data from the *Diagnostic and Statistical Manual of Mental Disorders*, 1994, 4th ed., revised. Copyright 1994 American Psychiatric Association.

banana a day diet. She thought she fell asleep in classes because she had stayed up too late, not because she was underfed. Such denial!

If you are anorexic or bulimic, I recommend that you seek help from a professional counselor experienced with eating disorders and get nutritional guidance from a registered dietitian. Extreme eating disorders usually reflect an inability to cope with life's day-to-day stresses. For example, one of my clients, a high-level executive, smothered her stress with peppermint ice cream, hot fudge sauce, and pecans. This

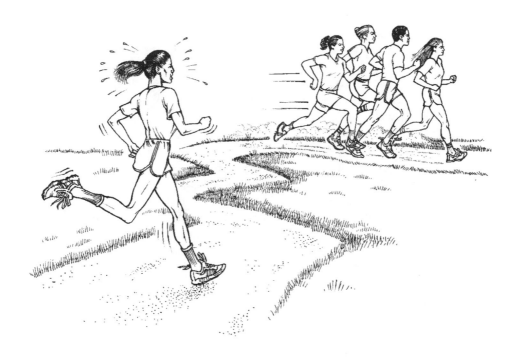

treat certainly diverted her attention from her problems, but it didn't resolve any of them. Afraid of gaining weight, she'd burn off the calories with a long workout that was pure punishment. She became injured from the excessive exercise, panicked at her inability to exercise, tried to eat next to nothing, became ravenous, binged, and then resorted to self-induced vomiting as a means to purge the calories because she could no longer do step aerobics. She came to me looking for help with food. I insisted that she also get psychological counseling to help her deal with stress and her feelings of being out of control.

CASE STUDIES

The following case studies are typical of the clients I treat. They may sound familiar and might help those of you who constantly struggle with food and exercise.

Case Study #1. A Runner With Disordered Eating Patterns

Pete, a 42-year-old runner, never was concerned about his weight until he began running in his late thirties. He felt fat compared to other runners and decided to diet. He'd force himself through a 10-mile run every morning, eat very little during the day, then devour any food in sight on arriving home from work. "I feel so guilty about the boxes of crackers, pretzels, and cookies I devour. After a binge, I won't eat dinner with my wife and children. Instead, I'll go for another run to burn off the excess calories. My kids get mad at me for eating all the cookies. My wife complains that I'm neglecting the family. I'm disappointed in myself for being such a failure. I'm embarrassed that I'm unable to do something as simple as lose a few pounds. I can't even eat normally now. I either diet or binge. I don't know if I should be seeing you or a psychologist."

To help Pete balance his food and exercise goals better and to normalize his disordered eating patterns, I measured his percent body fat (a very lean eight percent), and determined how many calories his body required each day—1,600 calories for his resting metabolic rate plus 800 calories for moderate daily activity plus 1,000 calories for purposeful exercise = 3,400 total calories per day (see chapter 14 for more calorie details). Then I devised a meal plan to stabilize his eating. Like many of my clients, he dieted too hard for someone with little excess fat to lose. His weight goal was well below the genetic weight that he could comfortably maintain, which explains one reason why weight loss was so difficult for him!

Pete unrealistically restricted his calories. He would run 10 miles in the morning, which burned about 1,000 calories. But he would eat nothing until lunch, at which time he limited himself to only 450 calories. No wonder he felt starved and stuffed himself with food the minute he arrived home for the evening! I advised him to stop dieting, start eating breakfast and lunch, and eat reasonably at night. He changed his habits and stopped his evening binges.

Pete followed my recommendations to eat 3,400 calories, divided more evenly throughout the day. When he returned two weeks later he reported with a big smile, "When I get home at night, I no longer act like a maniac in the kitchen, eating whatever I can get my hands on. I've decided to accept my body the way it is; nature just doesn't want me to be thinner. Eating a substantial breakfast and lunch helps me feel great. I have lots more energy at work. I'm less irritable. My running is improving. And, most important, I feel in control of my food."

Pete found peace with food by stopping his dieting and starting to eat appropriate meals at breakfast and lunch. He needed a better food plan to correct his food binges that stemmed from extreme hunger, not from life's stresses.

Case Study #2. A Triathlete With Bulimia

Mary, a 26-year-old advertising account executive and triathlete, had gained 8 pounds in two years' time despite being bulimic. She tended to overeat when work became overwhelming, and she felt like she couldn't do all that was expected of her. "I binge at night and then vomit. I'm exhausted from fighting with food and weight. I've stopped socializing with my friends because I'm afraid it'll present the opportunity to overeat and that I'll be unable to purge. Instead, I spend my time exercising twice a day trying to lose weight. I inevitably end up at the bakery, where I buy at least six bagels and God only knows what else. I'm a foodaholic and just can't seem to control my intake."

After listening to Mary's story, I recognized that she seemed addicted not only to food, but also to work and exercise. She constantly pushed herself to meet self-imposed deadlines, weight goals, and exercise demands. She constantly felt stressed and overextended. She lacked a healthy balance to her life.

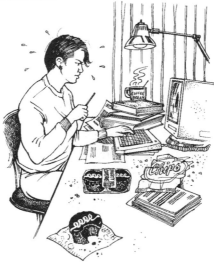

I asked if anyone in Mary's family had trouble with alcohol. She looked at me with surprise in her eyes, wondering how I guessed this family secret. Her father was an alcoholic.

At least one-third of my clients with eating disorders grew up in families with some type of dysfunction, most commonly related to alcohol. Though they themselves may not currently be addicted to alcohol, many are recovering alcoholics or drug abusers (Varner 1995). Or, they often express other addictive behaviors through overworking, overeating, overachieving, and overexercising. Surveys suggest that approximately one-third of children of alcoholics become bulimic (Brisman and Siegal 1984; Colins et al. 1985). They may purge by vomiting or by overexercising. Many disguise themselves as dedicated athletes, when actually they are compulsive exercisers. The traits and attitudes outlined in table 15.1 are characteristic of some people who grew up in an alcoholic or otherwise dysfunctional family.

Table 15.1　Athletes, Exercise, and Alcoholism

Athletes who suffer from disordered eating tend to have similar personality traits that affect their attitudes toward food, exercise, and weight. The traits may be the result of growing up in a family in which a parent was suffering from alcoholism or in an otherwise dysfunctional family where a parent may have been unavailable for the child. If you find yourself struggling with food and fitting the following description, you should understand that food is not a problem; it's a *symptom* of problems with life (Woititz 1983).

Characteristic trait	How commonly expressed
Drive for perfection	"I haven't missed a day of exercise in five years."
Desire for control	"I never touch white flour, refined sugar, red meat, or any food with more than 1 gram of fat."
Compulsive behavior	"I work out for two hours every day, regardless of holidays, injuries, or family crises."
Feelings of inadequacy	"I could have run even faster if I'd lost more weight."
Difficulty having fun	"You folks enjoy the movie. I have some work to catch up on."
Trouble with intimate relationships	"My wife gets angry with me for spending more time exercising than with my family."

Mary displayed all these traits. She had a strong drive to be perfect and a desire for control. Since childhood, she had tried to be perfect to compensate for her family's problems. Now, she was trying to eat the perfect diet, achieve the perfect weight, and maintain the perfect training schedule. She ran 10 miles every day, despite blizzards, illness, or fatigue (a "perfect" training schedule). She lived on calorie-free coffee, diet soda, and fat-free foods (the "perfect" diet), until ravenous hunger overwhelmed her good intentions. After a binge, she'd vomit (to bring control back to her life and compensate for her imperfect eating).

I helped Mary to get a better perspective on an appropriate weight by measuring her percent body fat, an appropriate diet by designing a meal plan, and an appropriate training program by referring her to a coach. I also advised her to read some books about adult children of alcoholics, seek guidance from an appropriate counselor, and perhaps join a support group such as Al-Anon or ACoA (Adult Children of Alcoholics). For additional readings, see appendix A.

"For years, I thought that food was the source of my struggles," she wrote in a follow-up letter. "It wasn't. Life was the problem. I'm now gentler on myself. I even let myself be imperfect. For example, I took three days off from training when I went on vacation! I'm eating well and exercising healthfully rather than pounding myself with megamiles to burn off calories. I feel better and am at peace with myself and my body."

Case Study #3. Ballet Dancer With Anorexia

> Shannon, a 16-year-old student at a highly competitive dance school, was sent to me by her doctor. She had an injury that was healing poorly. Shannon's mother forced her to come to the appointment and her first words were, "My mother made me come here. She thinks I don't eat enough. I agree, but I'm afraid to eat more because I don't want to get fat. I can't dance now that I'm injured, nor get as much exercise as I'd like."

Shannon weighed 97 pounds. Five months before, she had weighed 107 pounds, and at 64 inches, she could have appropriately weighed 120 pounds. She was limiting herself to only 1,000 calories per day, but deserved to eat about 1,800 calories. Because she was eating so little food, she was consuming inadequate amounts of protein, calcium, iron, zinc, and numerous other vitamins and minerals that her body needed to heal and be healthy.

Because Shannon was so afraid that she'd get fat if she were to eat more, I had to constantly remind her that food is fuel and health. She was currently unhealthy. She had stopped menstruating (one sign of poor health), and her injury was healing unusually slowly (a second sign). Shannon needed to eat a wider variety of food than bagels, apples, and carrots to balance her diet and provide the nutrients she was deficient in. She also needed to include more dietary fat (see chapters 1, 2, 8, and 14).

Shannon needed to fuel herself with more calories. I reminded her that she deserved to eat, even if she was not exercising. I asked her to take notice of all her friends who were nonexercisers. All ate, and most were very lean! Shannon required about 1,200 calories simply for her resting metabolic needs, plus another 600 for her daily activity at school. We established the following goals:

- Follow a food plan that would optimize her health.
- Fuel her body appropriately by gradually increasing calories at meals and snacks.
- Rebuild her body to an appropriate weight to optimize her strength and health.
- Reduce the risk of stress fractures and future osteoporosis by achieving regular menstrual periods.
- Attain peace with food and weight.

Shannon agreed to gradually increase her intake by 100 calories per week, adding more calories at breakfast and lunch until she had three 500-calorie meals that included at least three or four kinds of foods (such as cereal, milk, and fruit; sandwich bread, protein, and yogurt; fish, starch, vegetable, and milk). These dietary improvements would help her have more energy to concentrate better at school and to swim as an alternative exercise. I suggested that she practice eating more healthfully, just as she had practiced her ballet, and that she focus on how much better she felt when she fueled herself better.

Over the course of weeks, Shannon stopped rigidly controlling her food and started to eat more appropriately. My nutrition advice had provided helpful guidelines, but a key factor in her recovery was counseling. Shannon was counseled by a psychologist skilled with eating disorders and by a family therapist who met with her and her parents and sister. Through communicating and resolving many of the family's issues, Shannon was able to express her needs rather than withhold verbal communication and use food restriction as her nonverbal cry for help.

Within three months, Shannon started to menstruate—a good sign that she was adequately nourishing her body. She was feeling physically stronger, was happier with her family, and felt at peace with food and her body. She no longer felt she had to be perfect to earn her parents' love, nor did she need to be perfectly thin, eat the perfect diet, and be the perfect student and ballet dancer. She learned to enjoy being human, just like the rest of her family and friends. She let go of her fantasy that a perfect body would bring a perfect life. "I thought I'd be happier once I was thinner, but I was wrong. I've learned that happiness comes from loving myself from the inside out, not the outside in."

NUTRITION TIPS FOR THE ATHLETE WITH AMENORRHEA

If you are an athlete who previously had regular menstrual periods but have stopped menstruating, you are experiencing amenorrhea. Don't ignore it! Although you may think amenorrhea is desirable because you no longer have to deal with the hassles of monthly menstrual periods, amenorrhea can lead to problems that interfere with your health and ability to perform at your best. These problems include

- almost a three times higher incidence of stress fractures,
- premature osteoporosis that can affect your bone health in the not-too-distant future,
- possibly a higher risk of heart disease, and
- an inability to conceive easily should you want to start a family.

Amenorrhea is Complex

If you believe you lack periods only because you are too thin and are exercising too much, you are wrong. Studies have shown no body fat differences between athletic women who menstruate regularly and those who don't (Sanborn, Albrecht, and Wagner 1987). Many very thin athletes do have regular menses. Clearly, leanness and intense exercise are not the simple explanation to the complexities of amenorrhea.

But the question remains unanswered: Why are you amenorrheic when your peers, who have similar exercise programs and the same low percent body fat are not? Are you

- striving to maintain a weight lower than your natural set point,
- struggling harder to maintain your desired leanness, or
- eating inadequately to achieve your desired leanness?

If so, you are probably experiencing nutritional amenorrhea.

Resolving the Problem

The possible changes required to resume menses include exercising 5 to 15 percent less and eating a little more healthfully (Otis 1990). Some amenorrheic athletes have resumed menses with slightly reduced exercise and after gaining fewer than 5 pounds. A small amount of weight gain can be enough to achieve better health, yet does not result in your getting fat.

If you believe that poor eating may be part of the reason you have ceased menstruating, you should have a nutrition checkup with a registered dietitian or sports nutritionist. The following tips may also help you resume menses, or at least rule out nutrition-related factors.

1. Throw away the bathroom scale. Rather than striving to achieve a certain number on the scale, let your body weigh what it weighs. Weight is more than a matter of willpower; genetics play an important role. The information in chapters 13 and 14 can help you to determine an appropriate weight you can comfortably maintain without constantly dieting. Your physician or dietitian can also give unbiased professional advice.

2. If you have weight to lose, don't restrict calories by more than 20 percent. Women who go on severe diets commonly lose their menstrual periods. By following a healthy reducing program, you'll not only have greater success with long-term weight loss, but you'll also be able to enjoy enough energy to participate in your sports program.

3. If you are at an appropriate weight, practice eating like you did as a child. That is, eat when you are hungry and stop when you are content. If you are always hungry and constantly obsessing about food, you are undoubtedly trying to eat too few calories. Your body is complaining and requesting more food. Remember that you want to eat adequately to support your sports program. The information in chapter 14, plus advice from your doctor and dietitian, can help you determine an appropriate calorie intake.

Current research suggests that amenorrheic women who are maintaining their weights are indeed eating their required calories (Wilmore et al. 1992). However, they do so in nontraditional and chaotic eating patterns. For example, they may eat very little at breakfast and lunch only to overeat at night, or they restrict Monday through Thursday and then overeat on the weekends. If your weight is stable, you are somehow consuming the number of calories you need, so you might as well eat them on a regular schedule of wholesome, well-balanced meals. A registered dietitian can help you develop an appropriate food plan if you are struggling on your own.

4. Eat adequate protein. In one study, 82 percent of the amenorrheic women ate less than the recommended intake for protein (Nelson et al. 1986). Even if you are a vegetarian, remember that you still need adequate protein.

5. Eat at least 20 percent of your calories from fat. Amenorrheic athletes tend to avoid meat and other protein-rich foods because they are afraid of eating fat. For most active women, eating 40 to 60 grams of fat per day would be an appropriate low-fat diet. This clearly allows beef, peanut butter, cheese, nuts, and other wholesome foods that balance out a sports diet.

6. Include small portions of red meat two to four times per week. Surveys of runners show that those with amenorrhea tend to eat less red meat and are more likely to follow a vegetarian diet than their regularly menstruating counterparts are (Kaiserauer et al. 1989). Even though red meats can have a higher fat content than chicken or fish, an overall low-fat sports diet can accommodate some fat, and getting that fat via lean meats may help achieve regular menses.

7. Maintain a calcium-rich diet. If you are amenorrheic, you should regularly consume three to four 8-ounce servings of low-fat milk or yogurt (or other calcium-rich foods) daily to protect your bones. Your bones benefit from the protective effect of exercise, but this does not compensate for lack of calcium or lack of estrogen. Although you may cringe at the thought of spending so many calories on dairy foods, remember that milk is a wholesome food that contains many important nutrients (see chapters 1 and 2). If you are eating a diet that includes lots of bran cereal, fruits, and vegetables, you may have an even higher need for calcium; the fiber may interfere with calcium absorption.

Many amenorrheic women worry about their bone health and wonder if there is long-term damage. Probably. Women who resume menses do restore some of the bone density lost during the months of amenorrhea, but they do not restore all of it. Hence, your goal should be to minimize the damages of amenorrhea by eating appropriately and taking the proper steps to resolve the problem.

HOW TO HELP THE ATHLETE WITH AN EATING DISORDER

Perhaps you have friends, family, or teammates who struggle with food, and you wonder what you can do to help resolve the problem. Such was the case with Deb, a collegiate gymnast.

"I get scared when I see Alicia. She's nothing but skin and bones covered up with a baggy sweat suit. I rarely see her eat anything but sugar-free gum or lettuce topped with catsup for salad dressing. She never joins us at parties after meets because she has to study, or so she says. I think she's anorexic. What should I do?"

Deb was obviously concerned about her friend and teammate, Alicia, and was at a loss as to how to help her—if indeed Alicia was anorexic and did need help. Even health professionals can have trouble distinguishing between the "lean and mean" and the anorexic. Generally speaking, the anorexic athlete is a compulsive exerciser who trains frantically out of fear of gaining weight and who never takes rest days. In comparison, the lean and mean athlete trains hard with hopes of improving performance but also enjoys days with no exercise. Both push themselves to perfection—to be perfectly thin or to be the perfect athlete. Sometimes the two become intertwined.

Approximately half of anorexics become bulimic. Some purge by vomiting, others by excessive exercise. For example, some aerobics instructors who teach three or four classes per day plus do their own workouts may be bulimic, and they purge themselves of excess calories under the guise of teaching and training.

This constant battle with food endangers an athlete's physical and mental health and overall well-being. Unfortunately, too many coaches, parents, friends, and teammates shy away from the devastating stressfulness of this self-imposed struggle for ultimate thinness. After all, how can anyone who is training and seems happy be sick?

If you suspect that your friend, training partner, child, or teammate has a problem with food, don't wait until medical problems prove you right. Speak up in an appropriate manner. Anorexia and bulimia are life-threatening conditions that shouldn't be overlooked. Here are 10 tips for approaching this delicate subject.

1. Heed the Signs. You may notice that anorexics wear bulky clothes to hide their abnormal thinness or that their food consumption is abnormally restrictive and spartan in comparison to the energy expended. A runner, for example, may eat only a yogurt for dinner after having completed a strenuous 10-mile workout. Perhaps you'll never see them eating in public, at home, or with friends. They find some excuse for not joining others at meals. Or if they do, they may push the food around on the plate to fool you into thinking that they're eating. You may also notice other compulsive behaviors, such as excessive studying or working. The following lists describe other symptoms of anorexia.

Signs and Symptoms of Anorexia

- Significant weight loss
- Recurrent overuse injuries and stress fractures
- Loss of menstrual periods
- Loss of hair
- Growth of fine body hair, noticeable on the face and arms
- Cold hands and feet and extreme sensitivity to cold temperatures
- Lightheadedness
- Inability to concentrate
- Low pulse rate
- Hyperactivity, compulsive exercise beyond normal training
- Comments about how fat they are, distorted body image
- Expression of intense fear of becoming fat
- Wearing sweaters in summer heat due to feeling cold all the time
- Wearing layers of baggy clothing to hide thinness
- Nervousness at mealtime, avoidance of eating in public
- Food rituals, such as cutting food into small pieces and playing with it
- Antisocial behavior, isolation from family and friends
- Excessive working or studying, compulsiveness and rigidity
- High emotions: tearful, uptight, overly sensitive, restless

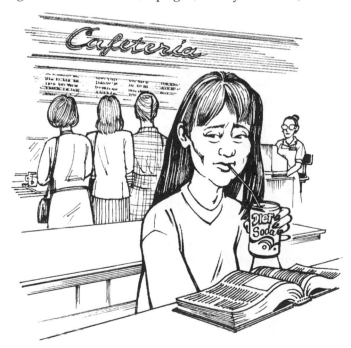

Bulimic behavior can be more subtle. The athlete may eat a great deal of food and then rush to the bathroom. You may hear water running to cover up the sound of vomiting. The person may hide laxatives or may even speak about a magic method of eating without gaining weight. She or he may have bloodshot eyes, swollen glands, and bruised fingers (from inducing vomiting). The following list describes other symptoms of bulimia.

Signs and Symptoms of Bulimia

- Weakness, headaches, dizziness
- Frequent weight fluctuations due to alternating binges and fasts
- Difficulty swallowing and retaining food, damage to throat
- Swollen glands that give a chipmunk-like appearance
- Frequent vomiting
- Bloodshot eyes
- Damaged tooth enamel from exposure to gastric acid when vomiting
- Strange behavior that surrounds secretive eating
- Running water in the bathroom after meals to hide the sound of vomiting
- Disappearance after meals, often to the bathroom to "take a shower"
- Extreme concern with body weight, shape, and physical appearance
- Ability to eat enormous meals without weight gain
- Petty stealing of food or of money to buy food for binges
- Compulsive exercise beyond normal training
- Depression

2. Express Your Concern Carefully. Approach these individuals gently but persistently, saying that you are worried about their health: "I'm concerned that your injuries are taking so long to heal." Talk about what you see: "I've noticed that you seem tired and your race times are getting slower and slower." Give evidence for why you believe they are struggling to balance food and exercise and ask if they want to talk about it.

Individuals who are truly anorexic or bulimic commonly deny the problem, insisting that they're perfectly fine. Continue to share your concerns about their lack of concentration, light-headedness, or chronic fatigue. These health changes are more likely to be stepping stones for accepting help, given that the athlete undoubtedly clings to food and exercise as attempts to gain control and stability.

3. Do *Not* Discuss Weight or Eating Habits. The athlete takes great pride in being perfectly thin and may dismiss your concern as jealousy. Avoid any mention of starving and binging as the issue, and focus on life issues not food issues.

4. Suggest Unhappiness as the Reason for Seeking Help. Point out how anxious, tired, or irritable the athlete has been lately. Emphasize that he or she doesn't have to be that way.

5. Be Supportive and Listen Sympathetically. Don't expect someone to admit right away that there's a problem. Give it time, and constantly remind the athlete that you believe in him or her. This will make a difference in recovery.

6. Offer a Written List of Professional Resources for Help. Although the athlete may deny the problem to your face, she or he may admit despair at another moment. If you don't know of local resources, ask the national organizations for the closest resource. Here's a list of organizations that may be able to help provide more information and help for someone with anorexia or bulimia.

American Anorexia/Bulimia Association, Inc.
293 Central Park West, Suite 1R;New York, NY 10024 212-501-8351
Offers written materials, referrals

American Dietetic Association
National Center for Nutrition and Dietetics
216 West Jackson Blvd, Suite 800
Chicago, IL 60609-6995   800-366-1655
Referral service for sports nutritionists skilled with handling eating disorders

Anorexia Nervosa and Related Eating Disorders (ANRED)
PO Box 5102; Eugene, OR 97045   503-344-1144
Offers written materials, referrals

National Anorexia Aid Society
1925 East Dublin Granville Rd; Columbus, OH 43229 614-436-1112
Focuses on prevention, written materials

Overeaters Anonymous
PO Box 92870; Los Angeles, CA 90009   213-542-8363
Refer to phone book for local chapters; free support groups

You can also call your local sports medicine clinic and ask to speak to their physician or nutritionist, your university health center or eating disorders program, or your local health center to consult with a pediatric or adolescent medicine specialist.

7. Limit Your Expectations. You alone can't solve the problem. It's more complex than food and exercise; it's a life problem. Share your concerns with others; seek help from a trusted family member, medical professional, or health service. Don't try to deal with the problem alone, especially if you are making no headway and the athlete is becoming more self-destructive.

8. Recognize That You May Be Overreacting. Maybe there is no eating disorder. Maybe the athlete is appropriately thin for enhanced sports performance. But how can you decide? To clarify the situation, insist the athlete have a mental health evaluation. If necessary, make the appointment and take the athlete there yourself. Only then will you get an unbiased opinion of the degree of danger, if any. The therapist may tell you to go home and stop worrying, or might detect misery and suicidal tendencies in the athlete and encourage immediate care.

9. Seek Advice From Health Care Professionals About Your Concerns. You may need to discuss your feelings with someone. Remember that you are not responsible for the other person's health, and you can only try to help. Your power comes from using guidance counselors, registered dietitians, medical professionals, or eating disorder clinics.

10. Be Patient. Recognize that the healing process can be long and arduous with many relapses and setbacks, but your reward will be that you can make a critical difference in that person's life. People die from anorexia and bulimia.

HOW TO HELP PREVENT EATING DISORDERS

Many athletes think—or feel pressured to believe—that by restricting their food intake to lose weight they will exercise better, look better, and enhance their overall performances. Ironically, restricting food in an attempt to improve performance can actually result in depleted fuel stores, muscle depletion, amenorrhea, stress fractures, fainting, weakness, fatigue, and eventually impaired performance. Some athletes may manage to do well for awhile without an obvious decline in performance, but then injuries and lack of energy will catch up with them.

Eating disorders would fade if people could learn to love their bodies. As a society, we must

- dispel the myth that thinness equals happiness and success,
- discourage the notion that the thinnest athlete is the best athlete,
- love our bodies for what they are rather than hate them for what they are not, and
- emphasize fit and healthy as more appropriate goals than slender and skinny.

16 *chapter*

Bulking Up Healthfully

> "I feel like an eating machine," complained Jim, a scrawny 21-year-old collegiate athlete. "But no matter how much I eat, my weight stays the same. I'll single-handedly devour a whole large pizza and then a pint of ice cream for dessert. Eating has become a chore, to say nothing of an expense. I'm tired of trying to gain weight."

> Martin, a high school football player, expressed similar concerns. "I want to bulk up before the football season and gain muscle but not fat. My coach wants me to gain 15 pounds. I've been trying all sorts of weight gain drinks, protein powders, and amino acid pills. Nothing seems to work."

When it comes to weight, most sports-active people contentedly maintain their desired weights or struggle to lose a few pounds. Others, however, wish they could add a few pounds. Many football and hockey players, bodybuilders, and teenage boys want to gain weight by building their muscles. Some very thin and spindly athletes even wish they could gain a little fat to fill out their physiques! For people struggling to gain

287

weight, eating can be a task, food a medicine. These individuals feel self-consciously thin, hate their skinny images, and seem to eat non-stop in hopes of putting a little meat on their bones. This chapter, along with the protein information in chapter 8, can give you the information you need to reach your goal healthfully.

HOW TO ADD WEIGHT

Theoretically, to gain 1 pound of body weight per week, you'd need to consume an additional 500 calories per day above your typical intake. Some people are hard gainers and require more calories than other people do to add weight. For example, some research subjects, who should have gained 11 pounds during a month-long overfeeding study, gained an average of only 6 pounds (Webb and Annis 1983). Researchers are mystified by this discrepancy. What happened to the excess calories that didn't turn into fat and didn't get burned off from the higher metabolism (a 9-percent increase in body heat production)?

In another study (Sims 1976), 200 prisoners with no family history of obesity volunteered to be gluttons. The goal was to gain 20 to 25 percent above their normal weights (about 30 to 40 pounds) by deliberately overeating. For more than half a year, the prisoners ate extravagantly and exercised minimally. Yet only 20 of the 200 prisoners managed to gain the weight. Of those, only two (who had an undetected family history of obesity or diabetes) gained the weight easily. One prisoner tried for 30 weeks to add 12 pounds to his 132-pound frame, but he couldn't get any fatter.

Current research suggests the body can adjust its metabolism to help maintain a predetermined genetic weight (Leibel, Rosenbaum, and Hirsch 1995). If you are a hard gainer, take a good look at your genetic endowment. If other family members are thin and sylphlike, you probably have inherited a genetic predisposition to thinness. You can alter your physique to a certain extent with diet, weight training, and aging, but you shouldn't expect miracles. Marathoner Bill Rodgers will never look like bodybuilder Charles Atlas, no matter how much eating and weight lifting he does!

Most scrawny athletes believe that the best way to gain weight is to eat a high-protein diet. False. You don't store excess protein as muscle. The pound of steak doesn't just convert into bigger biceps. You need extra calories, and those calories should come primarily from extra carbohydrates rather than extra protein. Carbohydrates fuel your muscles so the muscles can perform intense muscle-building exercise. By overloading the muscle not with protein but with weight lifting and other resistance exercise, the muscle fibers increase in size.

How to Balance Your Weight-Gain Diet

The best weight-gain diet follows the same guidelines for healthy eating as the Food Guide Pyramid. Because your muscles become saturated with glycogen when fed 3 to 5 grams of carbohydrate per pound of body weight, and your body uses less than 1 gram of protein per pound under growth conditions, your primary dietary goal is to satisfy these requirements for carbohydrates and proteins. Then, you can choose the balance of the calories in fat or additional carbohydrates.

Type of food	Portion of meal	Percent of calories	Target g/lb body weight
Carbohydrate	majority	60 to 70	3 to 5
Protein	accompaniment	10 to 15	0.7 to 0.9
Fat	small	balance of calories	

Example: Pablo, a high school soccer player, wanted to gain weight. He was five feet, eight inches, weighed 140 pounds, and wanted to gain 15 pounds. I calculated that he was maintaining his weight on about 3,000 calories per day, and I recommended he eat more to gain weight and try to hit the following targets.

Calories (increase by 20 percent)
20% × 3,000 calories = 600 more calories = 3,600 total = 4 meals at 900 calories each

Carbohydrate
65% × 3,600 = 2,340 calories carb = 585 g* = 4 g/lb body weight

Protein
15% × 3,600 = 540 calories pro = 135 g* = 1 g pro/lb body weight

Fat
20% × 3,600 = 720 calories fat = 80 g*—or more carbohydrates

I taught Pablo how to read food labels to learn more about the composition of the foods he was eating. He was surprised to learn that he could get most of his protein requirement with two 6-ounce cans of tuna (80 grams of protein) and one quart of low-fat milk (40 grams of protein). He no longer felt compelled to suffer through egg whites for breakfast and buy expensive high-protein weight-gain powders for snacks.

*Each gram of carbohydrate and protein contains 4 calories; each gram of fat contains 9 calories.

To date, research indicates that protein powders and amino acid supplements are a fruitless expense when it comes to gaining muscle weight. The only reason these may work for some athletes is because the protein beverage provides additional calories. One can just as easily eat another sandwich to get those calories. (See chapter 8 for additional information on protein supplements and building muscle.)

You are most likely to gain weight if you consistently eat larger-than-normal meals. I often counsel skinny athletes who swear they eat huge amounts of food.

For example, Tom, a soccer player swore that he ate at least twice what his friends did. However, he ate only two meals per day. Granted, he did eat a lot at those meals, but this merely compensated for the lack of breakfast and snacks.

Tom gained 3 pounds within three weeks after he started to consistently eat three meals per day plus an additional bedtime snack. "I now look at food as my weight-gain medicine. There are times when I'm

SPORTS PARENTS ASK...

Q. My 12-year-old son feels embarrassed that he is shorter than many of the girls his age. Will protein supplements help him grow faster?

A. No amount of extra protein will speed the growth process. Boys generally grow fastest between the ages of 13 and 14. After this growth spurt, he will have enough male hormones to add muscle mass and to start to grow a beard ("peach fuzz"). This growth spurt lasts longer in boys than in girls, and after the growth spurt boys continue to grow slowly until about age 20.

Q. My 11-year-old son wants to start lifting weights to bulk up. Should he?

A. Weight lifting (with light weights and a well-supervised program to prevent stress on immature bones and ligaments) can help your son get stronger. But it will not contribute to bulkier muscles until he has enough male hormones to support muscular development. Boys bulk up after they have finished their growth spurt. Remind him that patience is a virtue!

busy and tempted to skip lunch, but I remind myself that I have to take my medicine: two hefty sandwiches with two glasses of milk."

Adam, a six-foot, seven-inch high school basketball player, also chowed down on large portions. He felt embarrassed whenever he ate with his friends because he'd eat twice what they did. A large pizza was no challenge! When I calculated his calorie needs, he began to understand why he wasn't gaining weight. He needed about 6,000 calories per day to maintain his weight, plus more to gain weight. The pizza was 1,800 calories. Two pizzas would have been more appropriate.

I told Adam to feed his body what it needed and stop comparing his food intake to his shorter friends. I suggested that he explain to any teasers that his body was like a limousine that needed more gas to go the distance.

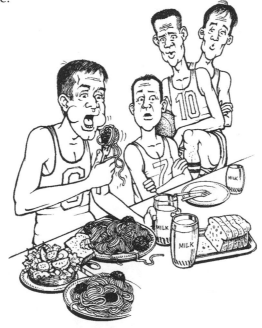

HOW TO BOOST YOUR CALORIES

If you have a busy day, finding the time to eat can be the biggest challenge to boosting your calories. You might need to pack a stash of portable snacks in your gym bag if most of your eating is done outside the home. To take in the extra calories needed to gain weight, you can eat frequently throughout the day, if that fits your lifestyle. Plan to have food on hand for every eating opportunity. Or you can try these tips:

- Eat an extra snack, such as a bedtime peanut butter sandwich with a glass of milk.

- Eat larger-than-normal portions at mealtime.
- Eat higher calorie foods.

If you eat foods that are compact and dense (for example, granola instead of puffed rice), more can fit into your stomach with less discomfort.

When you make your food selections, keep in mind that fats are the most concentrated form of calories. One teaspoon of fat (butter, oil, margarine, or mayonnaise) has 36 calories; the same amount of carbohydrate or protein has only 16 calories. Most protein-rich foods contain fat (such as the cream in cheese, the grease in hamburgers, or the oil in peanut butter), so these foods tend to be high in calories. However, some fats such as the saturated fat in cheese, beef, chicken skin, butter, and bacon are bad for your health. Try to limit your intake of these foods and focus on the healthful fats, such as walnuts, almonds, olive oil, old-fashioned (unprocessed) peanut butter, and oily fish such as salmon and sardines. You should still be eating the basic high-carbohydrate sports diet as described in chapters 1 and 7; you'll be adding extra unsaturated fats to that foundation. Too many fatty foods will fill your stomach but leave your muscles unfueled.

The following foods and beverages can help you healthfully boost your calorie intake:

Cold cereal. Choose dense cereals (as opposed to flaked and puffed types), such as granola, muesli, Grape-Nuts and Wheat Chex. Top with nuts, sunflower seeds, raisins, bananas, or other fruits.

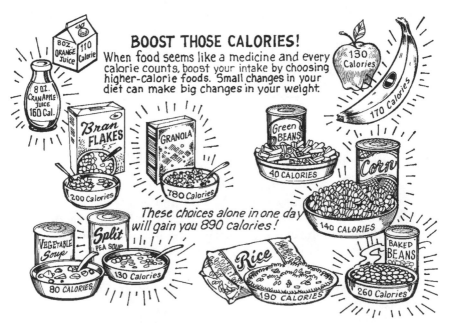

Hot cereal. Cooking with milk instead of water adds more calories and greater nutritional value. Add still more calories with mix-ins such as powdered milk, margarine, peanut butter, walnuts, sunflower seeds, wheat germ, and dried fruit.

Juices. Apple, cranberry, cranapple, grape, pineapple, and most of the juice blends (such as peach-orange-banana) have more calories than grapefruit, orange, or tomato juice. To increase the calorie value of frozen orange juice, add less water than the directions indicate.

Fruits. Bananas, pineapple, raisins, dates, dried apricots, and other dried fruits contain more calories than watery fruits such as grapefruit, plums, and peaches.

Milk. To boost the calorie value of milk, add 1/4 cup powdered milk to 1 cup of 2% percent milk. Or try malt powder, Ovaltine, Carnation Instant Breakfast, Nestle's Quik, and other flavorings. Mix these up by the quart to have them waiting for you in the refrigerator. You can also make blender drinks such as milk shakes and fruit smoothies. Fixing these is far less expensive than buying the canned liquid meal supplements that are typically just milk-based formulas with added vitamins.

Toast. Spread with generous amounts of peanut butter, margarine, and jam or honey.

Sandwiches. Select hearty, dense breads (as opposed to fluffy types), such as sprouted wheat, honey bran, rye, and pumpernickel. The bigger and more thickly sliced, the better! Spread with a moderate amount of margarine or mayonnaise. Stuff with tuna salad, chicken, or other fillings. Peanut butter and jelly makes an inexpensive, healthful, and high-calorie choice.

Soups. Hearty lentil, split pea, minestrone, and barley soups have more calories than brothy chicken and beef types, unless the broth is chock full of lots of veggies and meat. To make canned soups (such as tomato or chowder) more substantial, add evaporated milk in place of water or regular milk, or add extra powdered milk. Garnish with margarine, Parmesan cheese, and croutons. If you have high blood pressure, be sure to choose the reduced-sodium soups or homemade varieties.

Meats. Although beef, pork, and lamb tend to have more calories than chicken or fish, they also tend to have more saturated fat. Eat them in moderation and choose lean cuts. To boost calories, sauté chicken or fish in canola oil, olive oil, or margarine, and add wine sauces and bread crumb toppings.

Beans, legumes. Lentils, split pea soup, chili with beans, limas, and other dried beans are not only calorie dense but are also excellent sources of protein and carbohydrates. Hummus (made with chick-peas) is an easy snack or sandwich filling.

Vegetables. Peas, corn, carrots, winter squash, and beets have more calories than green beans, broccoli, summer squash, and other watery veggies. Add margarine, slivered almonds, and grated low-fat cheese. Add calories to the watery vegetables by stir-frying them in olive oil.

Salads. What may start out being low-calorie lettuce can be quickly converted into a substantial meal by adding cottage cheese, garbanzo beans (chick-peas), sunflower seeds, assorted vegetables, chopped walnuts, raisins, tuna fish, lean meat, croutons, and a liberal dousing of salad dressing made with heart-healthy oil, preferably olive or canola. (See chapter 5.)

Potatoes. Add generous amounts of margarine and extra powdered milk to mashed potatoes. Although you might be tempted to add lots of sour cream and gravy for extra calories, think again. You'd also be adding saturated fats that are unhealthful for your heart. Reduced fat sour cream and low-fat gravies would be better alternatives.

Desserts. By selecting desserts with nutritional value, you can enjoy treats as well as nourish your body. Try oatmeal-raisin cookies, Fig Newtons, chocolate pudding, stewed fruit compotes, low-fat frozen yogurt, or frozen fruit desserts. Blueberry muffins, corn bread with honey, banana bread, and other sweet breads and muffins can double as dessert.

Snacks. A substantial afternoon or evening snack is an excellent way to boost your calorie intake. If you don't feel hungry, just think of the food as the weight-gain medicine that you have to take. Some healthful snack choices include fruit yogurt, low-fat cheese and crackers, peanuts, sunflower seeds, almonds, granola, pretzels, English muffins, bagels (with low-fat cream cheese and jelly), bran muffins, pizza, peanut butter crackers, milk shakes, instant breakfast drinks, hot cocoa, fruit smoothies, bananas, dried fruits, and sandwiches.

Alcohol. Moderate amounts of beer and wine can stimulate your appetite and add extra calories, particularly when consumed with snacks such as peanuts and pretzels. Because alcohol offers little nutritional value, do not substitute it for juices, milk, or other wholesome beverages. (Never drink alcohol before an event; it has a dehydrating effect; it can create problems with hypoglycemia and hurt performance.)

The sample menus in table 16.1 implement some of these suggestions.

Table 16.1   Sample Weight Gain Menus

The trick to gaining weight is to consistently eat larger than normal portions, three meals per day, plus one or two snacks. These sample menus suggest healthful high-calorie, carbohydrate-rich sports meals.

	Approximate calories		Approximate calories
Breakfast			
16 oz orange juice	200	2 cups pineapple juice	280
6 pancakes	600	1 cup granola	500
1/4 cup syrup	200	1/4 cup raisins	120
1 pat margarine	50	2 cups low-fat milk	200
8 oz low-fat milk	100	1 large banana	130
Total	1,150	Total	1,230
Lunch			
4 slices hefty bread	400	1 7-inch pita pocket	240
1 6.5-oz can tuna	200	6-oz turkey breast	300
4 Tbsp lite mayo	150	2 Tbsp lite mayo	80
1 bowl lentil soup	250	2 cups apple juice	250
2 cups low-fat milk	200	1 cup fruit yogurt	250
2 oatmeal cookies	150	1 large muffin	300
Total	1,350	Total	1,420
Dinner			
1 medium cheese pizza	1,400	1 breast chicken	300
2 cups lemonade	200	2 large potatoes	400
Total	1,600	2 pats margarine	100
		1 cup peas	100
		2 biscuits	300
		2 Tbsp honey	100
		2 cups low-fat milk	200
		Total	1,500
Snacks			
2 slices hearty bread	200	2 bagels	440
2 Tbsp peanut butter	200	3 oz lite cheese	260
3 Tbsp jelly	150	2 cups crangrape juice	340
1-1/2 cups low-fat milk	150	Total	1,040
2 Tbsp chocolate powder	100		
Total	800		

Day's total: 4,900 calories
   60% carbohydrate (745 grams)
   15% protein (193 grams)
   25% fat (121 grams)

Day's total: 5,190 calories
   65% carbohydrate (830 grams)
   15% protein (180 grams)
   20% fat (123 grams)

PATIENCE IS A VIRTUE

By taking the prescribed 500 to 1,000 additional calories per day, you should see some weight gain. Be sure to include muscle-building resistance exercise (weight workouts, push-ups) to promote muscular growth rather than just fat deposits. Consult with the trainer at your school, health club, or gym for a specific exercise program that suits your needs. You might also want to have your body fat routinely measured, to be sure that your weight gain is indeed mostly muscle, not fat. Untrained men tend to initially gain about 3 pounds of muscle per month, and 20 pounds or more per year. The rate of gain in well-trained athletes is slower.

If you don't gain weight, look at your family members to see if you inherited a naturally trim physique. If everyone is thin, accept your fate and concentrate on improving your athletic skills. Rather than drain your energy fretting about being too thin, capitalize on being light, swift, and agile. You will likely be able to surpass the heavier hulks that lack your speed!

Also, keep in mind that most people gain weight with age. If you are still growing or are in your 20s, your turn to bulk up may still come! All too often, scrawny young athletes fatten up once they get out of school and start working.

Wes, a 30-year-old photographer and former football player, reported with a sigh, "I was skinny all through high school. In college, my football coach insisted that I gain weight by eating extra buttered bread, piles of french fries, and mounds of ice cream. I developed quite a liking for these foods. I continued to eat them even after I'd reached my weight-gain goals. Voilá—look at me now! I'm 60 pounds overweight and can barely walk, to say nothing of play football. I long for those days when I was lean and mean."

With a low-fat food plan, Wes did lose weight over the course of a year. That fall, he coached an after-school football program. Needless to say, he carefully advised the thin kids to be patient, eat healthfully, and develop smart, lifelong eating habits.

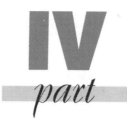

Recipes for Health and Fitness

Breads and Breakfasts

Rice and Potatoes

Pasta

Vegetables

Chicken and Turkey

Fish and Seafood

Beef and Pork

Eggs and Cheese

Tofu

Beans

Beverages

Snacks and Desserts

PRELIMINARY TIDBITS

Active people generally prefer to spend their time exercising rather than preparing meals. These recipes will enable you to spend minimal time preparing food for maximal nutrition. With them, you can produce meals that taste good and invest in health and top sports performance. All of the recipes are quick and easy to fix and use commonly available ingredients. Some have moderate amounts of sodium; athletes on a salt-restricted diet should eliminate or reduce the salt or salty foods in the recipes.

Many of the recipes are low-fat favorites contributed by athletes or food lovers. I've also adapted favorite higher-fat recipes to the more appropriate versions here. I've compiled a collection of foods that will be popular with all members of the family—athletes and support crew alike. My primary criterion for selection was whether the taste-testers requested a second helping.

How to Use the Nutrition Information With the Recipes

The calorie and nutrition information provided with each recipe represent approximate values. Remember that your total daily calorie intake should be about 60 percent carbohydrates, 25 percent fat, and 15 percent protein. To convert these targets into grams, multiply your daily calorie needs (see chapter 14) by the targets, and then divide the carbohydrate and protein products by 4 and the fat product by 9. For example, the calculations for an active woman who needs about 2,000 calories per day follow:

$$60\% \text{ carb} \times 2,000 \text{ calories} = 1,200 \text{ carb calories}$$
$$\div\ 4 = 300 \text{ grams carb}$$

$$25\% \text{ fat} \times 2,000 \text{ calories} = 500 \text{ fat calories}$$
$$\div\ 9 = 55 \text{ grams fat}$$

$$15\% \text{ protein} \times 2,000 \text{ calories} = 300 \text{ protein calories}$$
$$\div\ 4 = 75 \text{ grams protein}$$

Add up the grams of carbohydrates, proteins, and fats you consume daily to be sure that you balance your intake.

How to Cook Efficiently

Here are a few tips on efficient cooking:

1. Read a recipe completely before you start making it to be sure you understand the entire process clearly.

2. Be sure you have adequate amounts of all the ingredients on hand. Make a double recipe to freeze or to use later in the week.

3. Hang a grocery list in a convenient place so you can easily add items when your supply of a particular item begins to dwindle.

4. Use frozen or precut vegetables, prechopped garlic (in a jar in the produce section of the market), and dried onions instead of fresh.

5. For continental cooking, remember these approximate metric conversions:

1 teaspoon (tsp)	= 5 ml	1 quart (4 cups)	= 1 liter
1 tablespoon (Tbsp)	= 15 ml	1 pound (16 oz)	= 450 grams
1 cup (8 oz)	= 250 ml	2.2 pounds	= 1 kilo
350°F	= 180°C		

How to Spice Up Your Diet

Many busy people eat the same foods all the time. If that sounds like you, you can easily add variety to your limited repertoire by adding herbs, spices, and other seasonings. Use about 1/4 teaspoon of dry herbs (or 3/4 tsp fresh) for a dish that serves four people. Be conservative at first. It's better to use too little seasoning and have to add more than it is to have to double the recipe to dilute the flavor of too much seasoning. To enhance their flavor, crumble herbs between your fingers and heat them in oil. Add herbs during the last hour of cooking soups and stews. Store herbs in a cool place to retain their flavor; do not keep them near the stove.

Here are some harmonious combinations:

Basil	Tomato dishes, fish, salads
Cinnamon	Cooked fruits, winter squash, baked goods
Cloves	Hot cider or tea, cooked fruits, tomatoes, winter squash
Ginger	Cooked fruits, curry, chicken, stir-fry
Marjoram	Fish, meat, poultry, stuffing
Nutmeg	Apple desserts, puddings, winter squash
Oregano	Tomato dishes, fish, salads
Parsley	Soups, salads, vegetables, or as garnish for almost any plate

Poppy seeds Cottage cheese, noodles, cole slaw, baked goods
Rosemary Fish, meat, poultry, stuffing, vegetables
Sage Soups, stews, stuffing
Thyme Tomato dishes, stews, salads, vegetables

These additional flavor boosters are also worth stocking:

Sesame oil in chicken, fish, vegetables, soups
Dijon mustard in chicken, fish
Sun-dried tomatoes in pasta, tomato sauces
Salsa in fish, chicken, cheese, beans
Tabasco in stir-fry, soups, vegetables, pasta
Balsamic vinegar in salads, vegetables
Canned green chiles in eggs, tomato, cheese
Chicken broth in rice, vegetables
Hot chili oil in stir-fry, soups, vegetables, pasta

Microwave Cooking

Microwave ovens have revolutionized the way many people eat. I highly recommend them for active folks who want to eat well yet spend minimal time cooking and cleaning. With just a one-day cook-a-thon, you can have a week's worth of food ready to pop into the microwave oven. For example, on weekends, I might make a big pot of chili or curry or a chicken-rice casserole. I'll freeze some and leave the rest in the refrigerator, creating a ready supply of microwaveable entrées.

When cooking with the microwave, follow these tips:

• When cooking separate items such as pieces of meat or whole potatoes, arrange food with the thickest parts toward the outer edge of the dish. Leave a space in the center, allowing the microwaves to penetrate from all sides.

• Fish cooks well in microwave ovens. Sprinkle with seasonings as desired (pepper, lemon, oregano, basil, etc.), cover with waxed paper, and "zap."

• Cover vegetables loosely with waxed paper or plastic wrap to retain moisture. Veggies will continue to cook after the oven is off, so prevent overcooking by planning this into the preparation time. Since microwave cookery is quick and waterless, it retains a high percentage of a food's nutrients.

• Prick potatoes several times with a fork before baking them to reduce the risk of explosion due to steam buildup. Allow baked potatoes to stand for 5 minutes to finish cooking and improve their texture.

How to Freeze Foods Properly

When you cook, you can easily make a double batch and freeze the leftovers. Here are five tips for proper freezing:

1. Do not let food sit in the refrigerator for a few days and then freeze it. You might be freezing lots of bacteria, too.
2. Cool foods before freezing them. Hot food causes your freezer to work too hard.
3. Use the proper size container with a tight cover. Allow one-half to one inch of space above the food for expansion.
4. Label the container with the name of the food and the date you freeze it.
5. Use the food within 6 to 8 weeks.

How to Keep Food Safe

When you are planning for any event that involves packing food, here are some tips to keep meals safe so they won't spoil—nor spoil your event.

• Keep cold foods below 40°F and hot foods above 140°F. Bacteria multiply most rapidly in foods kept between these temperatures.

• Use insulated bags and coolers with reusable freezer packs to keep food safe longer. Make sure foods are very cold or frozen before you place them in the cooler. You can freeze sandwiches (without mayonnaise, lettuce, and tomatoes), individual containers of yogurt, or juice boxes in advance. They will be thawed but still cool several hours later.

• Pack the cooler so the foods you plan to eat first are located near the top. Store meat items near the bottom, where it's coolest. Allow space between items so cool air can circulate properly.

• Bring a separate cooler for beverages. Otherwise, every time someone opens the cooler for a beverage, the temperature inside will rise and warm the food items.

• Place your cooler or lunch bag in the coolest location possible. In the summer, do not put it in the trunk. Wrap it with a blanket or towels to keep out the heat. At the beach, you can make a cool spot by digging a large hole in the sand, placing the cooler inside, and then covering it with a folded towel to shade the top from the sunlight.

• After the event, throw away any food that has been outside of the cooler for more than 2 hours. Throw out leftover food that's inside the cooler, unless the cooler still has chunks of ice remaining in it. The safest rule is this: When in doubt, throw it out!

Breads and Breakfasts

Any way you slice them, breads are one of the favorite carbohydrates for active people. Here are some baking tips to help you prepare the yummiest of breads.

- The secret for light and fluffy quick breads, muffins, and scones is to stir the flour lightly and for only 20 seconds. Ignore the lumps! If you beat the batter too much, the gluten (protein) in the flour will toughen the dough.
- Breads made entirely with whole wheat flour tend to be heavy. In general, half whole wheat and half white flour is an appropriate combination. Many of these recipes have been developed using this ratio. You can alter the ratio as you like. When substituting whole wheat for white flour in other recipes, use 3/4 cup whole wheat for 1 cup white flour.

Breads made with 100-percent whole wheat flour do offer slightly more nutritional value than those made with white flour. However, if you or your family dislikes whole wheat products, compensate by consistently eating wholesome bran cereals, fruits, and vegetables. These will help replace the nutrients lost when whole wheat flour is refined into white flour. You needn't feel obligated to limit your intake to only 100-percent whole wheat breads.

- Most of these recipes have reduced sugar content. To reduce the sugar content of your own recipes, use one-third to one-half less sugar than indicated; the finished product will be just fine. If you want to exchange white sugar with honey, brown sugar, or molasses, use only 1/2 teaspoon baking powder per 2 cups flour, and add 1/2 teaspoon baking soda. This prevents an "off" taste.

- Most quick bread recipes instruct you to sift together the baking powder and flour. This method produces the lightest breads and best results. In some of these recipes, I direct you to mix the baking powder in with the wet ingredients and gently add the flour last. My method is easier, produces an acceptable product, and saves time and energy.

- To prevent breads from sticking, use nonstick baking pans or cooking spray or place a piece of waxed paper in the baking pan before pouring the batter. I've found that using waxed paper is foolproof. After the bread has baked, I let it cool for 5 minutes, tip it out of the pan, then peel off the paper.

- To hasten cooking time, bake quick breads in a 8" × 8" square pan instead of a loaf pan. They bake in half the time. You can also bake muffins in a loaf or square pan, eliminating the hard to wash muffin tins!

BREADS

APPLESAUCE RAISIN BREAD

WHOLE-WHEAT RAISIN QUICK BREAD

BANANA BREAD

OATMEAL-ORANGE BREAD

BASIC OATMEAL YEAST BREAD

IRISH SODA BREAD

SEEDY YEAST BREAD

MOIST CORNBREAD

HONEY BRAN MUFFINS

CINNAMON OAT BRAN MUFFINS

BRAN MUFFINS WITH MOLASSES AND DATES

BREAKFASTS

OAT BRAN DELUXE

GRIDDLE SCONES

GRANOLA

OATMEAL PANCAKES

COLD CEREAL DELIGHT

See also: French Toast with Cheese, Fruit Smoothie, Peanut Butter Ideas, Protein Shake, Maple Graham Shake, and suggestions in chapter 3.

APPLESAUCE RAISIN BREAD

This moist bread can double as a dessert.

Yield: 16 slices

1 16-ounce jar applesauce (1-1/2 cups)
1 egg or 2 egg whites
1/2 - 3/4 cup sugar
1/4 cup oil, preferably canola
2 teaspoons cinnamon
1 teaspoon salt
1 teaspoon baking powder
1 teaspoon baking soda
1 cup raisins
1-1/2 cups flour, preferably half whole wheat and half white

1.   Preheat the oven to 350°.
2.   Combine the applesauce, egg, sugar, oil, cinnamon, salt, baking powder, and baking soda. Mix well. Add raisins.
3.   Gently mix in flour. Stir 20 seconds or until just moistened.
4.   Pour into a 4" × 8" loaf pan that has been lightly oiled, treated with cooking spray, or lined with wax paper. Bake for 45 minutes, or until a toothpick inserted near the middle comes out clean.
5.   Let cool for 5 minutes before removing from the pan.

Nutrition Information: Total calories: 2,300
Calories per slice: 145

Nutrients	%	Grams
Carbohydrate	70	25
Protein	5	2
Fat	25	4

WHOLE-WHEAT RAISIN QUICK BREAD

This makes a large loaf—enough for breakfast and yummy peanut butter sandwiches for lunch! Using soured milk (made from milk and vinegar) contributes to a nice textured bread.

Yield: 16 slices

1-1/2 cups milk, preferably low-fat
2 tablespoons vinegar
1/2 cup molasses
1/2 cup sugar
1/4 cup oil
1/2 cup raisins
1 teaspoon salt
1-1/2 teaspoons baking powder
1-1/2 teaspoons baking soda
1/2 cup white flour
2-1/2 cups whole wheat flour

1. Preheat the oven to 350°.
2. In a bowl, make soured milk by mixing the milk and vinegar. Let stand 5 to 10 minutes.
3. Mix together the milk and remaining ingredients, except for the flour. Beat well.
4. Gently add the flour, stirring until just blended.
5. Pour into a 4" × 8" loaf pan, lightly oiled, treated with cooking spray, or lined with wax paper.
6. Bake for 50 to 60 minutes, or until a toothpick inserted near the center comes out clean.

Nutrition Information: Total calories: 3,000
Calories per slice: 185

Nutrients	%	Grams
Carbohydrate	75	35
Protein	5	2
Fat	20	4

BANANA BREAD

The key to good banana bread is to use well-ripened bananas that are covered with brown speckles.

Banana bread is my favorite "magic food" for premarathon carbohydrate-loading and for snacking during long-distance bike rides. Add some peanut butter and you'll have a delicious sandwich that'll keep you energized for a long time!

Yield: 12 slices

3 large well-ripened bananas
1 egg or 2 egg whites
2 tablespoons oil, preferably canola
1/3 cup milk
1/3 to 1/2 cup sugar
1 teaspoon salt
1 teaspoon baking soda
1/2 teaspoon baking powder
1-1/2 cups flour, preferably half whole wheat and half white

1. Preheat the oven to 350°.
2. Mash bananas with a fork.
3. Add egg, oil, milk, sugar, salt, baking soda, and baking powder. Beat well.
4. Gently blend the flour into the banana mixture and stir for 20 seconds, or until moistened.
5. Pour into a 4" × 8" loaf pan that has been lightly oiled, treated with cooking spray, or lined with wax paper.
6. Bake for 45 minutes, or until a toothpick inserted near the middle comes out clean.
7. Let cool for 5 minutes before removing from the pan.

Nutrition Information: Total calories: 1,600
Calories per slice: 135

Nutrients	%	Grams
Carbohydrate	70	24
Protein	10	3
Fat	20	3

OATMEAL-ORANGE BREAD

Nice for breakfast or snacks. Spread with orange marmalade for extra carbohydrates.

Yield: 12 slices

1 egg or 2 egg whites
1/4 cup honey
1/4 to 1/3 cup oil, preferably canola
1/2 cup milk, preferably low-fat
1/2 cup orange juice
1-1/2 cups uncooked rolled oats
1-1/2 teaspoons baking powder
1 teaspoon salt
1-1/2 cups whole wheat flour

Optional: 1 tablespoon grated orange rind; dash nutmeg; 1/2 cup chopped almonds; 1/2 cup raisins; 1/2 cup chopped apricots.

1. Preheat the oven to 400°.
2. Beat together the egg, honey, oil, milk, and orange juice.
3. Stir in the oats and let stand for 1 or 2 minutes. Add grated orange rind, if desired.
4. Add the baking powder, salt, and flour. Mix just until blended. Do not overbeat.
5. Pour the batter into a 4" × 8" loaf pan that has been lightly oiled, treated with cooking spray, or lined with wax paper.
6. Bake for 45 to 55 minutes, or until nicely browned.

Nutrition Information: Total calories: 2,050
Calories per slice: 170

Nutrients	%	Grams
Carbohydrate	60	25
Protein	10	4
Fat	30	5

BASIC OATMEAL YEAST BREAD

If you have never made your own yeast bread, don't be afraid to give it a try. Among other things, kneading the dough is good upper body exercise. While the dough rises, you can work out; while it bakes, you can stretch, shower, and change your clothes. The bread will be ready to enjoy warm from the oven when you are ready to eat.

Yield: 2 loaves, 32 slices

2 tablespoons yeast (2 packages)
1/2 cup lukewarm water (110°)
1 teaspoon sugar
1 cup oatmeal
1 tablespoon salt, as desired
2-1/2 cups boiling water
3 cups whole wheat flour
1/4 cup oil, preferably canola
1/4 cup honey or molasses
3 to 4 cups white flour

Optional: 2 tablespoons sesame seeds; 2 tablespoons powdered milk.

1. In a small bowl, sprinkle the yeast over the warm water. Stir in the sugar and set aside.
2. In a large bowl, combine the oatmeal, sesame seeds, powdered milk, and salt. Pour in the boiling water and mix well.
3. Add the whole wheat flour, and by now the dough should be cool enough to add the yeast without deactivating it.
4. Add the yeast mixture, oil, and honey. Beat well.
5. Gradually mix in the white flour. Turn the dough onto a floured board and knead until smooth and elastic, about 10 minutes.
6. Shape into 2 loaves. Place the loaves in 2 lightly oiled bread pans. Cover, let rise until almost double in bulk, about 30 to 45 minutes.
7. Bake at 350° for about 50 minutes, or until it is golden and sounds hollow when tapped with your fingers.

Nutrition Information: Total calories: 4,000
Calories per slice: 125

Nutrients	%	Grams
Carbohydrate	75	24
Protein	10	3
Fat	15	2

IRISH SODA BREAD

This bread's distinctive flavor comes from the caraway seeds, which add sweetness without sugar. For variety, bake this into muffins.

Yield: 12 wedges

2 cups flour, preferably half whole wheat and half white
2 teaspoons baking powder
1/2 teaspoon baking soda
1/2 teaspoon salt
2 teaspoons caraway seeds
1 cup raisins
1/3 cup oil, preferably canola
1 egg
1 cup milk, preferably low-fat

1. Preheat the oven to 375°.
2. In a mixing bowl, combine the flour, baking powder, baking soda, salt, and caraway seeds. Mix in the raisins.
3. Beat together the egg, oil, and milk; add to the flour mixture. Gently stir just until blended.
4. Put the dough into a 9" round cake pan that has been oiled, treated with cooking spray, or lined with wax paper, and form the dough into a round loaf.
5. Bake for 35 to 40 minutes, or until nicely browned.
6. Slice into wedges.

Nutrition Information: Total calories: 2,000
Calories per wedge: 165

Nutrients	%	Grams
Carbohydrate	55	23
Protein	5	2
Fat	40	7

SEEDY YEAST BREAD

This bread is delightfully chock-full of goodies and tastes delicious, especially toasted. Note, however, that all the sunflower, sesame, and poppy seeds boost both calories and fat. The bread can also be made without the seeds; try adding raisins or other dried fruit instead.

Yield: 16 slices

1 tablespoon yeast
1-1/2 cups warm water
1/2 cup molasses
1/2 cup oil, preferably canola
2-1/2 cups raw bran (not cereal type)
2 teaspoons salt, as desired
1/2 cup sesame seeds
1/2 cup poppy seeds
1/2 cup sunflower seeds
3-1/2 cups whole wheat flour

1. Mix the yeast, warm water, and molasses; let stand for 5 minutes.
2. Add the oil, raw bran, salt, seeds, and 2-1/2 cups whole wheat flour. Mix well, then turn out onto floured surface; knead in the rest of the flour until the dough is smooth and elastic, about 10 minutes. You might need more or less flour, depending on the particular brand.
3. Place the dough in a lightly oiled bowl, cover with plastic wrap, and let rise in a warm place for about an hour or until doubled. To shorten preparation time, omit this step and let the bread rise once, in the pan, before baking.
4. Punch the dough down, shape it into a loaf, and put it into a lightly oiled 4" × 8" loaf pan. Cover and let rise again until almost doubled.
5. Bake at 350° for about 55 minutes, or until it sounds hollow when tipped out of the pan and tapped with your fingers.

Nutrition Information: Total calories: 3,800
Calories per slice: 240

Nutrients	%	Grams
Carbohydrate	50	30
Protein	10	6
Fat	40	10

MOIST CORNBREAD

The cream style corn in this bread makes the final product very moist, unlike many corn breads that are dry and crumble easily. When made with the cheese and beans, it becomes a hearty lunch.

Yield: 9 squares

1 cup yellow cornmeal
2 teaspoons baking powder
1/2 teaspoon salt
1 egg or 2 egg whites
3/4 cup milk, preferably low-fat
1/4 cup oil, preferably canola
1 16-ounce can cream-style corn

Optional: 1 tablespoon chili powder; 4 ounces shredded cheddar cheese, preferably low-fat; 1 cup kidney or pinto beans.

1. Preheat the oven to 350°.
2. In a medium bowl, combine cornmeal, baking powder, salt, and chili powder if desired.
3. Optional: Sprinkle cheese and beans onto the cornmeal mixture and gently mix in.
4. Beat together the egg, milk, oil, and cream-style corn. Add to the cornmeal mixture; stir just until blended. Do not overbeat.
5. Pour into an 8" × 8" baking pan that has been oiled, treated with cooking spray, or lined with wax paper. Bake about 40 minutes, or until golden and a toothpick inserted near center comes out clean. Let stand for 10 minutes before cutting into squares.

Nutrition Information: Total calories: 1,620
Calories per square: 180

Nutrients	%	Grams
Carbohydrate	55	25
Protein	10	5
Fat	35	7

HONEY BRAN MUFFINS

Bakery muffins are often made with more fat and less bran than is optimal for health. These muffins are a super alternative. When you make them, bake a double batch, storing several in the freezer, so they'll always be ready and waiting to be eaten for breakfast, lunch, and snacks. Add raisins for extra carbohydrates.

Yield: 12 muffins

1/2 cup buttermilk or plain yogurt (or 1/2 cup milk mixed with
     1 teaspoon vinegar and set aside for 5 to 10 minutes)
1-1/2 cups All-Bran
1 cup hot water
1/3 cup honey
1/4 cup oil, preferably canola
1/2 teaspoon salt
1 egg or 2 egg whites, beaten
1 teaspoon baking soda
1-1/2 cups flour, preferably half whole wheat and half white

Optional: 1/2 cup raisins; 1/2 cup chopped nuts; 2 tablespoons poppy seeds or sunflower seeds.

1. Preheat the oven to 400°. Line muffin tin with paper baking cups or use a nonstick muffin pan.
2. Combine the bran cereal, hot water, honey, oil, salt, and egg. Let stand for 1 or 2 minutes.
3. Add buttermilk or yogurt, then the flour with the baking soda stirred into it. Mix gently until just blended. Do not overbeat!
5. Fill the muffin cups 2/3 full.
6. Bake for 20 to 25 minutes, or until a toothpick inserted near center comes out clean.

Nutrition Information: Total calories: 1,900
Calories per muffin: 160

Nutrients	%	Grams
Carbohydrate	65	26
Protein	5	2
Fat	30	5

CINNAMON OAT BRAN MUFFINS

These muffins are a tasty way to boost your oat bran intake. I often add chopped apples, pears, peaches, or other fruits to the batter for variety.
Yield: 12 muffins

1-1/2 cups oat bran, uncooked
1/4 cup brown sugar
1 teaspoon cinnamon
1 teaspoon salt, as desired
2 teaspoons baking powder
1 egg or 2 egg whites
2 tablespoons oil, preferably canola
1-3/4 cup milk, preferably low-fat
1 cup flour, preferably half whole wheat and half white

Optional: 1 cup chopped fruit (apples, peaches, pears, etc.);
1/2 cup chopped nuts; 1/2 cup raisins or chopped dried fruit.

1. Preheat the oven to 400°. Line muffin tin with paper baking cups or use a nonstick pan.
2. In medium bowl, combine the oat bran, brown sugar, cinnamon, salt, and baking powder. Mix well.
3. Beat the egg with the oil; add the milk, then combine with the oat bran mixture. Gently blend in the flour, mixing until just moistened.
4. Fill the muffin cups 2/3 full. Bake about 20 minutes, or until a light golden brown.

Nutrition Information: Total calories: 1,550
Calories per muffin: 130

Nutrients	%	Grams
Carbohydrate	60	20
Protein	15	5
Fat	25	4

BRAN MUFFINS
WITH MOLASSES AND DATES

These muffins are sweet and moist, despite having no added fat. The acid in the yogurt and molasses, when combined with the baking soda, makes the muffin batter puff up and contributes to a light texture.

Yield: 9 muffins

1/2 cup chopped dates
1 cup boiling water
1 egg or 2 egg whites
1/3 cup molasses
1 cup yogurt or buttermilk
3/4 cup unprocessed bran (not the cereal)
1/2 teaspoon salt
1 teaspoon baking soda
1 cup whole wheat flour

Optional: 1/2 teaspoon cinnamon; 1 teaspoon grated orange rind; 1 teaspoon vanilla extract; cinnamon and sugar.

1. Preheat the oven to 350°, and lightly oil the muffin cups or treat them with cooking spray.
2. Soak the chopped dates in the boiling water while you prepare the other ingredients.
3. In a large bowl, mix together the egg, molasses, yogurt, bran, and salt.
4. Drain the dates and add them to the batter.
5. Gently stir in the wheat flour, baking soda, cinnamon, orange rind, and vanilla as desired.
6. Fill the muffin cups 2/3 full. Sprinkle the top of each muffin with cinnamon and sugar if desired. Bake for 18 to 20 minutes, or until a toothpick inserted near the center comes out clean.

Nutrition Information: Total calories: 1,330
Calories per muffin: 150

Nutrients	%	Grams
Carbohydrate	85	30
Protein	10	4
Fat	5	1

OAT BRAN DELUXE

Oat bran is a favorite breakfast before my morning run. It not only settles well and provides sustained energy, but also may help to lower blood cholesterol levels. The following suggestions add variety to oat bran (and oatmeal) breakfasts.

Yield: 1 serving

2/3 cup oat bran
2 cups water or low-fat milk
1/4 teaspoon salt, as desired

Your choice of mix-ins: Fresh or dried apple, banana, pineapple, raisins, dates, apricots, applesauce, canned fruit; chopped almonds, walnuts, sunflower seeds, sesame seeds, peanut butter. Flavorings: cinnamon, vanilla, maple syrup, honey, molasses, jam, brown sugar, or even garlic powder!

1. Cook oat bran according to package directions. (Make a double serving so that you'll have adequate calories for a sports breakfast.)
2. To add calcium and protein, cook the cereal in milk, fortify it with extra powdered milk, top it with yogurt, or serve it with milk.
3. For a substantial meal that will stick to your ribs, add mix-ins that contain protein or healthful fat such as milk, nuts, and peanut butter.

Nutrition Information: Calories for plain oat bran (2/3 cup, uncooked) with 1/2 cup low-fat milk: 285

Nutrients	%	Grams
Carbohydrate	60	44
Protein	25	17
Fat	15	5

GRIDDLE SCONES

These look like plump pancakes, but they are eaten like biscuits and are especially tasty with strawberry jam! I generally make them on top of the stove, but you can also bake them in the oven at 425° for about 20 minutes.

Yield: 10 scones

1 cup plain yogurt (or 1 cup low-fat milk mixed with 2 teaspoons vinegar and set aside for 5 minutes)
2 cups flour, preferably half whole wheat and half white
2 tablespoons sugar
2 teaspoons baking powder
1/2 teaspoon baking soda
1/4 cup oil, preferably canola

Optional: 1/2 cup raisins, currants, blueberries, or other fruit; 1/2 teaspoon cinnamon.

1. In a medium bowl, mix together the flour, sugar, baking powder, baking soda, and salt.
2. Add the yogurt (or milk) and oil. Stir gently to make a soft dough.
3. Heas¿1 nonstick griddle or lightly oiled skillet over medium heat. Drop in the dough by tablespoons; pat into biscuit shapes.
4. Cover and let brown on one side for about 4 minutes. Flip, partially cover, and brown on the other side. (Don't pat them with the spatula or they'll end up heavy and flat rather than light and fluffy.)
5. Wrap the scones in a clean towel to keep them warm.

Nutrition Information: Total calories: 1,500
Calories per scone: 150

Nutrients	%	Grams
Carbohydrates	55	20
Protein	10	4
Fat	35	6

GRANOLA

Homemade granola is good not only for breakfast but also for a yogurt topping, hiking food, or wholesome snack. Add extra dried fruits, rather than nuts and sunflower seeds, to boost the carbohydrate value.

Yield: 10 (1/2-cup) servings

4 cups rolled oats, old-fashioned or quick
1/4 to 1/2 cup brown sugar, maple syrup, or honey
1/4 cup oil, preferably canola
1/4 cup water

Optional: 1 teaspoon vanilla, 1 to 2 teaspoons cinnamon; 1 cup raisins, chopped dates, dried apricots, apples, or other dried fruit; 1/2 cup sunflower or sesame seeds; 1/2 cup wheat germ; 1/2 cup millet or kasha; 1/2 cup chopped almonds, cashews, or walnuts.

1. Preheat the oven to 300°.
2. In a large bowl, combine the oats and sugar (and cinnamon, if desired). Combine the oil and water (and vanilla, if desired); mix well with the oats.
3. Spread in a large baking pan.
4. Bake for 10 minutes, stir to allow even toasting, then bake 10 minutes more.
5. While the mixture is still hot, stir in the optional ingredients as desired. Let cool.
6. Store in an airtight container.

Nutrition Information: Total calories: 2,000
Calories per 1/2 cup: 200

Nutrients	%	Grams
Carbohydrate	55	28
Protein	10	5
Fat	35	8

OATMEAL PANCAKES

The pancakes are light and fluffy prizewinners, perfect for carbo-loading or recovering from a hard workout. For best results, let the batter stand for 5 minutes before cooking.

Yield: 6 6" pancakes

1/2 cup uncooked oats (quick or old fashioned)
1/2 cup yogurt or buttermilk
1/2 to 3/4 cup milk
1 egg or 2 egg whites, beaten
1 tablespoon oil, preferably canola
2 tablespoons packed brown sugar
1/2 teaspoon salt, as desired
1 teaspoon baking powder
1 cup flour, preferably half whole wheat and half white

Optional: dash cinnamon.

1. In a medium bowl, combine the oats, yogurt, and milk. Set aside for 15 to 20 minutes to let the oatmeal soften.
2. When the oatmeal is through soaking, beat in the egg and oil and mix well. Add the sugar, salt, and cinnamon, then the baking powder, baking soda, and flour. Stir until just moistened.
3. Heat a lightly oiled or nonstick griddle over medium-high heat (375° for electric frying pan).
4. For each pancake, pour about 1/4 cup batter onto the griddle.
5. Turn when the tops are covered with bubbles and the edges look cooked. Turn only once.
6. Serve with syrup, honey, applesauce, yogurt, or other topping of your choice.

Nutrition Information: Total calories: 1,000
Calories per serving (2 pancakes): 330

Nutrients	%	Grams
Carbohydrate	65	52
Protein	15	13
Fat	20	8

With 2 tablespoons of maple syrup: Calories per serving: 460

Nutrients	%	Grams
Carbohydrates	75	84
Protein	10	13
Fat	15	8

COLD CEREAL DELIGHT

Hot fruit on cold cereal converts breakfast into a dessert! Any combination of fruit and cereal works well; this is my favorite.

Yield: 1 serving

1 cup Life cereal
1/2 cup All-Bran
1/4 cup low-fat granola
1/2 cup blueberries or other fruit
1 cup low-fat milk

1. In a microwaveable bowl, combine the cereals.
2. Sprinkle with the blueberries or other fruit of your choice.
3. Heat in the microwave oven for 20 to 40 seconds, until the blueberries are warm, then pour the cold milk over the warm blueberries. Dig in!

Nutrition Information: Total calories: 500

Nutrients	%	Grams
Carbohydrates	70	85
Protein	20	20
Fat	10	7

Rice and Potatoes

Carbohydrate-rich meals are the key to a high-energy sports diet. The following recipes can help you fuel your muscles for training and competing.

RICE RECIPES

QUICK AND EASY RICE IDEAS   **HONEY NUT RICE**
LOW-FAT FRIED RICE   **CINNAMON RAISIN RICE**
COMPANY RICE SALAD   **ORANGE RICE**

See also: Orange Chicken, Chicken and Rice With Plum Sauce, Sweet 'n Spicy Orange Beef, Beans and Rice.

POTATO RECIPES

QUICK AND EASY POTATO IDEAS   **MEAL-IN-ONE POTATO**
QUICK POTATO WEDGES   **GREEK STUFFED POTATO**
MIGHTY MASHED POTATO   **IRISH TACOS**
OVEN FRENCH FRIES

See also: Egg-Stuffed Baked Potato, Potato Snacks.

RICE

Rice is the world's third leading grain, after wheat and corn. Brown rice is made into white rice when the fiber-rich bran is removed during the refining process. This also removes some of the nutrients, but you can compensate for this loss (if you prefer white to brown rice) by eating other whole grains such as bran cereals and whole wheat breads at your other meals. Here are some tips for cooking rice:

- Because of its tough bran coat and germ, brown rice needs about 45 to 50 minutes to cook; white rice needs only about 20 to 30 minutes.
- Consider cooking rice in the morning while you are getting ready for work, so that it will be waiting to be reheated when you get home.
- When cooking rice, cook double amounts to have leftovers that you can freeze or refrigerate.
- Portions: 1 cup raw white rice = 3 cups cooked = 700 calories; 1 cup raw brown rice = 3 to 4 cups cooked = 700 calories.
- Rice is popularly cooked by two methods:

  1. Bring a saucepan of water to a full boil, stir in 1/3 to 1/2 cup rice per person plus 1 to 2 teaspoons of salt, as desired. Simmer about 20 minutes, or until a grain of rice is tender when you bite into it. Drain into a colander, rinse it under hot tap water to remove the sticky starch, and put it back into the saucepan. Keep the rice warm over low heat, fluffing it with a fork. Or,
  2. For each 1 cup of rice, put 2 cups of water into a saucepan, and 1 teaspoon salt, as desired. Bring to a boil, then cover and turn the heat down low. Let the rice cook undisturbed until it is tender and all the water has been absorbed. Then, stir gently with a fork. (Stirring too much may result in a sticky mess.) This method retains more of the vitamins that otherwise get lost into the cooking water.

QUICK AND EASY RICE IDEAS

Here are a few rice suggestions for hungry athletes.

Cook rice in these liquids:

- Chicken or beef broth
- Mixture of orange or apple juice and water
- Water with seasonings: cinnamon, soy sauce, oregano, curry, chili powder, or whatever might nicely blend with the menu.

Combine rice with these foods:

- Leftover chili
- Low- or no-fat Italian dressing and mustard
- Toasted sesame seeds
- Steamed vegetables
- Chopped mushrooms and green peppers, either raw or sautéed
- Nonfat sour cream, raisins, tuna, and curry powder
- Raisins, cinnamon, and applesauce

LOW-FAT FRIED RICE

This is a low-fat version of what you might get in a Chinese restaurant. Use your imagination and add whatever vegetables or protein-rich foods are handy.

Yield: 2 main dish servings

1 tablespoon oil
2 scallions with greens, chopped (or 1 small onion)
1 cup sliced mushrooms
1 egg, or egg substitute, or 2 egg whites, as desired
2 cups cooked rice (about 2/3 cup, uncooked)
1 tablespoon soy sauce

Optional vegetables: broccoli, celery, peas, snow peas, bok choy, Chinese cabbage, water chestnuts. *Optional protein:* shrimp, beef, chicken, ground turkey, tofu, nuts, sesame seeds. *Optional seasonings:* garlic, sesame oil, cayenne pepper.

1. Heat the oil in a large skillet or wok over medium-high heat.
2. Add the scallions and mushrooms (and other vegetables and proteins, as desired); stir-fry 2 or 3 minutes.
3. Push the vegetables aside. Pour the egg into the skillet and scramble it.
4. Stir in the rice, gently separating the grains. Add the soy sauce; stir thoroughly until heated.

Nutrition Information: Total calories: 680
Calories per serving: 340

Nutrients	%	Grams
Carbohydrate	60	30
Protein	10	9
Fat	30	10

COMPANY RICE SALAD

Water chestnuts and artichoke hearts can spiff up plain rice and make it into a special treat. Although this is designed to be a cold salad, it can be served warm.

Yield: 4 side servings

2 cups water
1 cup uncooked rice, brown or white
1 teaspoon salt, as desired
1 7-ounce can sliced water chestnuts
1 6-ounce jar marinated artichoke hearts

1. Bring the water to a boil. Add the rice; add salt as desired. Stir.
2. Cook, covered, until tender: 20 to 25 minutes for white rice or 45 to 50 minutes for brown rice. Add more water if needed.
3. Gently mix in the water chestnuts and marinated artichoke hearts (including marinade).
4. Chill.

Nutrition Information: Total calories: 640
Calories per serving: 160

Nutrients	%	Grams
Carbohydrate	70	28
Protein	10	4
Fat	20	4

HONEY NUT RICE

The honey adds a touch of sweetness, the nuts a bit of crunch.

Yield: 4 side servings

> 2 cups water
> 1 cup rice, brown or white
> 1 tablespoon honey
> 1 teaspoon salt, as desired
> 1/4 cup chopped walnuts or almonds

Optional: 1/2 cup golden raisins or chopped apricots.

1. Bring the water to a boil.
2. Add the rice, honey, and salt. Stir.
3. Cover and cook over low heat until tender: 20 to 25 minutes for white rice, 45 to 50 minutes for brown rice. Add more water if needed.
4. Add the nuts and raisins (optional).

Nutrition Information: Total calories: 680
Calories per serving: 170

Nutrients	%	Grams
Carbohydrate	70	30
Protein	5	2
Fat	25	5

CINNAMON RAISIN RICE

This goes nicely with chicken, fish, and especially Mexican bean dishes.

Yield: 4 side servings

> 1 cup uncooked rice, brown or white
> 2 cups water
> 1 to 2 teaspoons cinnamon
> 1/2 cup raisins
> 1 teaspoon salt, as desired

1. In a saucepan, combine the rice, water, cinnamon, raisins, and salt.
2. Bring to a boil, cover, and cook over medium-low heat for 20 to 25 minutes for white rice, 45 to 50 minutes for brown rice. Add more water if needed.

Nutrition Information: Total calories: 640
Calories per serving: 160

Nutrients	%	Grams
Carbohydrate	95	38
Protein	5	trace
Fat	—	—

ORANGE RICE

This goes nicely with chicken, pork, or fish dishes.

Yield: 4 side servings

1-1/2 cups water
1/2 cup orange juice
1 cup uncooked rice, brown or white

Optional: 1 teaspoon salt or 2 chicken bouillon cubes; 1 teaspoon sugar, dash of nutmeg, or dash of cloves.

1. Bring the water, juice, and salt or bouillon (if desired) to a boil.
2. Add the rice and optional seasonings; stir. Cover and cook over low heat until tender: 20 to 25 minutes for white rice or 45 to 50 minutes for brown rice. Add more water if needed.

Nutrition Information: Total calories: 460
Calories per serving: 115

Nutrients	%	Grams
Carbohydrate	90	26
Protein	10	2
Fat	—	—

POTATOES

The potato is a carbohydrate-rich vegetable that actually offers more vitamins and minerals than plain rice or pasta does. To help you include more potatoes in your sports diet, here are some tips.

• Potatoes come in different varieties. Some varieties are suited for baking (russets), others for boiling (red or white rounds). Ask the produce manager at your grocery store for guidance.

• Potatoes are best stored in a cool, humid (but not wet) place that is well ventilated, such as your cellar. Do not refrigerate potatoes because they will become sweet and off-colored.

• Rather than peel the skin (under which is stored most of the vitamin C), scrub the skin well and cook the potato skin and all. Yes, even mashed potatoes can be made with unpeeled potatoes!

• One pound of potatoes equals three medium or two large potatoes. The large, "restaurant size" potato has about 200 calories.

• To bake a potato in the oven, allow about 40 minutes at 400° for a medium potato, closer to an hour for a large potato. Because potatoes can be baked at any temperature, you can adjust the cooking time to whatever else is in the oven.

• You can tell that the potato is done when you can easily pierce it with a fork.

• To cook a potato in the microwave oven, prick its skin in several places with a fork, place it on some paper toweling on the bottom of the microwave, and cook it for about 4 minutes if it is medium-sized, or 6 to 10 minutes if it's large. Cooking time will vary according to the size of the potato, the power of your oven, and the number of potatoes being cooked. Turn the potato over halfway through cooking. Remove the potato from the oven, wrap it in a towel, and allow it to finish cooking outside the oven for about 3 to 5 minutes.

QUICK AND EASY POTATO IDEAS

To spice up your potato, try the following toppings.

• Plain yogurt
• Imitation butter granules (such as Molly McButter) and milk
• Mustard
• Mustard and Worcestershire sauce
• White and flavored vinegars
• Soy sauce

- Pesto
- Chopped chives and green onion
- Herbs such as dill and parsley
- Steamed broccoli or other cooked vegetables
- Chopped jalapeño peppers
- Low- or no-fat salad dressing
- Nonfat sour cream, chopped onion, and grated low-fat cheddar cheese
- Cottage cheese and garlic powder
- Cottage cheese and salsa
- Soup broth
- Milk mashed into the potato
- Lentils or lentil soup
- Baked beans or refried beans
- Applesauce

QUICK POTATO WEDGES

The microwave oven makes cooking easy for hungry potato lovers!

Yield: 1 serving

> 1 large baking potato, washed and pierced with a fork
> Seasonings as desired: garlic powder, oregano, chili powder; Parmesan cheese

1. Cook the potato in the microwave oven for 6 to 10 minutes, then let it stand for about 3 to 5 minutes to finish cooking.
2. Using a potholder to protect your hands, cut the potato in half, then into wedges.
3. Spray the wedges with cooking spray, then sprinkle on seasonings of your choice.
4. Broil the wedges in the toaster oven for about 2 minutes, or until golden.

Nutrition Information: Calories per serving: 225

Nutrients	%	Grams
Carbohydrate	90	52
Protein	10	4
Fat	—	—

MIGHTY MASHED POTATO

This dish is "mighty" because it is fortified with protein and calcium from powdered milk. It's also rich in fiber from the potato skins, which are left on to save time and retain nutrients. For more protein, add a scoop of cottage cheese.

Yield: 1 serving

> 1 large (8-ounce) potato with peel, diced
> 1/2 cup water
> 1/3 cup milk powder
> Salt and pepper, as desired

Optional: chopped onion; low-fat cottage cheese or cheddar or other hard cheese; mashed tofu.

1. Cook the potato in water in a covered pan for about 15 to 20 minutes, or until tender when pierced with a fork. Do *not* drain the cooking water.
2. With a potato masher or big spoon, mash together the potato and the cooking water.
3. Add the milk powder and seasonings as desired.

Nutrition Information: Total calories: 225
Calories per serving: 225

Nutrients	%	Grams
Carbohydrate	80	44
Protein	20	12
Fat	—	—

OVEN FRENCH FRIES

This french fry recipe is healthy and potassium rich, and no one will know it is low in fat! For a flavor boost, dip the fries in salsa, nonfat yogurt mixed with fresh herbs, or ketchup.

Yield: 1 serving

1 large baking potato, cleaned, unpeeled
1 teaspoon oil, preferably canola or olive
Cooking spray
Salt and pepper to taste

Optional: red pepper flakes; dried basil, oregano, minced garlic; Parmesan cheese.

1. Cut each potato lengthwise into 10 or 12 pieces. Place in a large bowl; cover with cold water and let stand for 15 to 20 minutes. (This soaking can be eliminated, but it shortens the cooking time and improves the final product.)
2. Drain the potatoes and dry them on a towel. Drizzle them with the oil and sprinkle with the salt and pepper, as desired. Toss to coat evenly.
3. Spray a baking sheet thoroughly with cooking spray and place the potatoes evenly on it.
4. Bake at 425° for 15 minutes. Turn the potatoes over, sprinkle with the optional seasonings, as desired, and continue baking for another 10 to 15 minutes. Serve immediately. Be careful; the potatoes will be very hot!

Nutrition Information: Calories per serving: 260

Nutrients	%	Grams
Carbohydrate	80	52
Protein	5	4
Fat	15	4

MEAL-IN-ONE POTATO

A baked potato is a particularly convenient food for those who exercise before dinner. If the potato bakes while you work out, it will be ready when you are! You'll likely want two, so make enough.

Yield: 1 serving

1 large baking potato
2/3 cup cottage cheese, low-fat or nonfat, as desired

Optional seasonings: scallions, onions; Italian seasonings, garlic powder; crumbled blue cheese, Parmesan cheese.

1. Bake the potato at 425° for 45 to 60 minutes or cook it in the microwave oven for about 8 minutes and let stand for 3 to 5 minutes.
2. Slit it open by cutting an X on top and puff it up.
3. Spoon on the cottage cheese mixed with seasonings of your choice.

Nutrition Information: Calories per serving: 275

Nutrients	%	Grams
Carbohydrate	55	83
Protein	35	95
Fat	10	3

Per ounce of blue cheese used, add 100 calories, 8 grams of fat, and 6 grams of protein.

Per tablespoon of Parmesan, add 25 calories, 1.5 grams of fat, and 2 grams of protein.

GREEK STUFFED POTATO

While you're at it, make extra for tomorrow's lunch or dinner—if these last that long!

Yield: 2 servings

2 large baking potatoes, 8 ounces each
1 10-ounce box frozen chopped spinach, thawed and squeezed dry
2 ounces feta cheese, crumbled

Optional: 2 tablespoons Parmesan cheese; salt, pepper, garlic powder.

1. Bake the potatoes at 425° for 45 to 60 minutes or cook them in the microwave oven for about 8 minutes and then let stand for 3 to 5 minutes.
2. When the potatoes are done, scoop their insides into a small bowl, being careful not to burn your fingers! (Try holding the potato with a clean towel or potholder.)

3. Add the spinach, cheeses, and seasonings to your taste. Mix.
4. Fill the potato skins with the mixture and bake them in the oven 10 minutes longer to blend the flavors.

Nutrition Information: Total calories: 520
Calories per serving: 260

Nutrients	%	Grams
Carbohydrate	60	78
Protein	20	13
Fat	20	8

IRISH TACOS

These potatoes will make you say "O' lé!"

Yield: 2 servings

2 large baking potatoes (8 ounces each)
1/2 15-ounce can pinto beans
1/2 cup salsa or chili sauce
2 ounces shredded cheddar cheese, preferably low-fat

Optional toppings: chopped scallions, tomatoes, lettuce; salsa.

1. Bake the potatoes in a conventional oven at 425° for 45 to 60 minutes or cook them in a microwave oven for about 8 minutes and let them stand for 1 to 2 minutes.
2. Heat the beans with the salsa or chili sauce.
3. Split the cooked potatoes and puff them up. Spoon on the beans with salsa; top with the cheese.

Nutrition Information: Total calories: 800
Calories per serving: 400

Nutrients	%	Grams
Carbohydrate	70	70
Protein	25	25
Fat	5	2

Pasta

Without a doubt, pasta is among the most popular sports foods for busy athletes. Perhaps the following recipes will add some variety to the standard spaghetti and tomato sauce meals.

PASTA RECIPES

QUICK AND EASY PASTA IDEAS
PASTA WITH SPINACH AND PINE NUTS
HONEY-GINGER NOODLES
SPICY CHINESE NOODLES
PASTA WITH SPINACH AND COTTAGE CHEESE
PASTA AND BEANS
STUFFED SHELLS
PASTA WITH PESTO SAUCE
PASTA WITH SHRIMP AND ASPARAGUS
CREAMY PASTA AND VEGGIES
SESAME PASTA WITH BROCCOLI
PASTA SALAD PARMESAN
SWEET WALNUT NOODLES

See also: Hamburger-Noodle Feast, Easy Cheesy Noodles, Lazy Lasagna.

How to Cook Pasta

If you eat lots of pasta, you might as well know how to cook it perfectly: tender yet firm when bitten with the teeth—"al dente" as the Italians say. The following pasta tips are taken from my nutrition guide and cookbook for runners, *The New York City Marathon Cookbook* (Clark, N. 1994. 830 Boylston St., Brookline, MA 02167; $20).

• Use a big pot filled with water so the individual pieces of pasta can float freely. Allow 10 minutes for the water to reach a rolling boil.

• Allow 4 quarts (4 liters) of water per pound of dry pasta. Plan to cook no more than 2 pounds of pasta at a time; otherwise, you may end up with a gummy mess.

• To keep the water from boiling over, add 1 tablespoon of oil to the cooking water. You can also add 1 to 2 tablespoons of salt, as desired, to heighten the flavor of the pasta.

• Bring the water to a vigorous, rolling boil before you add the pasta. Then add the pasta in small amounts that will not cool the water too much and cause the pieces to clump. When cooking spaghetti or lasagna, push down the stiff strands as they soften, using a long-handled spoon.

• If the water stops boiling, cover the pan, turn up the heat, and bring the water to a boil again as soon as possible.

• Cooking time will depend on the shape of the pasta. Pasta is done when it starts to look opaque. To tell if it is done, lift a piece of pasta (with a fork) from the boiling water, let it cool briefly, then carefully pinch or bite it (being sure not to burn yourself). The pasta should feel flexible but still firm inside.

• When the pasta is done, drain it into a colander set in the sink, using potholders to protect your hands from the steam. Shake the pasta briefly to remove excess water, then return it to the cooking pot or to a warmed serving bowl.

• To prevent the pasta from sticking together as it cools, toss the pasta with a little oil or sauce.

Twenty-Six Varieties

Pasta comes in at least 26 shapes, ranging from plain spaghetti strands to bow ties. All the shapes are made from the same wheat-and-water dough, sometimes tinted with vegetable juice (spinach, tomato). The best pasta is made from durum wheat that has been ground into fine granules called semolina or into durum flour. Durum wheat has a high gluten (protein) content that gives the pasta a firm texture. Whole wheat pasta, in comparison, tends to have more fiber and be softer; soy pastas still softer.

When trying to decide which shape of pasta to use for a meal, the rule of thumb is to use twisted and curved shapes (such as twists and shells) with meaty, beany, and chunky sauces. The shape will trap more sauce than the straight strands of spaghetti or linguini would.

Although pasta is an international favorite food of runners, you may struggle with understanding what the shapes are called. Here is the translation into English for runners who are not fluent in the most common shapes of pasta:

Capellini d'angelo	Angel hair
Conchiglie	Shells
Conchigliette	Little shells
Farfalle	Butterflies or bow ties
Fettucini	Flat, wide spaghetti
Fusilli	Twisted spaghetti strands
Linguini	Thinner than fettucini; wider than spaghetti
Manicotti	Big tubes
Penne	Skinny tubes with pointed ends
Rigatoni	Tubes
Rotelle	Twists
Route	Cartwheels
Stelline	Little stars
Vermicelli	Thin, flat spaghetti
Ziti	Small tubes

The quickest cooking pastas include angel hair, alphabets, and the little stars. With these, the time-consuming part is getting the water to boil. If desired, you can cook the pasta in half the amount of water, and it will cook OK—in less time.

QUICK AND EASY PASTA IDEAS

The following quick and easy pasta toppings are a change of pace from the standard tomato sauce straight from the jar.

Steamed, chopped broccoli
Salsa
Salsa heated in the microwave, then mixed with cottage cheese
Red pepper flakes
Low-fat Italian salad dressing mixed with a little Dijon mustard
Low/no-fat salad dressings of your choice
Low/no-fat Italian salad dressing with tamari, chopped garlic, steamed vegetables
Nonfat sour cream and Italian seasonings
Cottage cheese, Parmesan, and Italian seasonings
Parmesan cheese and a sprinkling of herbs (basil, oregano, Italian seasonings)
Chicken breast sautéed with oil, garlic, onion, and basil
Chili with kidney beans (and cheese)
Lentil soup (thick)
Spaghetti sauce with a spoonful of grape jelly (adds a sweet 'n sour taste)
Spaghetti sauce with added protein: canned chicken or tuna, tofu cubes, canned beans, cottage cheese, ground beef or turkey

PASTA WITH SPINACH AND PINE NUTS

Pine nuts are a tasty addition to many dishes, including this one! Because they are expensive, you might want to use chopped walnuts instead. Note that the addition of nuts boosts the fat content, but at least with a healthful type of fat.

Yield: 5 servings

1/2 cup pine nuts or chopped walnuts
12 ounces fresh spinach, washed, or 1 10-ounce box frozen spinach
1 to 4 cloves garlic, crushed, or 1/8 to 1/2 teaspoon garlic powder
1 pound pasta, such as linguini
3 to 4 tablespoons oil, preferably olive or canola
Salt and pepper, as desired

1. Toast the pine nuts (or walnuts) by baking them in a shallow dish for about 8 minutes in a 300° oven.
2. Meanwhile, cook the pasta according to the directions on the package and prepare the spinach by washing the leaves and cutting off the stems.
3. Heat the oil in a large skillet. Add the spinach and garlic, and toss until the spinach is just wilted, about 2 to 3 minutes.
4. Add the drained pasta to the spinach; toss together. Add salt to taste and half of the pine nuts.
5. Serve, and scatter the rest of the pine nuts on top.

Nutrition Information: Total calories: 2,750
Calories per serving: 550

Nutrients	%	Grams
Carbohydrate	52	75
Protein	15	21
Fat	33	20

HONEY-GINGER NOODLES

These noodle are delicious hot, cold, plain, with steamed vegetables, or on top of a salad. The original recipe (in *The New York City Marathon Cookbook*) calls for Japanese Udon Noodles, but standard pastas such as spaghetti, vermicelli, or linguini work nicely. This goes well with chicken, fish, or tofu.

Yield: 4 servings

> 1 pound dry pasta such as spaghetti, linguini, or fettucini
> 2 to 4 cloves of garlic, or 1/4 to 1/2 teaspoon garlic powder
> 2" piece of fresh ginger (about 1 square inch)
> 1/4 cup tamari sauce or soy sauce
> 1/4 cup honey
> 1/4 cup oil, preferably sesame

Cook noodles according to directions. Mix remaining ingredients in a blender or food processor for 1 to 2 minutes until smooth. Toss into warm noodles. Serve hot or cold.

Nutrition Information: Total calories: 1,600
Calories per serving: 400

Nutrients	%	Grams
Carbohydrate	60	61
Protein	15	12
Fat	25	12

SPICY CHINESE NOODLES

If you were to call this Peanut Butter Pasta, folks might groan. Call it Spicy Chinese Noodles, and they'll come back for seconds! When serving this to guests, be sure that no one is allergic to nuts. This dish can fool even the most cautious eaters.

Yield: 4 side servings

8 ounces dry pasta
1/3 cup peanut butter, preferably chunky
3 tablespoons soy sauce
3 tablespoons vinegar
1 tablespoon sugar, as desired
1 or 2 dashes of cayenne pepper, as desired

Optional: lightly steamed green pepper strips, snow peas, chopped scallions; garlic powder.

1. Cook the pasta according to the directions on the package. Drain.
2. While the pasta is cooking, combine in a small saucepan the peanut butter, soy sauce, vinegar, sugar, and cayenne.
3. Mix together the pasta and the peanut butter sauce. Add vegetables, as desired. If the pasta is dry, add a little water to thin the sauce.

Nutrition Information: Total calories: 1,500
Calories per serving: 375

Nutrients	%	Grams
Carbohydrate	55	50
Protein	15	15
Fat	30	12

PASTA WITH SPINACH AND COTTAGE CHEESE

This pasta meets three important requirements for a top sports diet: simple, nutritious, and tasty! If you are in a rush, note that angel hair pasta cooks the quickest!

Yield: 2 servings

6 ounces pasta, preferably angel hair
1 10-ounce box frozen chopped spinach
1 cup cottage cheese, preferably low-fat
1/4 cup grated Parmesan cheese

Optional seasonings: dash of cayenne; sprinkling of garlic powder, oregano, basil.

1. Cook the pasta according to the directions on the package.
2. While the pasta is cooking, thaw and cook the spinach in the microwave oven or on the stove top.
3. Drain the cooked spinach, add the cottage cheese, Parmesan, seasonings; mix well and then add the cooked pasta.

Nutrition Information: Total calories: 950
Calories per serving: 475

Nutrients	%	Grams
Carbohydrate	60	71
Protein	30	36
Fat	10	5

PASTA AND BEANS

When you add beans to pasta, your muscles will get the benefit of extra carbohydrates as well as more protein. This recipe works well with black, white, and pinto beans. Take your choice! Rather than draining the liquid from canned beans, you can add it to the pasta. Just beware that the black beans' liquid gives a brown color to the pasta. It's tasty, but not very attractive!

Yield: 5 servings

8 ounces uncooked pasta, preferably shells
1 12-ounce jar salsa
1 11-ounce can corn
1 15-ounce can black, white, or pinto beans, drained and rinsed
    if desired

Optional: grated low-fat cheddar cheese.

1. Cook the pasta according to the directions on the package.
2. Combine the salsa, corn, and beans in a large pot and heat.
3. Add the cooked, drained pasta and mix well.

Nutrition Information: Total calories: 2,350
Calories per serving: 470

Nutrients	%	Grams
Carbohydrates	50	60
Protein	46	54
Fat	4	2

STUFFED SHELLS

This recipe works well with either spinach or chopped broccoli. The nutmeg adds a nice, different flavor—a change from the traditional Italian seasonings.

Yield: 4 servings

6 ounces large pasta shells (1/2 box)
1 10-ounce box frozen chopped spinach (or broccoli)
8 ounces part-skim ricotta cheese
1 tablespoon flour
2 tablespoons grated Parmesan
1/4 teaspoon nutmeg
1 cup spaghetti sauce

Optional: 1/4 teaspoon oregano, salt, pepper, garlic powder.

1. Cook the shells according to the directions on the box. Drain.
2. Steam the spinach until tender; drain well.
3. To the drained spinach, add the ricotta, flour, Parmesan, nutmeg; add oregano, garlic, salt, and pepper as desired. Mix well.
4. Stuff each cooked shell with about 1 tablespoon of the ricotta–spinach mixture.
5. Put stuffed shells in a nonstick 9" × 9" baking pan with a little spaghetti sauce on the bottom. Spoon the rest of the spaghetti sauce over the shells.
6. Cover and bake 25 minutes at 350°.

Nutrition Information: Total calories: 1,300
Calories per serving: 325

Nutrients	%	Grams
Carbohydrate	55	45
Protein	20	16
Fat	25	9

PASTA WITH PESTO SAUCE

In restaurants, pesto can be a deceptively high-fat meal. This recipe uses less oil, so it's better for carbo-loading but still not as high in carbohydrates as you might think.

Basil is an excellent source of vitamins C and A and potassium. If you prefer a flavor milder than basil (or if you have no basil), simply replace all or part of it with a 10-ounce box of frozen chopped spinach.

Yield: 4 servings

8 ounces dry pasta
1 cup loosely packed fresh basil leaves (or 1/4 to 1/3 cup dried, chopped basil, or 1 box frozen chopped spinach, cooked)
1/4 cup (1 ounce) walnuts
1/4 cup Parmesan cheese, grated
1-1/2 tablespoons oil, preferably olive
1 to 2 cloves garlic, or 1/8 teaspoon garlic powder
Salt and pepper as desired

1. Cook the pasta according to package directions.
2. In a blender, combine the basil (or spinach), walnuts, cheese, oil, garlic, and seasonings. Cover and blend until smooth.
3. Combine with the cooked pasta. Serve either hot or cold.

Nutrition Information: Total calories: 1,400
Calories per serving: 350

Nutrients	%	Grams
Carbohydrate	55	48
Protein	15	13
Fat	30	11

PASTA WITH SHRIMP AND ASPARAGUS

Expensive but elegant, this can be a party dish or a nice treat for a quick dinner.

Yield: 2 big servings

1/2 pound dry pasta such as ziti, penne, or shells
1 10-ounce box frozen asparagus (spears or pieces), or 2/3
    pound fresh asparagus
1 clove garlic, minced, or 1/8 teaspoon garlic powder
1/2 cup water
2 tablespoons olive oil
1/2 pound cooked shrimp

Optional: 2 to 4 scallions, chopped; 4 tablespoons chopped fresh parsley; 2 teaspoons lemon juice; 2 to 4 ounces crumbled feta cheese.

1. Cook the pasta according to the directions on the box.
2. While the pasta is cooking, cut the asparagus spears into 1" pieces.
3. Put the asparagus, garlic, (scallions), and water in a large nonstick skillet. Cover, bring to a boil, and then simmer over medium heat for about 4 minutes, or until tender-crisp.
4. Add the oil and shrimp (parsley, lemon juice); heat through.
5. Add the drained pasta; toss well.

Nutrition Information: Total calories: 1,400
Calories per serving: 700

Nutrients	%	Grams
Carbohydrate	55	96
Protein	25	44
Fat	20	15

CREAMY PASTA AND VEGGIES

Simple as can be! Any leftovers are excellent for tomorrow's lunch, warm or cold.

Yield: 3 servings

8 ounces dry pasta
1 cup fat-free sour cream or fat-free creamy salad dressing
4 cups vegetables of your choice such as broccoli, fresh
    tomatoes, mushrooms, sliced carrots, green pepper
Seasonings as desired: garlic powder, salt, pepper, oregano,
    parsley, basil, Parmesan cheese

1. Cook the pasta according to the directions on the package. Drain.
2. While the pasta is cooking, steam the vegetables until tender-crisp.
3. Mix the fat-free sour cream with the cooked pasta; add the cooked vegetables and seasonings.

Nutrition Information: Total calories: 1,095
Calories per serving: 365

Nutrients	%	Grams
Carbohydrate	80	73
Protein	16	15
Fat	4	2

SESAME PASTA WITH BROCCOLI

Sesame paste (tahini) is the secret ingredient in this recipe. Not only does it have a wonderful flavor but it's also a good source of vitamin E. Look for tahini in the ethnic food section of the supermarket or at the health food store. If you can't find it, substitute peanut butter diluted with 1 or 2 tablespoons of boiling water.

Yield: 4 side servings; 2 main dish servings

8 ounces dry pasta
2 cups fresh or frozen broccoli, chopped
1/4 cup tahini (sesame butter) or peanut butter

Optional: cayenne pepper, garlic powder; vegetables of your choice such as celery, scallions.

1. Cook pasta according to directions on the package. Drain.
2. While pasta is cooking, steam broccoli until tender-crisp.
3. Add tahini to drained pasta, mix well. Add cooked broccoli and the water in which it was cooked if the pasta is "dry."
4. Add a dash of cayenne or garlic powder, as desired.

Nutrition Information: Total calories: 1,300
Calories per 1/4 recipe: 325

Nutrients	%	Grams
Carbohydrate	60	50
Protein	15	12
Fat	25	9

PASTA SALAD PARMESAN

The Parmesan cheese adds a light "bite" to this colorful salad.

Yield: 4 side servings

8 ounces dry pasta, preferably shells, spirals, or elbows
2 cups broccoli florets or peas, steamed
2 tablespoons olive oil
1/2 cup Parmesan cheese
2 cups cherry tomatoes, halved
Seasonings as desired: 1/2 teaspoon basil, 1/4 teaspoon garlic powder, 1/2 teaspoon salt, pepper

Optional: 2 scallions, sliced, or 1/2 onion, chopped; red or green peppers, diced; 2 tablespoons poppy seeds.

1. Cook the pasta according to the directions on the package. Drain.
2. While pasta cooks, steam the broccoli; chop the scallions or onion (optional).
3. Combine the cooked pasta, broccoli, (scallions), olive oil, basil, garlic powder, and salt. Mix well. Sprinkle on the cheese and toss again.
4. Chill before serving.

Nutrition Information: Total calories: 1,440
Calories per serving: 360

Nutrients	%	Grams
Carbohydrate	60	54
Protein	15	13
Fat	25	10

SWEET WALNUT NOODLES

This is a delightfully different side dish that is exceptionally tasty when served with spinach (or mixed with cooked chopped spinach), chicken, or fish. Despite their high fat content that adds calories to this dish, walnuts are thought to protect against heart disease and are an overall positive addition to your diet.

Yield: 5 servings

2 to 3 tablespoons butter, margarine, or olive oil
1/4 cup sugar
1/2 to 1 cup (2 to 4 ounces) walnuts (or other nuts), crushed
   with a rolling pin or bottle
8 ounces wide egg noodles

Optional: 1 10-ounce package frozen chopped spinach, cooked and drained.

1. Cook noodles according to the directions on the package.
2. Meanwhile, in a small saucepan, melt the butter over low heat. Add the crushed walnuts and cook them for 3 minutes over medium heat. Add the sugar, then remove the pan from the heat.
3. Drain the noodles, mix in the walnut mixture (and spinach), and toss well.

Nutrition Information: Total calories: 1,600
Calories per serving: 320

Nutrients	%	Grams
Carbohydrate	55	44
Protein	10	8
Fat	35	12

Vegetables

Vegetables are perfectly delicious when served plain, without added flavorings. The trick is to cook them until tender-crisp and still flavorful. Limp, overcooked veggies can lose their appeal as well as some of their nutrients.

Most vegetables contain negligible amounts of protein and fat but are filled with carbohydrates and packed with vitamins and minerals.

The first five recipes offer basic advice about cooking methods. Nutrition information is provided only for the final four recipes. Tables 1.4 and 7.4 provide more nutrition information.

VEGETABLE RECIPES

STEAMED VEGETABLES
STIR-FRIED VEGETABLES
CHINESE VEGETABLES: AN INTRODUCTION
BAKED VEGETABLES
MICROWAVED VEGETABLES
WINTER SQUASH SOUP FOR ONE
"CREAMY" SPINACH
STIR-FRIED BROCCOLI WITH SESAME SEEDS
CARROTS IN ORANGE JUICE

See also: Pasta With Spinach and Cottage Cheese, Pasta With Pesto Sauce, Stuffed Shells, Sesame Pasta With Broccoli, Sweet Walnut Noodles, Pasta With Shrimp and Asparagus, Low-Fat Fried Rice, Greek Stuffed Potato, Fish and Broccoli Soup, Egg-Drop Soup

STEAMED VEGETABLES

Here are some basic guidelines for steaming vegetables.

1. Wash the vegetables thoroughly to remove soil. Cut into the desired size.
2. Put 1/2" of water in the bottom of a pan with a tight lid. Bring to a boil, then add the vegetables. Cover tightly, or put the vegetables in a steamer basket and put the basket into a saucepan with 1" of water (or enough to prevent the water from boiling away). Cover tightly and bring to a boil.
3. Cook over medium heat until tender-crisp, about 3 to 10 minutes.
4. Drain the vegetables, reserving the cooking liquid for soup, sauces, or even for drinking as vegetable broth.

Optional: Sprinkle vegetables with herbs before or after cooking. I often add basil and oregano to zucchini squash, ginger to carrots, and garlic powder to green beans. Be creative!

STIR-FRIED VEGETABLES

Vegetables stir-fried until tender-crisp are very flavorful, but they do have more fat than steamed vegetables. If you are watching your weight, be sure to add the least possible amount of oil.

Olive and canola oils are among the heart-healthiest choices for stir-frying. For a wonderful flavor, add a little sesame oil (available in the Chinese food section of larger supermarkets or health food stores).

Although a wok is popular for stir-frying, any large frying pan or saucepan can do the job. I prefer a cast-iron skillet.

To stir-fry vegetables, follow these instructions.

1. Wash, drain well (to prevent oil from spattering when the vegetables are added), and cut the vegetables of your choice into bite-sized pieces or 1/8" slices. Whenever possible, slice the vegetables diagonally to increase the surface area; this allows faster cooking. Try to make the pieces uniform so they will cook evenly. Some popular vegetable stir-fry combinations are carrots, broccoli, and mushrooms; onions, green peppers, zucchini, and tomatoes; and Chinese cabbage and water chestnuts.
2. Heat the wok, skillet, or large frying pan over high heat. Add 1 to 3 teaspoons of canola, olive, or sesame oil—just enough to coat the bottom of the pan. For interesting flavor, try adding a slice of ginger root or minced garlic to the oil. Stir-fry for a minute to flavor the oil.

3. First add vegetables that take the longest to cook (carrots, cauliflower, broccoli); a few minutes later, add the remaining veggies (mushrooms, bean sprouts, cabbage, spinach). Constantly lift and turn the pieces to coat with oil. Add a little bit of water (1/4 to 1/2 cup) and cover and steam the vegetables. Adjust the heat to prevent scorching.

4. Don't overcrowd the pan. Cook small batches at a time. The goal is to cook the vegetables until they are tender but still crunchy, about 2 to 5 minutes. You might add in soy sauce or stir-fried beef, chicken, ground turkey, tofu, or other protein of your choice to make this into a main course.

5. Thicken the juices, as they do in Chinese restaurants, by stirring in a mixture of 2 teaspoons cornstarch and 1 tablespoon water. Add more water or broth if the broth is too thick. Garnish the vegetables with toasted sesame seeds or toasted nuts (almonds, cashews, peanuts), or mandarin orange sections or pineapple chunks, if desired.

CHINESE VEGETABLES: AN INTRODUCTION

If you are bored by the same old veggies—broccoli, green beans, carrots, corn, and peas—be adventurous! Try some of the Chinese vegetables found at larger grocery stores or Chinese markets. They tend to have a mild flavor that even picky eaters enjoy.

My favorites include these:

• **Bok choy.** Slender white stalks with dark green, leafy tops. Bok choy is sweet and mild tasting, good either raw or cooked. Cut off the root end, separate the stalks, and slice diagonally. Cut the leaves into 1" strips. Stir-fry, steam, or add to soups or vegetable dishes.

• **Chinese cabbage.** Flat, white ribs with pale, cabbage-colored leaves. It has a mild flavor and can be stir-fried, steamed, or added to soups, salads, or vegetable dishes.

• **Napa.** A light cabbage-colored vegetable that comes in a bunch like celery but has broad stalks with crinkled leaves. It has a mild, sweet flavor and is good stir-fried or in salads, soups, or vegetable dishes.

• **Chinese pea pods.** The flat, green pods are deliciously sweet and crunchy. Eat the whole pod! Rinse in water, trim the stems, and enjoy the pods raw in salads, as a snack, or in stir-fry dishes.

• **Bean sprouts.** These crunchy little strands are a fun addition to stir-fried dishes, salads, soups, and casseroles. Raw or cooked, they have a mild flavor and a nice crunch.

• **Water chestnuts.** Canned, sliced water chestnuts are a crunchy addition to stir-fry dishes, salads, or entrées. They're also a low-calorie snack alternative to munching on celery stalks!

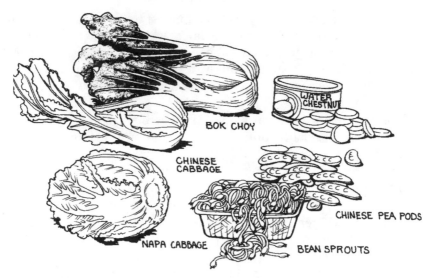

To prepare any of these Chinese vegetables

- stir-fry them according to the recipe for Stir-Fried Vegetables,
- add them to chicken broth and enjoy them in the form of a Chinese vegetable soup, or
- eat them raw in salads.

These vegetables blend well with the recipes for Low-Fat Fried Rice, Egg-Drop Soup, Fish and Broccoli Soup, and Scallops Baked in Foil.

BAKED VEGETABLES

If you're baking potatoes, chicken, or a casserole, you might as well make good use of the oven and bake the vegetables, too! Wrap them in foil to save yourself cleanup time.

1. Wrap the vegetables in foil or put them in a covered baking dish (with a small amount of water). Some popular combinations include eggplant halves sprinkled with garlic powder, zucchini or summer squash halves covered with onion slices, carrot chunks, or sweet potato slices and apples.
2. Bake at 350° for 20 to 30 minutes (depending on the size of the chunks) until tender-crisp.
3. When you open the foil, be careful of escaping steam so that you don't get burned.

MICROWAVED VEGETABLES

Microwave cookery is ideal for vegetables because it cooks them quickly and without water, retaining a greater percentage of nutrients than with conventional methods.

1. Wash the vegetables and cut them into bite-sized pieces. Put them on a plate and cover them with plastic wrap. If the vegetables vary in thickness (like stalks of broccoli do), arrange them in a ring with the thicker portions toward the outside of the dish. Try sprinkling the vegetables with herbs (basil, parsley, oregano, garlic powder), soy sauce, or whatever suits your taste.
2. Microwave until tender-crisp. The amount of time will vary according to your particular oven and the amount of vegetables you are cooking. You'll learn by trial and error! Start off with 3 minutes for a single serving; larger quantities take longer. The vegetables will continue cooking after they are removed from the oven, so plan that into the time allotment.

WINTER SQUASH SOUP FOR ONE

When you are hankering for something sweet for lunch or supper, this will do the job with wholesome carbohydrates rich in beta carotene. To make this soup into a more substantial meal, add some cooked ground turkey and leftover rice.

Yield: 1 serving

1 10-ounce box frozen winter squash
1 cup milk
2 to 3 teaspoons brown sugar
1/2-1 teaspoon salt, as desired

Optional: a few dashes of ginger or nutmeg; cooked ground turkey; leftover rice.

1. In a saucepan or a microwaveable dish, heat the squash with the milk.
2. Add the brown sugar, salt, seasonings, and other add-ins, as desired. Stir until blended.
3. Pour into a bowl or mug and enjoy.

Nutrition Information: Calories per serving: 220

Nutritients	%	Grams
Carbohydrate	75	40
Protein	20	11
Fat	5	2

"CREAMY" SPINACH

This is a nice side vegetable served with chicken or fish. The nutmeg adds a distinctive, pleasant taste. The spinach could also be the topping for a pizza (using an English muffin, tortilla, or pita round for the crust), sprinkling cheese on top, and heating the pizza in a toaster oven until the cheese is melted.

Yield: 2 servings

1 10-ounce box frozen chopped spinach
2 dashes nutmeg
2 to 4 tablespoons fat-free or low-fat sour cream
Salt and pepper, as desired

1. Cook the frozen spinach according to the directions on the box. Drain it well by squeezing out all the excess water.
2. Add the nutmeg, sour cream, and salt and pepper as desired.

Nutrition Information: Total calories: 120
Calories per serving: 60

Nutrients	%	Grams
Carbohydrate	75	11
Protein	25	4
Fat	—	—

STIR-FRIED BROCCOLI WITH SESAME SEEDS

This dish is particularly good with broiled chicken or fish. Cooking with the oil and sesame seeds adds about 130 calories; weight watchers might want to stick to plain steamed vegetables.

Yield: 2 servings

2 stalks (1 pound) fresh broccoli
2 teaspoons oil, preferably olive, canola, or sesame
2 to 4 tablespoons water
1 to 2 tablespoons sesame seeds
Salt and pepper as desired

1. Wash the broccoli, separate the florets from the stems, and cut the florets into bite-sized pieces.
2. Strip off the tough outer layer of the stems with a sharp knife. Slice the peeled stem into diagonal pieces.
3. Heat the oil in a heavy skillet or wok. Add the stems and stir fry for 2 minutes. Add the florets, stir, and then add the water. Cover and steam for 2 to 4 minutes, or until tender-crisp.
5. Sprinkle with sesame seeds, salt, and pepper as desired.

Nutrition Information: Total calories: 270
Calories per serving: 135

Nutrients	%	Grams
Carbohydrate	35	12
Protein	20	7
Fat	45	7

CARROTS IN ORANGE JUICE

This recipe is suitable for the stove top or the oven. This combination of carrots with a hint of orange flavor goes nicely with chicken and fish.

Yield: 3 servings

1 pound carrots, sliced on the diagonal into 1/3" thick ovals
1/2 cup orange juice

Optional: dash of ginger, cloves, or nutmeg; 1 teaspoon honey.

1. Put the carrots in a small saucepan or casserole with a tight cover. (You might want to first peel the carrots if you are concerned about the appearance of the final product. When cooked, the peels have a slightly darker, wrinkled look.)
2. Add the orange juice and seasonings, as desired. Cover and either simmer on top of the stove about 20 minutes or bake in the oven with the rest of the meal for about 1/2 hour.

Nutrition Information: Total calories: 225
Calories per serving: 75

Nutrients	%	Grams
Carbohydrate	90	17
Protein	10	2
Fat	—	—

Chicken and Turkey

The white and dark meat of chicken and turkey are excellent examples of muscle physiology. They represent two different types of muscle fibers.

- The white breast meat is primarily fast-twitch muscle fibers. These are used for bursts of energy. Athletes such as gymnasts, basketball players, and others who do sprint types of exercise tend to have a high percentage of fast-twitch fibers.

- The dark meat in the legs and wings is primarily slow-twitch muscle fibers that function best for endurance exercise. Marathoners, long-distance cyclists, and other endurance athletes tend to have a high percentage of slow-twitch fibers.

The dark meat (endurance muscle fibers) of poultry contains more fat than the white meat (sprint fibers) because the fat provides energy for greater endurance; the dark meat also has slightly more fat calories than light meat:

Chicken breast white meat has 120 calories per 3 ounces cooked.
Chicken thigh dark meat has 150 calories per 3 ounces cooked.

The dark meat also has more iron, zinc, B vitamins, and other nutrients. I recommend that people who don't eat beef select skinless dark meat poultry to boost their intake of these important nutrients. Because the highest source of fat in chicken is in the skin, be sure to remove the skin prior to cooking. This eliminates the temptation to eat it!

For easy cleanup when baking chicken, use a nonstick pan or a regular baking pan treated with cooking spray, or line the pan with aluminum foil.

CHICKEN

BASIC STEAMED CHICKEN
BAKED CHICKEN WITH MUSTARD
CHICKEN IN DIJON SAUCE
ORANGE CHICKEN
HONEY-BAKED CHICKEN
BAKED CHICKEN CHINESE STYLE
CHICKEN AND RICE WITH PLUM SAUCE
CHICKEN 'N CHEESE
CHICKEN STIR-FRY WITH APPLES AND CURRY

See also: Mexican Baked Chicken and Pinto Beans, Stir-Fried Vegetables, Easy Enchiladas, Sweet and Sour Tofu.

TURKEY

ROAST TURKEY
TURKEY 'N CHEESE CALZONE
TURKEY BURGERS I
TURKEY BURGERS II

See also: Low-Fat Fried Rice, Winter Squash Soup for One, Tortilla Roll-Ups, Easy Enchiladas, Sloppy Joefus, Eggplant-Tofu Parmesan, Chili, Tortilla Lasagna.

BASIC STEAMED CHICKEN

This basic recipe lends itself to 101 creative touches, some of which are listed below.

Yield: 1 serving

> Water
> 1 piece chicken, skinned

1. Put 1/2 inch of water in a saucepan.
2. Add the chicken, cover tightly, and bring just to a boil. Turn down heat.
3. Gently simmer over medium-low heat for 20 to 25 minutes, or until the juices run clear when the chicken is poked with a fork.

Variations:

- Replace water with orange juice, white wine, or stewed tomatoes.
- Add seasonings: a chicken bouillon cube, soy sauce, curry, basil, or thyme.
- Cook rice along with the chicken (add extra water).
- Make stuffing with the chicken broth and stuffing mix.
- Add vegetables in the last 5 minutes.

Nutrition Information: Calories per serving: 160 (based on 4 ounces cooked breast meat)

Nutrients	%	Grams
Carbohydrate	—	—
Protein	80	31
Fat	20	4

BAKED CHICKEN WITH MUSTARD

This chicken recipe is so simple but still tastes good enough for a special dinner. This recipe also works well with fish.

Yield: 1 serving

1 piece chicken, skinned
1 to 2 teaspoons mustard
2 teaspoons grated Parmesan cheese

1. Place the chicken in a nonstick baking pan or a pan that has been treated with cooking spray or lined with foil.
2. Spread the chicken with mustard; sprinkle with Parmesan cheese.
3. Bake uncovered at 350° for 20 to 30 minutes.

Nutrition Information: Calories per serving: 190 (based on 4 ounces cooked breast meat)

Nutrients	%	Grams
Carbohydrate	—	—
Protein	65	32
Fat	35	7

CHICKEN IN DIJON SAUCE

Delightfully different, this is my favorite "company chicken" recipe. It goes nicely with rice and carrots.

Yield: 4 servings

4 chicken breasts, skinned
1 cup water
2 chicken bouillon cubes
2 tablespoons Dijon (spicy) mustard
1/2 cup white wine (optional)
2 tablespoons flour
1/2 cup evaporated skim milk or low-fat milk

1. In a large saucepan, put the chicken, water, bouillon, mustard, and wine (optional).
2. Cover and bring to a boil; simmer over medium-low heat for 20 minutes, or until the juices run clear when the chicken is poked with a fork.
3. Mix the flour with the milk. (Evaporated milk offers a richer flavor.)
4. Skim off any fat on top of the broth. Thicken the broth into a nice sauce by slowly stirring in the flour and milk mixture.
5. Cover and cook over low heat for 5 minutes to allow the flavors to blend.

Nutrition Information: Total calories: 800
Calories per serving: 200 (based on 4 ounces cooked breast meat)

Nutrients	%	Grams
Carbohydrate	15	9
Protein	65	32
Fat	20	4

ORANGE CHICKEN

This is one variation of the recipe for Steamed Chicken. I sometimes add another cup of water and cook rice along with the chicken.

Yield: 4 servings

4 pieces chicken, skinned
1 cup orange juice
1 tablespoon cornstarch mixed in 2 tablespoons water

Optional: 1/4 teaspoon cinnamon or ginger; 1 tablespoon honey or brown sugar; salt or chicken bouillon cube, as desired; pepper.

1. Put the chicken and orange juice in a saucepan. Add seasonings as desired.
2. Cover, bring to a boil, and then simmer over medium-low heat for 20 minutes.
3. Skim the fat from the broth; thicken the broth by stirring in the cornstarch and water mixture until the broth is the desired consistency.

Nutrition Information: Total calories: 800
Calories per serving: 200 (based on 4 ounces cooked breast meat)

Nutrients	%	Grams
Carbohydrate	15	9
Protein	65	31
Fat	20	4

HONEY-BAKED CHICKEN

When you are tired of plain baked chicken, this offers a nice flavor change.

Yield: 1 serving

1 piece chicken, skinned
2 teaspoons honey
1/4 teaspoon curry powder

1. Place the chicken in a nonstick baking pan or a pan that has been treated with cooking spray or lined with foil.
2. Spoon on the honey, coating the chicken with a thin layer.
3. Sprinkle with curry powder.
4. Bake uncovered at 350° for 20 to 30 minutes.

Nutrition Information: Calories per serving: 200 (based on 4 ounces cooked breast meat)

Nutrients	%	Grams
Carbohydrate	10	5
Protein	65	31
Fat	25	6

BAKED CHICKEN CHINESE STYLE

Easy but tasty. For more flavor, let the chicken marinate overnight.

Yield: 4 servings

1/4 cup soy sauce
3/4 teaspoon dry mustard
1/4 teaspoon ground ginger
4 chicken breasts, skinned

Optional: 1 small clove garlic, minced, or 1/8 teaspoon garlic powder; 1 tablespoon oil; 1/8 teaspoon black pepper.

1. In a small bowl or zippered bag, combine the soy sauce, mustard, ginger, and optional seasonings, as desired.
2. Place the chicken in the bag, a nonstick baking pan, or a pan that has been treated with cooking spray or lined with foil and coat the chicken on all sides with the marinade. Let stand for 5 to 30 minutes or overnight.
3. Bake the chicken at 350° for 20 to 30 minutes, turning once or twice and brushing with the sauce.

Nutrition Information: Total calories: 670 (based on 16 ounces cooked breast meat)
Calories per serving: 165

Nutrients	%	Grams
Carbohydrate	4	1
Protein	80	33
Fat	16	3

CHICKEN AND RICE WITH PLUM SAUCE

Chinese plum sauce, sometimes called duck sauce, is available in the ethnic food section of the supermarket. It has a sweet taste that deliciously complements chicken and rice.

Yield: 4 servings

1/2 cups water
1/2 cup Chinese plum sauce
1 teaspoon salt or 2 teaspoons soy sauce, as desired
1 cup uncooked rice, brown or white
4 pieces chicken, skinned

1. In a medium-sized covered pot, bring the water to boil. Add the plum sauce, salt, and rice; return to a boil. If you are using brown rice, add it to the water and cook it for 20 minutes before adding the chicken.

2. Add the skinless chicken pieces. Cover and simmer over medium-low heat for 20 to 25 minutes, or until both the rice and chicken are cooked. Add more water if needed.

3. Serve with a green vegetable, such as peas or spinach. If you like, add the vegetable to the cooking pot in the last 5 minutes; you'll save yourself a dish to wash!

Nutrition Information: Total calories: 1,500 (based on 16 ounces cooked chicken breast)
Calories per serving: 375

Nutrients	%	Grams
Carbohydrate	55	52
Protein	35	32
Fat	10	4

CHICKEN 'N CHEESE

To make this into a chicken cordon bleu, add a slice of lean ham along with the cheese. To make a simple dinner for 4, bake the chicken in a covered pan with 2-1/2 cups of water or chicken broth and 1-1/2 cup of rice per 4 pieces of chicken.

Yield: 1 serving

1 6-ounce boneless chicken breast, skin removed
1/2 ounce string cheese

1. Roll the chicken around the string cheese. Secure with toothpicks.
2. Bake uncovered in a nonstick pan at 350° for 25 minutes.

Nutrition Information: Calories per serving: 200

Nutrients	%	Grams
Carbohydrate	—	trace
Protein	70	34
Fat	30	7

CHICKEN STIR-FRY WITH APPLES AND CURRY

For curry lovers, this dinner is easy to prepare and goes nicely with rice.

Yield: 3 servings

1 tablespoon oil, preferably olive or canola
1/2 cup celery, sliced on the diagonal
1 green pepper, sliced into strips
2 apples, diced
1 pound boneless chicken breasts, skinned and cut into 1" pieces
1 teaspoon curry

Optional: 1/4 teaspoon cumin; 1 teaspoon ground cloves; salt and pepper as desired; 1/3 cup raisins; 1/2 cup pineapple chunks.

1. Heat the oil in a large skillet or wok. Stir-fry the celery, peppers, and apples 3 to 5 minutes, or until tender-crisp. Keep covered, stirring every half minute. Remove to a platter.
2. To the skillet add the chicken; stir-fry 2 or 3 minutes, adding a little more oil if needed.
3. Add the vegetables and apples back into the skillet. Sprinkle with curry and seasonings as desired. Serve over rice.

Nutrition Information: Total calories: 750
Calories per serving: 250

Nutrients	%	Grams
Carbohydrate	15	9
Protein	45	28
Fat	40	11

ROAST TURKEY

When I know I have a busy week ahead of me, I'll roast a turkey on Sunday so there will be plenty of food for quick sandwiches or simple dinners. Although roasting a turkey may seem a monumental task, it's really very simple, whether the turkey is stuffed or unstuffed. The oven does all the work. You simply enjoy the aromas—and then the leftovers!

The general rule of thumb when buying turkey is to allow 3/4 pound per person if the turkey weighs less than 12 pounds and 1/2 to 3/4 pound per person if the turkey weighs more than 12 pounds.

1. Rinse the turkey inside and out under running water. Remove and discard any separable fat from around and under the skin near the body cavity.
2. *Optional:* Prepare stuffing mix according to package directions, except eliminate or reduce the butter. Stuff the mix into the turkey cavity.
3. Fold the flap of neck skin up and over the top of the back and fasten it with either a skewer or a large safety pin.
4. Tie the legs together over the body opening.
5. Place on a rack (if you have one) in a shallow roasting pan.
6. Cover the turkey with a tent of aluminum foil and place in a preheated, 325° oven.

Approximate cooking times for a whole turkey, unstuffed (add 5 minutes per pound if stuffed):

Less than 15 pounds—15 to 20 minutes per pound
More than 15 pounds—13 to 15 minutes per pound

To determine doneness, poke the turkey with a fork. The turkey is done if its juices run clear; a meat thermometer should register 180°. If the drumsticks easily move back and forth, it's overdone! Plan an extra 15 to 20 minutes into the cooking schedule to allow the turkey to rest before being carved; it'll slice more easily.

Nutrition Information: Calories per serving (4 ounces cooked breast meat): 160

Nutrients	%	Grams
Carbohydrate	—	trace
Protein	90	35
Fat	10	2

Calories per serving (4 ounces cooked thigh meat): 185

Nutrients	%	Grams
Carbohydrate	—	trace
Protein	65	31
Fat	35	7

Low-fat gravy
Yield: 2 cups

1. After the turkey has cooked, spoon off the grease from the roasting pan.
2. Add 2 cups of water to the roasting pan, scraping the browned drippings into this water.
3. Pour this water (gravy base) into a small saucepan. Let the fat rise to the top; skim it off. Bring the gravy base to a boil.
4. Mix 1/4 cup of flour into 1/2 cup of cold water.
5. Gradually add the flour and water mixture to the gravy base until the gravy reaches the desired thickness. Turn the heat down to low. Season with salt and pepper as desired.

Nutrition Information: Total calories: 120
Calories per 1/4 cup gravy: 15

Nutrients	%	Grams
Carbohydrate	90	3
Protein	10	trace
Fat	—	trace

TURKEY 'N CHEESE CALZONE

This makes a yummy hot sandwich, perfect for serving with vegetable soup on a cold winter's day. It's easiest to make if you buy premade pizza dough from the supermarket or pizza shop. Be creative with the fillings, using ham, lean roast beef, chicken, beans, vegetables, or whatever happens to be on hand.

Yield: 4 servings (from 1 pound of dough)

Dough for 1 pizza, about 1 pound
4 ounces sliced deli turkey
4 ounces (4 rolls) string cheese

Optional: chopped broccoli, green pepper, onion, and other vegetables for the topping; different low-fat cheeses such as Swiss or cheddar; seasonings as desired.

1. Cut the pizza dough into 4 pieces and shape each piece into a rectangle slightly longer than the string cheese.
2. Roll the sliced turkey around the cheese, then place it on the dough. Add extra fillings (vegetables, seasonings) as desired.
3. Fold the dough over the filling and pinch it tightly together to make a very firm seal (to prevent the cheese from oozing out during baking).
4. Place on a nonstick baking pan and bake at 400° for 10 to 12 minutes, or until the crust is golden.

Nutrition Information: Total calories: 1,300
Calories per serving: 325

Nutrients	%	Grams
Carbohydrate	50	41
Protein	25	20
Fat	25	9

TURKEY BURGERS I

Ground turkey is a fine alternative to a ground beef and is a good source of iron and zinc. These burgers are especially tasty on a roll with a little cranberry sauce.

Yield: 1 serving

> 6 ounces ground turkey (yields about 4 ounces cooked)
> Salt and pepper as desired

Optional: Add a drop of sesame oil to the skillet.

1. Shape the ground turkey into patties.
2. Cook over medium heat in a nonstick skillet.

Nutrition Information: Calories per serving: 180

Nutrients	%	Grams
Carbohydrate	—	trace
Protein	55	33
Fat	45	5

TURKEY BURGERS II

Adding oatmeal makes the burgers juicier than when they're made with plain ground turkey.

Yield: 4 servings

> 1/3 cup oatmeal, uncooked
> 1/2 cup chicken broth, canned, homemade, or from bouillon cubes
> 1 pound ground turkey
> 1 egg, or egg substitute, or 2 egg whites
> 2 tablespoons grated onion
> Salt and pepper as desired

Optional: two dashes nutmeg; 1/4 teaspoon allspice.

1. In a medium bowl, combine the oatmeal, broth, turkey, egg, onion, and seasonings.
2. Shape into 4 patties. Cook over medium-high heat in a nonstick skillet for about 5 minutes per side.

Nutrition Information: Total calories: 750
Calories per serving: 190

Nutrients	%	Grams
Carbohydrate	10	5
Protein	55	26
Fat	35	7

Fish
and Seafood

Fish meals tend to be more popular in restaurants than at home, because many people don't know how to buy or prepare fish. The following tips will take the mystique out of fish cookery; fish is one of the easiest foods to prepare!

Buying Fish

Fresh fish, when properly handled, has no fishy odor whether it is raw or cooked. The odor comes with aging and bacterial contamination. Whenever possible, ask to smell the fish you want to buy. Signs of freshness to look for are bulging eyes, reddish gills, and shiny scales that adhere firmly to the skin. After buying fresh fish, use it quickly, preferably within a day. Keep it in the coldest part of the refrigerator.

When buying commercially frozen fish, be sure the box is firm and square, showing no sign of thawing and refreezing. To thaw, defrost the fish in the refrigerator or microwave oven. Do not refreeze.

For each serving, allow one pound of whole fish (such as trout or mackerel) or 1/3 to 1/2 pound fish fillets or steaks (such as salmon, swordfish, halibut, or sole). To rid your hands of any fishy smell, rub them with lemon juice or vinegar. Wash cooking utensils with 1 teaspoon of baking soda per quart of water.

Cooking Tips

Here are a few tips to help you prepare your "catch."

- If possible, cook fish in its serving dish; fish is fragile, and the less it is handled the more attractive it is.
- Seasonings that go well with fish include lemon, dill, basil, rosemary, and parsley (and paprika for color).
- To test for doneness, gently pull the flesh apart with a fork. It should flake easily and not be translucent.
- Use leftover fish, warm or cold, in sandwiches as a change from chicken or turkey.

Broiling. Place fish on a broiling pan that has been lightly oiled or treated with cooking spray to prevent sticking, sprinkle with a little olive oil and seasonings (if desired), and place 4 to 6 inches from the heat source. Thin fillets (such as sole or bluefish) can be cooked in 5 minutes (without turning); thicker fillets (such as salmon or swordfish) may require about 5 or 6 minutes per side.

Baking. Set the fish in a baking dish that has been lightly oiled or treated with cooking spray, season as desired, cover, and bake at 400° for 15 to 20 minutes, depending on thickness.

Poaching. Set the fish in a nonstick skillet, cover the fillets with water, white wine, or milk; season as desired, cover and gently simmer on the stove top for about 10 minutes.

Microwaving. If possible, place the thickest part of the fillet toward the outside of the dish, overlapping thin portions to prevent overcooking. Season as desired, cover with waxed paper, and microwave for the minimum amount of time to prevent the fish from turning tough and dry. Remove from the oven before the fish is totally cooked and allow it to stand for 5 minutes to finish cooking before serving. Whitefish fillets may need 4 minutes, salmon steaks 6 to 7 minutes.

FISH AND SEAFOOD RECIPES

ORIENTAL STEAMED FISH	**BROILED FISH DIJON**
CRUNCHY FISH FILLETS	**CURRIED TUNA SALAD**
FISH FLORENTINE	**SCALLOPS BAKED IN FOIL**
FISH AND BROCCOLI SOUP	**SALMON STEW**
FISH IN FOIL MEXICAN STYLE	

See also: Pasta With Shrimp and Asparagus, Baked Chicken With Mustard, Egg-Drop Soup.

ORIENTAL STEAMED FISH

The scallions add a nice gentle flavor. If you have none, use a small onion instead.

Yield: 2 servings

1 teaspoon oil, preferably sesame
1 pound fresh fish
2 scallions, chopped
1 tablespoon soy sauce
2 tablespoons water

1. Heat the oil in the bottom of a skillet that has a tight lid.
2. Add the fish. Cover with the scallions and soy sauce. Add the water.
3. Cover and cook over low heat for 15 minutes, or until the fish flakes easily.

Nutrition Information: Total calories (made with cod): 420
Calories per serving: 210

Nutrients	%	Grams
Carbohydrate	5	3
Protein	80	42
Fat	15	3

CRUNCHY FISH FILLETS

Many cereals make a nice topping for this fish dish. Try bran flakes or crushed shredded wheat for variety.

Yield: 2 servings

1 pound fish fillets
Salt and pepper as desired
2 teaspoons olive oil
1/3 cup crispy rice cereal or cornflake crumbs

Optional: sprinkle with parsley flakes or Parmesan cheese.

1. Preheat the oven to 450°.
2. Wash and dry the fish fillets. Cut into individual servings.
3. Season with salt and pepper as desired; coat with the oil.
4. Dip the fish fillets into the cereal crumbs.
5. Arrange the fillets on a lightly oiled baking dish and bake for 12 minutes; don't turn.

Nutrition Information: Total calories (made with cod): 480
Calories per serving: 240

Nutrients	%	Grams
Carbohydrate	15	8
Protein	65	40
Fat	20	5

FISH FLORENTINE

This goes nicely with rice or sesame noodles.

Yield: 2 servings

1 10-ounce box frozen chopped spinach
1/2 cup (2 ounces) shredded mozzarella cheese
1 pound fish fillets
Salt, pepper, and lemon juice as desired

1. Preheat the oven to 400°.
2. Thaw the spinach and squeeze our†excess moisture. Spread on bottom of a small baking dish.
3. Sprinkle with the cheese and top with the fish. Season as desired.
4. Cover with foil. Bake for 20 minutes, or until the fish flakes easily.

Nutrition Information: Total calories (made with cod): 560
Calories per serving: 280

Nutrients	%	Grams
Carbohydrate	10	6
Protein	70	50
Fat	20	6

FISH AND BROCCOLI SOUP

Because fish cooks so quickly, it makes a simple soup in no time at all. I like this because it's simple to make, tasty, and low in calories. For a heartier meal, add rice or ramen noodles.

Yield: 1 serving

1 cup chicken broth (homemade, canned, or from a bouillon cube)
1/3 pound white fish, cut into 1" cubes
1 cup fresh or frozen broccoli, chopped

Optional: 1 tablespoon cornstarch mixed in 1 tablespoon water; 3/4 cup cooked rice or ramen noodles; 1/4 teaspoon sesame oil.

1. Heat the chicken broth.
2. *Optional:* Stir in cornstarch mixed with water to slightly thicken the broth.
3. Add the cut fish and chopped broccoli along with the sesame oil, if desired. Bring to a boil, then turn down the heat.
4. Simmer for about 5 minutes or until the broccoli is tender-crisp and the fish is translucent.

Nutrition Information: Calories per serving: 200

Nutrients	%	Grams
Carbohydrate	25	15
Protein	70	33
Fat	5	1

FISH IN FOIL MEXICAN STYLE

Fish always comes out moist and flavorful when cooked in foil.

Yield: 2 servings

2 18"-long pieces of heavy duty foil
1 pound white fish fillets
1/2 cup salsa

Optional: 1 diced green pepper and 1 diced small onion, sautéed in 1 teaspoon olive oil; 1/8 teaspoon garlic powder; salt and pepper; low-fat grated cheddar cheese.

1. If desired, sauté the onion and pepper in olive oil.
2. In the middle of the foil, place 1/2 pound of fish. Cover with 1/4 cup salsa, (peppers and onions and other ingredients or seasonings, as desired.)
3. Wrap by bringing together two edges, folding them over, then folding up the ends and crimping the edges.
4. Bake or grill the packets for 15 to 20 minutes. Lift with a spatula, and open carefully, being sure to not burn yourself on escaping steam.

Nutrition Information: Total calories: 400
Calories per serving: 200

Nutrients	%	Grams
Carbohydrate	5	4
Protein	85	42
Fat	10	2

BROILED FISH DIJON

Simple but tasty with that classic Dijon flavor.

Yield: 2 servings

1 pound fish fillets
1 to 2 tablespoons lite mayonnaise
1 to 2 tablespoons Dijon mustard

1. Combine the mayonnaise and mustard, and then spread the mixture on top of the fish.
2. Broil the fish 4" to 6" from the heat source for about 5 minutes, or until it flakes easily with a fork.

Nutrition Information: Total calories (made with cod): 400
Calories per serving: 200

Nutrients	%	Grams
Carbohydrate	—	—
Protein	85	42
Fat	15	3

CURRIED TUNA SALAD

Tasty in a salad or stuffed into a pita pocket. To further reduce the fat content, replace part or all of the mayonnaise with plain yogurt.

Yield: 2 servings

2 tablespoons lite mayonnaise
1/4 teaspoon curry
1/2 8-ounce can pineapple tidbits, drained
1 7-ounce can tuna, drained and broken into chunks

Optional: 2 tablespoons chutney, chopped.

1. In a small bowl, combine the mayonnaise, curry, and pineapple (and chutney, if you like).
2. Add the flaked tuna. If time permits, cover and chill the mixture to allow the flavors to blend.
3. Serve on a bed of lettuce or in a sandwich.

Nutrition Information:　Total calories: 440
Calories per serving: 220

Nutrients	%	Grams
Carbohydrate	35	20
Protein	50	28
Fat	15	4

SCALLOPS BAKED IN FOIL

Moist and tasty, this is an easily prepared but elegant meal that leaves you with little cleanup.

Yield: 2 servings

Heavy duty foil
4 cups vegetables, such as a combination of broccoli, bok choy, snow peas, sliced mushrooms, and water chestnuts
1 pound scallops
Salt and pepper as desired

1. Cut two sheets of foil, each about 18" square.
2. Cut the vegetables into bite-sized pieces.
3. Mix together the vegetables, scallops, and seasonings as desired.
4. Divide the mixture onto the foil squares. For each square, bring opposite sides of the foil up over the food, fold them together, and then fold the other ends toward the center and crimp to seal.
5. Place the foil packets on a baking sheet. Bake in 450° oven for 20 minutes.
6. Place each package on a plate. (Do not try to lift them by the foil; use a spatula!)
7. Cut open the top to make a "bowl"; be careful not to burn yourself on the steam. Serve with rice.

Nutrition Information: Total calories: 560
Calories per serving: 280

Nutrients	%	Grams
Carbohydrate	35	25
Protein	65	45
Fat	—	—

SALMON STEW

Salmon is among the best sources of fish oil, the omega-3 fats that protect against heart disease. Eat it often, and enjoy your good health as well as a good meal! This stew goes nicely with cornbread or crackers.
Yield: 3 servings

1 15-ounce can stewed tomatoes
1 7-ounce can salmon, drained
1 12-ounce can corn
1 5-ounce can evaporated skim milk with 1 can water
Salt and pepper as desired

Optional: 1/2 teaspoon sugar, 1 teaspoon dill.

1. In a saucepan, heat the tomatoes, salmon, and corn (with liquid).
2. Add the evaporated milk, water, and seasonings as desired. Warm until heated; do not boil.

Nutrition Information: Total calories: 810
Calories per serving: 270

Nutrients	%	Grams
Carbohydrate	55	37
Protein	30	10
Fat	15	4

Beef and Pork

Despite popular belief, lean beef and pork can be a part of a heart-healthy diet. They are excellent sources of protein, iron, and zinc—nutrients important for everyone, particularly athletes. The main health concern about red meat is its fat content. The solution is to choose lean cuts, trim the fat, and eat smaller portions.

These are the leanest cuts of beef:

- Top round roast and steak
- Bottom round roast
- Eye of the round
- Boneless rump roast
- Tip roast and steak
- Round, strip, and flank steak
- Lean stew beef

And here are the leanest cuts of pork:

- Sirloin roast and chops
- Loin chops
- Top loin roast
- Tenderloin
- Cutlets

Finally, the leanest cuts of ham:

- Lean and extra-lean cured ham (labeled 93- to 97-percent fat free)
- Center-cut ham
- Canadian bacon

For more information about low-fat meat cookery, refer to chapter 8. For more information about iron and zinc, refer to the section on minerals in chapter 12.

BEEF RECIPES

HAMBURGER-NOODLE FEAST
GOULASH
TORTILLA ROLL-UPS
SWEET 'N SPICY ORANGE BEEF
STIR-FRY BEEF AND BROCCOLI

See also: Low-Fat Fried Rice, Lazy Lasagna, Easy Enchiladas, Sloppy Joefus, Chili, Tortilla Lasagna.

PORK RECIPES

PORK CHOPS BAKED WITH APPLE AND SWEET POTATO
PORK CHOPS IN APPLE CIDER
STIR-FRY PORK WITH FRUIT

See also: Low-Fat Fried Rice, Sweet and Sour Tofu.

HAMBURGER-NOODLE FEAST

Perfect for feeding a crowd, this simple casserole will keep everyone well fueled.

Yield: 6 large servings

1 pound uncooked noodles
1 pound extra-lean hamburger
2 large onions, chopped
1 24-ounce jar spaghetti sauce
1 10-ounce box frozen corn
1 10-ounce box frozen peas
1/4 pound grated cheddar cheese, preferably low-fat

Optional: peppers, mushrooms, celery; 1 to 2 teaspoons chili powder and 1/2 teaspoon cumin for a Mexican flavor; 1 teaspoon oregano for more of an Italian flavor.

1. Cook the noodles according to package directions, draining them when they are slightly underdone because later they will be baked in the oven.

2. In a skillet, brown the hamburger and chopped onion. Drain the fat.
3. Add the spaghetti sauce and simmer for a few minutes to blend the flavors.
4. In a large casserole dish, combine the noodles, meat sauce, and still frozen corn and peas; mix well.
5. Top with grated cheese. Cover and bake at 350° for 30 minutes.

Nutrition Information: Total calories: 3,450
Calories per serving: 575

Nutrients	%	Grams
Carbohydrate	55	80
Protein	30	43
Fat	15	10

GOULASH

Most goulash recipes call for stew beef, but I usually make this with lean hamburger to reduce the cooking time. Serve with noodles and peas to boost the carbohydrate content of the meal.

Yield: 4 servings

1 pound extra-lean hamburger
1 large onion, chopped
1/2 teaspoon garlic powder or 1 clove garlic, minced
1 8-ounce can tomato sauce
1/8 teaspoon ground cloves
1/2 teaspoon basil
1 tablespoon molasses
Salt and pepper as desired

1. In a large skillet, brown the hamburger, onion, and garlic. Drain any grease.
2. Add the tomato sauce and seasonings. Cover, simmer from 20 minutes to 2 hours (longer time yields better flavor).

Nutrition Information: Total calories: 720
Calories per serving: 180

Nutrients	%	Grams
Carbohydrate	20	10
Protein	55	25
Fat	25	5

TORTILLA ROLL-UPS

This quick and easy casserole is a popular family food. You can also make it with ground turkey or diced chicken. For a vegetarian meal, replace the beef with kidney beans or pinto beans, and add chopped vegetables such as mushrooms, peppers, and onion.

Yield: 3 servings, 2 tortillas each

3/4 pound extra-lean ground beef (or ground turkey)
1 cup low-fat cottage cheese
1 tablespoon flour
1/2 teaspoon oregano
1/2 teaspoon basil
1/4 teaspoon garlic powder
Salt and pepper as desired
1 to 1-1/2 cups spaghetti sauce
6 6" flour or corn tortillas

Optional: 4 ounces shredded mozzarella cheese.

1. In a skillet, cook the beef (or turkey) until browned; drain the fat.
2. Stir in the cottage cheese and flour. Add the seasonings as desired.
3. Put a thin layer of spaghetti sauce in the bottom of a 9" × 9" baking pan.
4. Spoon about 1/3 cup meat mixture onto each tortilla; roll up jelly roll style. Place the tortillas, seam down, in the spaghetti sauce in the baking pan.
5. Pour the remaining sauce over the tortillas.
6. Cover with foil; bake in a 350° oven for 30 minutes.
7. If desired, uncover and sprinkle with mozzarella; bake for 3 to 5 minutes longer, or until cheese melts.

Nutrition Information: Total calories: 1,500
Calories per serving: 500

Nutrients	%	Grams
Carbohydrate	45	54
Protein	30	41
Fat	25	13

SWEET 'N SPICY ORANGE BEEF

Here's a welcome treat after a hard workout when you're hankering for something sweet but healthful. This goes nicely with cooked carrots and peas.

Yield: 3 servings

1 cup uncooked rice
1 pound extra-lean ground beef
1/4 cup orange marmalade
1/4 teaspoon red pepper flakes or a few dashes cayenne pepper

Optional mix-ins: cooked peas, diced celery, green peppers, pineapple chunks.

1. Cook the rice according to package directions.
2. In a skillet, cook the beef until browned; drain fat.
3. To the beef, add the marmalade, red pepper flakes, and cooked rice. Mix well. Add mix-ins as desired.

Nutrition Information: Total calories: 1,500
Calories per serving: 500

Nutrients	%	Grams
Carbohydrate	55	70
Protein	35	42
Fat	10	6

Stir-Fry Beef and Broccoli

For a richer flavor, marinate the beef for an hour or overnight. For simplicity, use frozen chopped broccoli in place of the fresh. Serve over rice.

Yield: 4 servings

1 pound extra-lean round steak or flank steak, thinly sliced
1 teaspoon oil
1 pound (2 large stalks) broccoli, cut into florets
1/2 cup water
2 tablespoons soy sauce
2 teaspoons cornstarch mixed into 1 tablespoon water

Optional: 2 tablespoons soy sauce and 1 tablespoon sherry as marinade; sliced onions, mushrooms, and carrots; 1 teaspoon sesame oil; dash hot pepper.

1. Slice the beef into thin strips. If time permits, place in the optional marinade and refrigerate for 1 hour or overnight.
2. Heat a large skillet, wok, or nonstick frying pan until very hot. Add 1 teaspoon oil, then the beef. Stir quickly, browning the beef on all sides. Remove the beef to a serving platter.
3. Add the broccoli to the frying pan along with 1/2 cup water and 2 tablespoons soy sauce. Cover and steam until tender-crisp, about 5 minutes.
4. Return the beef to the pan; stir in cornstarch and water mixture; cook until the liquid reaches a desired consistency.

Nutrition Information: Total calories: 840
Calories per serving (without rice): 210

Nutrients	%	Grams
Carbohydrate	20	10
Protein	65	35
Fat	15	4

PORK CHOPS BAKED WITH APPLE AND SWEET POTATO

Open this foil packet carefully to avoid getting burned by the steam.

Yield: 1 serving

1 lean pork loin cutlet, trimmed (about 5 ounces)
1 medium sweet potato
1 small apple

Optional: 1 tablespoon raisins; dash of cinnamon; salt and pepper as desired.

1. Slice the sweet potato thinly. Quarter, core, and slice the apple into eight pieces.
2. On a large piece of foil, put sweet potato slices, a pork chop, and then apple slices. If desired, sprinkle with raisins, cinnamon, salt, and pepper.
3. Wrap well; bake at 350° for 40 minutes.

Nutrition Information: Calories per serving: 450

Nutrients	%	Grams
Carbohydrate	50	55
Protein	30	34
Fat	20	10

PORK CHOPS IN APPLE CIDER

Apples and pork are a tasty combination; both go well served with rice. For a simple dinner, cook some rice along with the pork, adding extra cider, water, or both.

Yield: 1 serving

1 extra-lean pork chop or pork cutlet, trimmed (about 5 ounces, raw)
1/3 cup apple cider

Optional: 1/2 onion, sliced; 1 apple, sliced; salt, pepper, and basil as desired.

1. In a saucepan or small skillet, combine the pork and cider, along with onion, apple, and seasonings as desired.
2. Cover and simmer over medium-low heat for 20 minutes.
3. Skim the fat from the broth. If desired, thicken the broth with 1 teaspoon cornstarch mixed with 1 tablespoon water.

Nutrition Information: Calories per serving: 250

Nutrients	%	Grams
Carbohydrate	15	10
Protein	50	10
Fat	35	30

STIR-FRY PORK WITH FRUIT

This is a popular family food that appeals to children and adults alike. Pineapple is a nice alternative or addition to the mandarin oranges.

Yield: 4 servings

1 teaspoon oil
1 pound boneless pork cutlets, trimmed and sliced into thin strips
1/2 cup water
1/4 cup vinegar
2 tablespoons molasses
2 tablespoons soy sauce
1 medium apple, diced
1/4 cup raisins
1 11-ounce can mandarin orange slices
1 tablespoon cornstarch mixed in 1 tablespoon water

Optional: pineapple chunks; green pepper chunks; 1/4 cup chopped walnuts.

1. Heat the oil in a large skillet or wok. Add the sliced pork and stir-fry until browned.
2. Add the water, vinegar, molasses, soy sauce, diced apple, raisins, and mandarin oranges; add the peppers and pineapple as desired.
3. Bring to a boil; cover and simmer for 5 minutes.
4. Thicken the broth by slowly adding the cornstarch and water mixture and cooking until thickened to desired consistency.
5. Sprinkle with chopped walnuts, if desired.

Nutrition Information:

Total calories: 1,200
Calories per serving: 300

Nutrients	%	Grams
Carbohydrate	40	30
Protein	35	25
Fat	25	8

Eggs and Cheese

EGGS

Eggs have both positive and negative nutritional features. On the positive side, they are an economical and highly nutritious source of protein. They are nutrient dense, supplying a lot of vitamins and minerals and all essential amino acids. They store well in the refrigerator, are easy to cook, and are handy for breakfast, lunch, or dinner.

On the negative side, egg yolks are very high in cholesterol. One medium egg yolk contains about 210 milligrams of cholesterol, as compared to 30 milligrams in an ounce of cheese and 60 milligrams in a small serving of chicken. When cooking and baking, you can substitute two egg whites (with a trace of cholesterol) for one egg yolk in most recipes, or use cholesterol-free eggs or egg substitutes.

Health professionals still debate whether or not the cholesterol in eggs contributes to high blood cholesterol; a lot depends on your genetics. To date, the heart-healthy diet recommended by the American Heart Association limits intake to three egg yolks per week. One way to reduce your intake is to save eggs for quick and easy dinners, instead of eating them for breakfast.

CHEESE

Cheese also has positive and negative nutritional aspects. Cheese is a good source of protein, riboflavin, and calcium. It is economical and versatile, it keeps well, and it can be an enjoyable part of breakfast, lunch, dinner, snacks, and even desserts.

However, full-fat cheeses are high in saturated fat, sodium, and calories. Fortunately for our health, the food industry is now making several brands of low-fat cheeses. You can lower the fat content of your favorite hard cheese by melting it in the microwave oven. From 1 ounce of full-fat cheddar, you can drain off about a teaspoon of fat (about 4 grams, or half the original amount).

Cheese tastes best when eaten at room temperature, but it's easiest to grate, shred, or slice when it's cold or even partially frozen. I grate and freeze the odds and ends of cheese that accumulate in the refrigerator. It's ready and waiting whenever I want a quick handful to garnish a hot meal or bowl of chili or to add to a casserole.

EGG RECIPES

FRENCH TOAST WITH CHEESE
EGG-STUFFED BAKED POTATO
EGG-DROP SOUP

See also: Low-Fat Fried Rice

CHEESE RECIPES

EASY CHEESY NOODLES
PIZZA FONDUE
LAZY LASAGNA
EASY ENCHILADAS

See also: Moist Cornbread, Pasta With Spinach and Cottage Cheese, Stuffed Shells, Pasta Salad Parmesan, Turkey 'n Cheese Calzone, Meal-in-One Potato, Greek Stuffed Potato, Tortilla Roll-Ups, Eggplant-Tofu Parmesan, Cheesy Bean and Rice Casserole, Potato Snacks.

FRENCH TOAST WITH CHEESE

This is quick and easy for brunch or dinner. When served with maple syrup, it's my favorite recovery food after a long Sunday run.

Yield: 1 serving

1 egg or 2 egg whites, beaten
1/3 cup low-fat milk
Salt and pepper as desired
2 slices whole grain bread
1 to 2 slices cheese, preferably low-fat

Optional: maple syrup; orange marmalade.

1. Beat the eggs and milk; add salt and pepper.
2. Over a medium setting, heat a nonstick skillet.
3. Soak the bread in the egg and milk mixture; place in the skillet.
4. Cook until golden, turning once.
5. Sandwich the cheese between the two slices of French toast before serving.
6. If desired, serve with maple syrup or marmalade.

Nutrition Information: Total calories (no syrup): 325
(with 3 tablespoons syrup): 525

Nutrients	Without syrup %	Without syrup Grams	With syrup %	With syrup Grams
Carbohydrate	35	28	60	128
Protein	30	26	20	26
Fat	35	12	20	12

EGG-STUFFED BAKED POTATO

If you let the potato bake while you exercise, dinner will be ready when you are! Or, prepare it in the microwave oven. One of these potatoes alone may not provide adequate calories for a dinner. Plan to supplement this meal with soup and salad, or eat two potatoes.

Yield: 1 serving

1 large baking potato (1/2 pound; 3-1/4")
1 egg
1 ounce shredded cheese, preferably low-fat
Salt and pepper as desired

Optional: 1 to 2 tablespoons milk.

1. Prick the potato in several places with a fork. Bake in a 400° oven for an hour or until done; the potato should be tender if pierced with a fork. Or cook the potato for about 8 minutes in a microwave oven, letting it rest for an additional 3 minutes.
2. Cut an X on top of the baked potato. Fluff up the insides and make a well.
3. Optional: For moistness add 1 tablespoon of milk.
4. Break the egg into the well. Top with cheese and salt and pepper as desired.
5. Return to the oven until the egg is cooked, about 10 minutes. Or microwave at medium power for 1 to 2 minutes, being sure to pierce the yolk (otherwise, it will explode).

Nutrition Information: Calories per serving: 270

Nutrients	%	Grams
Carbohydrate	50	34
Protein	25	17
Fat	25	8

EGG-DROP SOUP

Easy to make and low in calories. I often add cooked rice or ramen noodles to boost the carbohydrates.

Yield: 1 serving

1 cup chicken broth (homemade, canned, or from bouillon cubes)
2 teaspoons cornstarch mixed with 2 tablespoons cold water
1 egg

Optional: dash of soy sauce, hot pepper, or sesame oil; spinach leaves; broccoli, thinly sliced; bean sprouts; Chinese cabbage, shredded; bok choy, chopped; scallions, chopped; rice, cooked; ramen noodles, cooked; chicken, turkey, or fish (leftovers, or precooked in the broth).

1. Bring the broth to a boil.
2. Beat the egg slightly, adding soy sauce if desired.

3. Thicken the broth by slowly stirring in the cornstarch and water mixture.
2. Stir the boiling soup quickly. While it swirls, slowly add the beaten egg. Remove from the heat. Do not stir.
3. If desired, add vegetables. They will cook in the heat of the soup, remaining crunchy but becoming warmed.

Nutrition Information: Calories per serving: 125

Nutrients	%	Grams
Carbohydrate	25	8
Protein	25	8
Fat	50	7

EASY CHEESY NOODLES

Another family favorite, served as a main dish with a green vegetable and salad or as a side dish with chicken or fish. Different types of cheese—Parmesan, low-fat cheddar, or Swiss—offer different flavors.

Yield: 4 servings

8 ounces dry egg noodles
1 tablespoon olive oil
6 ounces shredded cheese, preferably low-fat

Optional: salt, pepper, garlic powder, Italian seasonings, parsley; diced tomatoes, steamed broccoli, peas, or other vegetables.

1. Cook the noodles according to package directions. drain.
2. Mix in the oil, seasonings to taste, and shredded cheese.

Nutrition Information: Total calories: 1,300
Calories per serving: 325

Nutrients	%	Grams
Carbohydrate	56	45
Protein	22	18
Fat	22	8

PIZZA FONDUE

This family favorite serves well as a friendly, informal meal. It's also ideal for camping trips or picnics if you have a small camp stove. To boost the carbohydrate content, eat more bread and less fondue.

Yield: 5 servings

1 16-ounce jar spaghetti or pizza sauce
8 ounces grated mozzarella cheese
2 tablespoons flour
1 loaf French or Italian bread, broken into chunks

Optional: celery chunks, green pepper cubes, mushroom caps.

1. Heat the spaghetti sauce in a fondue pot or medium-sized saucepan.
2. Shake together the grated cheese and flour. (This step is optional, but helps to thicken the sauce.)
3. Gradually melt the cheese into the spaghetti sauce, stirring constantly.
4. Keep the fondue warm by placing the pot on a pot stand, heating tray, or camp stove.
5. Using forks, dip chunks of bread or raw veggies into the pizza fondue. Enjoy!

Nutrition Information: Total calories: 2,200
Calories per serving: 550

Nutrients	%	Grams
Carbohydrate	55	77
Protein	20	27
Fat	25	15

LAZY LASAGNA

The recipe eliminates one big step—precooking the noodles! The noodles cook during the baking process, absorbing the water added to the tomato sauce. This recipe may seem skimpy on cheese, but it's designed for people who want to carbo-load, not fat-load. Many lasagnas with thick cheese layers are extremely high in fat and protein.

Yield: 8 servings

16 ounces part-skim ricotta or low-fat cottage cheese, or a combination of the two
1 tablespoon flour
1/4 to 1/2 cup water if needed to thin the cheese mixture
48 ounces spaghetti sauce diluted with 3 cups water
1 16-ounce box lasagna noodles

Optional: 1 to 2 10-ounce boxes frozen spinach or chopped broccoli; 4 ounces shredded low-fat mozzarella for topping; 2 teaspoons oregano, 1 teaspoon basil, 1/8 teaspoon garlic powder, or salt and pepper as desired for the cheese mixture; mix-ins of 1 pound browned hamburger, ground turkey, or kidney beans; 1 to 2 cups sliced mushrooms, chopped onions, diced green peppers, and other vegetables.

1. Cook the spinach, broccoli, or other vegetables as desired; drain.
2. In a large bowl, mix the vegetables with the ricotta, desired seasonings, and the flour; add water if the mixture is too thick to spread easily.
3. In a nonstick oblong pan (9" × 13"), alternate 4 layers of the diluted sauce, uncooked lasagna noodles, and ricotta mixture, ending with sauce.
4. Top with cheese, if desired.
5. Cover tightly with foil and bake at 350° for 75 minutes. Let stand for 10 minutes before serving.

Nutrition Information: Total calories: 3,600
Calories per serving: 450

Nutrients	%	Grams
Carbohydrate	60	68
Protein	15	17
Fat	25	12

EASY ENCHILADAS

Many Mexican dishes are ladened with fat. Here's a lower fat version of a popular meal. For variety, add lean ground beef, ground turkey, beans, or tofu to the sauce.

Yield: 3 servings

1 8-ounce can enchilada sauce
1 4-ounce can chopped green chiles
1 8-ounce jar salsa
2 cups fat-free sour cream
6 ounces low-fat cheddar cheese, grated
1 8-ounce bag baked corn tortilla chips

1. In a saucepan, combine the enchilada sauce, chiles, salsa, fat-free sour cream, and 4 ounces of the grated cheese. Heat.
2. Spray a 13″ × 9″ pan with cooking spray, then line the pan with the tortilla chips. Pour on the enchilada sauce. Sprinkle the top with the remaining 2 ounces of grated cheese.
3. Bake uncovered at 350° for 10 to 15 minutes, or until bubbly.

Nutrition Information: Total calories: 1,500
Calories per serving: 500

Nutrients	%	Grams
Carbohydrate	60	75
Protein	20	25
Fat	20	11

Tofu

Tofu, also known as bean curd, is made from an extract of soybeans. It is a complete protein that contains all the essential amino acids. Tofu has no cholesterol and is relatively low in calories and sodium. Surprisingly, about half the calories in tofu do come from fat—unsaturated fat, that is. Tofu is a popular alternative to meat, and can be a source of calcium for people allergic to milk. It is protective against heart disease and cancer and is a very healthful addition to your diet.

Tofu is found in most supermarkets in the refrigerated vegetable or dairy sections. You can buy soft or firm tofu cakes that are packaged in water; be sure to check the "sell by" date, and buy the freshest brand. Soft or silken tofu is preferable for blending into a smooth cream; firm tofu is good to crumble or slice. To store tofu, drain off the water, place the tofu in a container with a tight lid, cover with fresh cold water, and keep it in the refrigerator. If you change the water every other day, it will keep up to a week without spoiling.

Tofu itself has very little flavor; it takes on the flavors of the foods with which it's prepared. For example, tofu mixed with soy sauce takes on a soy flavor; with chili, a chili flavor. Due to this versatility, tofu lends itself to many recipes: spaghetti, salads, chili, Chinese stir-fry, and even salad dressings. To achieve an interesting, spongy texture, freeze the tofu for at least two days. After it has thawed, squeeze out the water (as if it were a kitchen sponge), tear the tofu into chunks, and add them to spaghetti sauce, chili, soups, or other dishes.

TOFU RECIPES

PAN-FRIED TOFU SLICES
SWEET AND SOUR TOFU
HOT AND SOUR SOUP
SCRAMBLED TOFU
SLOPPY JOEFUS
EGGPLANT-TOFU PARMESAN
TOFU SALAD DRESSING

See also: Chili, Stir-Fried Vegetables, Egg-Drop Soup, Easy Enchiladas, Protein Shake, Mighty Mashed Potato.

PAN-FRIED TOFU SLICES

This pan-fried tofu can be eaten as a main course or in sandwiches.

Yield: 1 serving

1/3 cake firm tofu, sliced
1 teaspoon oil, preferably sesame or olive
Seasonings as desired: salt, pepper, garlic powder, curry, cumin

1. Slice the tofu into 1/4"-thick pieces. Season as desired.
2. Heat the oil in a skillet using a moderate setting. Add the tofu.
3. Cook about 5 minutes per side, until golden and crispy.

Nutrition Information: Calories per serving: 200

Nutrients	%	Grams
Carbohydrate	5	2
Protein	40	20
Fat	55	12

SWEET AND SOUR TOFU

This pungent recipe is suitable for adding to stir-fried chicken or pork. For a mild sauce, start out using less sugar or vinegar. Serve with rice.

Yield: 4 servings

1 cup pineapple juice
1/4 cup soy sauce
1/4 cup honey or sugar
1/4 cup vinegar
1/4 cup catsup
2 tablespoons cornstarch mixed into 2 tablespoons water
2 pounds firm tofu, sliced into 1" cubes
2 green peppers, cut into strips
1 20-ounce can pineapple chunks

Optional: sliced carrots, celery, water chestnuts, other fruits or vegetables.

1. In a saucepan, combine the juice, soy sauce, honey, vinegar, and catsup. Bring to a boil, then add the cornstarch and water mixture. Cook over low heat for 3 minutes, or until thickened.
2. Stir in the tofu, green peppers, and pineapple chunks. Cook over low heat for 5 minutes.
3. Serve over rice.

Nutrition Information: Total calories: 2,000
Calories per serving: 500

Nutrients	%	Grams
Carbohydrate	45	13
Protein	25	30
Fat	30	17

HOT AND SOUR SOUP

Who says you have to eat at a Chinese restaurant to enjoy this soup?

Yield: 4 servings

5 cups chicken broth, canned, homemade, or from bouillon cubes
1 tablespoon soy sauce
2 tablespoons cider vinegar
1/8 teaspoon cayenne pepper
1 16-ounce cake firm tofu, diced
4 tablespoons cornstarch
4 tablespoons water

Optional: 1 egg, beaten; 1 teaspoon sugar; 1 tablespoon sherry; 1 teaspoon sesame oil; 2 cups chopped Chinese vegetables or raw spinach; 2 tablespoons finely sliced scallion greens.

1. Combine the chicken broth, soy sauce, vinegar, and pepper (and sherry) in a large pot and bring to a boil.
2. Add the tofu and vegetables and simmer for 5 minutes.
3. In a small bowl, combine the cornstarch and water to form a paste. Add the paste to the soup and stir until the broth is thickened.
4. *Optional:* Add the egg slowly, gently stirring it into the soup. (Add the sesame oil and scallions, as desired.)

Nutrition Information: Total calories: 600
Calories per serving: 150

Nutrition	%	Grams
Carbohydrate	25	10
Protein	35	12
Fat	40	7

SCRAMBLED TOFU

Scrambled tofu can be made in several ways, depending on your mood. Serve either with rice and vegetables or stuffed into a pita pocket.

Yield: 4 servings

2 teaspoons margarine or olive oil
1 small onion, diced
1 green pepper, diced
1 pound firm tofu, crumbled

Optional: raisins, chopped walnuts, and curry powder; sesame seeds, sesame oil (instead of margarine), and soy sauce; garlic powder; salt; pepper.

1. Melt the margarine in a skillet; add the onion and green pepper. Sauté until tender.
2. Add the crumbled tofu and seasonings; heat thoroughly.

Nutrition Information: Total calories: 750
Calories per serving: 190

Nutrients	%	Grams
Carbohydrate	12	5
Protein	38	18
Fat	50	10

SLOPPY JOEFUS

This is a tasty version of the original Sloppy Joe, made with browned hamburger or ground turkey.

Yield: 3 servings

1 pound firm tofu, crumbled
1 bottle chili sauce
3 bulky rolls or English muffins

Optional: grated low-fat mozzarella or cheddar cheese.

1. Pour the chili sauce into a saucepan.
2. Crumble the tofu into the chili sauce; heat over medium heat.
3. Toast the rolls or English muffins; top with the tofu mixture.
4. If desired, sprinkle with cheese.

Nutrition Information: Total calories: 1,350
Calories per serving: 445

Nutrients	%	Grams
Carbohydrate	50	55
Protein	25	28
Fat	25	12

EGGPLANT-TOFU PARMESAN

This dish tastes even better the second day, when the flavors have melded. It's a good sandwich filling when stuffed into a pita pocket. As a main dish, serve with rice. Lean hamburger or ground turkey can be used in place of, or in addition to, the tofu.

Yield: 4 servings

1 large (2-pound) eggplant, cut lengthwise into 1/2" slices
1 24-ounce jar spaghetti sauce
1 pound firm tofu, crumbled
1/2 cup grated Parmesan cheese

1. Place the eggplant slices on a flat pan and broil for about 5 minutes on each side, until golden and tender.
2. Arrange half the slices in a flat baking dish coated with a thin layer of spaghetti sauce.
3. Add layers of tofu, Parmesan, and sauce.
4. Add second layers of eggplant, tofu, and sauce. End with a sprinkling of Parmesan.
5. Bake covered at 350° for 25 minutes, or until heated.

Nutrition Information: Total calories: 1,440
Calories per serving: 480

Nutrients	%	Grams
Carbohydrate	30	27
Protein	30	27
Fat	40	16

TOFU SALAD DRESSING

This is an excellent way to boost the protein value of a tossed salad. Be creative with added seasonings—Italian, curry, Mexican, sweet and sour. Whatever your favorite dressing, you can adapt it to this tofu base.

Yield: 4 servings (1/2 cup each)

1 cake silken tofu (about 16 ounces)
Water or vinegar
Seasonings to taste:

- garlic, oregano, basil, or parsley
- curry and sweetener
- crumbled blue cheese
- chili, cayenne, or cumin

1. In a blender, whip the tofu until it's smooth. Add the water or vinegar to make it the desired consistency.
2. Add seasonings to taste. Blend well. Store in a covered container.

Nutrition Information: Total calories: 560
Calories per serving: 140

Nutrients	%	Grams
Carbohydrate	5	2
Protein	45	15
Fat	50	8

Beans

Beans—protein-rich foods with little fat and no cholesterol—are some of nature's greatest foods. They help lower blood cholesterol, control blood sugar, fight cancer, reduce problems with constipation, build muscles with their protein, fuel muscles with their carbohydrate, and nourish muscles with lots of B vitamins, iron, zinc, magnesium, copper, folic acid, and potassium.

Many athletes snicker at beans because of their potential to produce intestinal gas and discomfort. Beans can contribute to gas production because they contain types of fiber and sugar the body can't break down. Instead of being digested or absorbed in the small intestine like other foods are, they pass into the large intestine where they're broken down by bacteria that are naturally part of the intestinal flora. There they ferment, forming carbon dioxide and other gases that can make you feel distended, crampy, or gassy. This flatulence is highly individual, depending on the bacteria that inhabit your large intestine. Some people can eat beans with no problems; others experience great physical and social distress. If beans cause you intestinal problems, eat small amounts. You can also try Beano™, a product that when added to beans helps reduce gas formation.

Because beans are a healthful source of both protein and carbohydrate, vegetarian meals such as chili, hummus, bean and rice casseroles, and other bean meals are perfect for a sports diet. When beans are the only protein source, be sure to eat them in large quantities to consume adequate protein (see chapter 8). Or if you are a meat-eater who wants to become more of a vegetarian, replace part or all of the meat in recipes with more beans, such as replacing ground beef in chili or lasagna with kidney beans.

The following recipes offer some quick and easy suggestions to help you enjoy these high-protein, low-fat, carbohydrate-rich additions to your sports diet. Canned beans or home-cooked dried beans are nutritionally similar. I generally use the canned; they're quicker and more convenient.

Here are some popular types of beans:

Bean	Description	Popular uses
Navy	Small white ovals	In soups, stews, and Boston baked beans; great pureed
Kidney	Kidney-shaped	Often used in chili or three-bean salads
Pinto	Light brown medium ovals	Refried in stews, dips, and many Tex-Mex dishes
Great northern	Large white ovals	Soups, stews
Garbanzo	Medium tan, bumpy balls	Salads, hummus

If you prefer home cooked beans, here are some tips:

• Beans (except for lentils) should be soaked overnight or for 6 to 8 hours in water at room temperature. This soak shortens the cooking time, and improves the flavor, texture, and appearance of the beans. Soaking also reduces the beans' gas-causing qualities.

If you want to speed the soaking process, add beans to a large pot of boiling water, boil them for 2 minutes, cover, then remove them from the heat and let stand for an hour. Drain and rinse them and then they'll be ready to cook.

• Beans cook nicely in a crock-pot (5 to 10 hours, moderate heat) or pressure cooker (10 to 35 minutes), depending upon how much time you have to cook.

• Be sure to use a large enough kettle. Beans expand!

• Cook enough beans for more than one meal. They refrigerate and freeze well. For convenience, freeze them in individual portions.

• Because beans lack the amino acid methionine, serve them with methionine-rich rice or corn to enhance their protein value.

For more complete information about preparing homemade beans and creating bean dishes, read cookbooks that specialize in vegetarian cookery. Appendix A has some additional reading suggestions.

RECIPES

QUICK AND EASY BEAN IDEAS
BEANS AND RICE
CHILI
BLACK AND WHITE CHILI
MEXICAN BAKED CHICKEN AND PINTO BEANS
MEXICAN SALAD
TORTILLA LASAGNA
CHICKEN BLACK BEAN SOUP
CHEESY BEAN AND RICE CASSEROLE
BEANS BAKED WITH APPLES
BARBECUE BEAN CASSEROLE
HUMMUS

See also: Pasta and Beans, Irish Tacos, Tortilla Roll-Ups, Easy Enchiladas.

QUICK AND EASY BEAN IDEAS

- In a blender, mix black or pinto beans, salsa, and cheese. Heat in the microwave and use as a dip or on top of tortillas or potatoes.
- Sauté garlic and onions in a little oil; add canned beans (whole or mashed), and heat together. Eat with rice or rolled in a tortilla.
- Add beans to salads, spaghetti sauce, soups, and stews for a protein booster.
- Make an easy burrito: top a tortilla with 1/2 can vegetarian refried beans, 1/2 cup cottage cheese, salsa, chopped lettuce, and tomato as desired. Roll into a burrito, and heat in the microwave oven.
- Combine black beans, refried beans, and salsa to taste. Spoon onto a tortilla. Top with more salsa and cheese, as desired.

BEANS AND RICE

Use black beans with brown rice or red beans with white rice. Any combination works well and provides a high-carbohydrate, low-fat meal that is a good source of protein.

Yield: 2 big servings

1 to 2 tablespoons oil
1/2 cup chopped onion
2 cups cooked rice, brown or white
1 16-ounce can or 2 cups cooked pinto, kidney, or other beans
    of your choice
Salt and pepper as desired

Optional: 1/2 cup chopped celery; 1 red or green pepper, diced; 1 or 2 jalapeño peppers, seeded and finely diced; 1 large tomato, diced; 1 cup corn; 1 tablespoon chili powder; 1 tablespoon chopped parsley; 1/4 teaspoon garlic powder or 2 cloves minced fresh garlic; several dashes hot sauce.

1. In a large skillet, heat the oil and sauté the onion (and garlic) until tender.
2. Add the rice and beans (and other seasonings) and simmer for 5 minutes to blend the flavors.

Nutrition Information: Total calories: 960
Calories per serving: 480

Nutrients	%	Grams
Carbohydrate	70	84
Protein	15	18
Fat	15	8

CHILI

As is true of most casseroles, the flavor of chili improves with age. Make a big batch and enjoy it more as the week goes on! For variety, serve it as a Mexican Salad. Moist Cornbread is a nice accompaniment.

Rather than making chili with beef, try ground turkey. For vegetarian chili, replace the meat with corn, tofu, or shredded cheese.

Yield: 4 servings

1 large onion, chopped
1 pound lean hamburger or ground turkey
2 16-ounce cans kidney beans
1 16-ounce can crushed tomatoes
2 tablespoons chili powder

Optional: 2 teaspoons cumin; salt, pepper, and garlic powder to taste; 1 tablespoon molasses, 1 pound diced tofu, 1 to 2 cups corn, or cheese shredded on top for protein; chopped mushrooms, green peppers, broccoli, green beans, or raisins as mix-ins.

1. In a large skillet, brown the chopped onion with the hamburger or turkey. Drain the grease. If using tofu, sauté it with the onion in a little bit of olive oil.
2. Add the beans, tomatoes, seasonings, and optional mix-ins.
3. Cover. Simmer for 15 minutes to 2 hours—the longer, the better.

Nutrition Information: Total calories (with meat): 1,900
Calories per serving: 475

Nutrients	%	Grams
Carbohydrate	50	30
Protein	40	47
Fat	10	5

BLACK AND WHITE CHILI

This is a simple variation of the standard chili recipes that use kidney beans. The cumin enhances the flavor. If you have none, you can make the recipe without it. Better yet, dash to the store and discover the pleasure of this flavorful herb.

Yield: 3 servings

1 teaspoon oil, preferably olive or canola
1 medium onion (1 cup), diced
2 cups chicken broth, canned or from bouillon cubes
1 6-ounce can tomato paste
1 or 2 4-ounce cans green chiles, chopped
1 teaspoon cumin
1 16-ounce can black beans, drained and rinsed
1 16-ounce can navy beans, drained and rinsed

Optional: 1 pound ground turkey.

1. In a large soup pot, heat the oil over medium-high heat, add the onions (and ground turkey, as desired); cook for 5 minutes.
2. Add the broth, tomato paste, chiles, cumin, and beans. Bring to a boil.
3. Reduce heat to low, simmer for 10 to 15 minutes, stirring occasionally.

Nutrition Information: Total calories: 1,140
Calories per serving: 380

Nutrients	%	Grams
Carbohydrate	65	62
Protein	20	19
Fat	15	6

MEXICAN BAKED CHICKEN AND PINTO BEANS

A spicy favorite! When cooking for myself, I wrap one piece of chicken, a quarter of a can of beans, and 1/4 cup of salsa in a piece of foil, bake it in the oven, and have no dishes to wash!

Yield: 4 servings

2 16-ounce cans pinto beans
4 pieces chicken, skinned
1 cup salsa

1. Drain the beans and put in the bottom of a baking dish.
2. Put the skinless chicken on top; cover with the salsa.
3. Cover and bake in a 350° oven for 25 to 30 minutes. If desired, bake uncovered the last 10 minutes to thicken the pan juices.

Nutrition Information: Total calories: 1,400
Calories per serving: 350

Nutrients	%	Grams
Carbohydrate	40	35
Protein	35	30
Fat	25	10

MEXICAN SALAD

This cool, low-fat version of taco salad is an appealing summertime alternative to a bowl of steaming hot chili. I pack it into a plastic container for lunch at work or enjoy it for a no-cook dinner.

Yield: 1 serving

1 to 2 cups chopped lettuce
1 cup chili, cold (see above recipes)

Optional: 1/2 tomato, chopped; 1 ounce shredded cheese, preferably low-fat cheddar; 1/4 onion, chopped; salsa to taste.

1. On a plate, put as much chopped lettuce as you'd like to eat.
2. Cover with the chili.
3. If desired, add the optional ingredients.

Nutrition Information: Calories per serving: 325

Nutrients	%	Grams
Carbohydrate	50	40
Protein	40	32
Fat	10	4

TORTILLA LASAGNA

Tortillas are easy, precooked alternatives to lasagna noodles, and they taste great.

Yield: 4 servings

1 16-ounce container cottage cheese
1 16-ounce can kidney or pinto beans
1 tablespoon flour
1/4 teaspoon dried red pepper or 1/8 teaspoon cayenne
Salt, pepper, and garlic powder, as desired
1 tablespoon chili powder, as desired
6 tortillas, flour or corn
Sauce:
1 32-ounce can *crushed* tomatoes
2 tablespoons chili powder
1/4 teaspoon red pepper flakes
1 tablespoon molasses

Optional: 1 10-ounce package frozen chopped spinach or broccoli, cooked; 1 cup chopped mushrooms, peppers, or other vegetables; 1 cup corn; 1 pound lean ground beef or turkey, browned and drained.

1. Mix together the cottage cheese, beans, flour, seasonings, and vegetables as desired.
2. Make sauce by combining the tomatoes and seasonings.
3. Preheat the oven to 375°.
4. In a 9" × 9" nonstick pan or casserole dish, alternate layers of sauce, tortillas, and cheese mixture. Top with sauce.
5. Bake, covered, for 30 minutes. Let stand about 5 minutes before cutting into squares.

Nutrition Information: Total calories: 1,800
Calories per serving: 450

Nutrients	%	Grams
Carbohydrate	60	68
Protein	25	28
Fat	15	7

CHICKEN BLACK BEAN SOUP

Beans provide a hearty foundation for wholesome soups. This recipe uses canned beans as a quick alternative to cooking dried beans. To make this recipe into an even heartier meal, add leftover cooked pasta (or cook pasta in the soup during the last 8 to 12 minutes).

Yield: 4 servings

4 boneless, skinless chicken breasts
5 cups water or broth
2 carrots, peeled and sliced
2 tomatoes, chopped
1/2 onion, chopped
3 to 5 cloves garlic, crushed
2 16-ounce cans black beans, rinsed and drained
1 teaspoon dried oregano

Optional: 2 to 4 cups cooked pasta shells or bow ties; 2 ounces grated low-fat cheddar cheese; hot red pepper flakes; 1/2 cup marsala wine.

1. In a large soup pot, cover the chicken breasts, vegetables, garlic, beans, and seasonings in water. Bring the water to a boil, reduce the heat, and simmer for about 20 minutes, or until done.
2. Remove the chicken pieces from the broth and set them aside to cool. Keep the broth warm over low heat. (Optional: Add the cooked pasta.)
3. Dice the chicken into small pieces. Return it to the soup and heat through.
4. Garnish with grated cheese and red pepper flakes, as desired.

Nutrition Information: Total calories: 1,200
Calories per serving: 300

Nutrients	%	Grams
Carbohydrate	45	33
Protein	45	34
Fat	10	3

CHEESY BEAN AND RICE CASSEROLE

This is a hearty, stick-to-your-ribs winter meal that's a welcome treat after skiing. The green chiles add a spicy zip!

Yield: 4 servings

3 cups cooked rice
1 16-ounce can kidney or pinto beans, drained
1 large onion, chopped
1 clove minced garlic or 1/8 teaspoon garlic powder
1 cup low-fat cottage cheese
1 tablespoon flour
3 ounces grated cheddar cheese, preferably low-fat

Optional: 1 4-ounce can green chile peppers, chopped.

1. In a large mixing bowl, combine rice, beans, onion, garlic, cottage cheese, and flour (and chile peppers).
2. Pour the mixture into a casserole dish; top with the grated cheese.
3. Bake covered at 350° for 30 minutes.

Nutrition Information: Total calories: 1,600
Calories per serving: 400

Nutrients	%	Grams
Carbohydrate	60	60
Protein	25	25
Fat	15	7

BEANS BAKED WITH APPLES

A simple variation from plain old canned beans. Add other fruits such as raisins, pineapple, and pears for variety.

Yield: 3 servings

1 16-ounce can baked beans   1 tablespoon mustard
1 tablespoon molasses   1 large apple, chopped
1 tablespoon vinegar

1. Mix all the ingredients in a saucepan.
2. Simmer gently on the stove top for 10 to 15 minutes.

Nutrition Information: Total calories: 690
Calories per serving: 230

Nutrients	%	Grams
Carbohydrate	75	45
Protein	15	10
Fat	10	3

BARBEQUE BEAN CASSEROLE

Served hot in the winter, these beans are a hearty side dish or entrée. In summer, I sprinkle them cold on a salad, along with a scoop of low-fat cottage cheese, to boost the salad's protein value. If you want to make a smaller quantity, the recipe works well with only one or two types of beans.

Yield: 8 servings

1 16-ounce can red kidney beans
1 16-ounce can pinto beans
1 16-ounce can chick-peas
3/4 cup barbecue sauce
2 tablespoons brown sugar
2 teaspoons mustard

1. Drain the beans.
2. In a saucepan or casserole dish combine the beans, barbecue sauce, sugar, and mustard.
3. Simmer on the stove top over low heat for 15 to 60 minutes (longer time yields better flavor). Or, bake them in a 350° oven for 30 to 60 minutes; uncover the last 15 minutes to thicken the sauce.

Nutrition Information: Total calories: 1,600
Calories per serving: 200

Nutrients	%	Grams
Carbohydrate	70	35
Protein	20	10
Fat	10	2

HUMMUS

This tasty spread is a higher-carbohydrate alternative to peanut butter. You might find, as I did, that hummus becomes a favorite sandwich filling (spread inside pita halves), snack (rolled into a tor-tilla), or dip for cucumber slices, green pepper strips, celery sticks, or pita wedges.

The secret ingredient in hummus is tahini, or sesame paste. You can buy tahini in the ethnic food section of supermarkets or health food stores. Store leftover tahini in the refrigerator. Try tahini mixed with plain pasta, too!

Yield: about 2 cups

> 1 16-ounce can chick-peas
> 1 tablespoon lemon juice, bottled or fresh
> 1 clove garlic or 1/4 teaspoon garlic powder to taste
> 2 tablespoons tahini or peanut butter
> Salt and pepper as desired

Optional: dash of cayenne; 1 tablespoon parsley; 1/4 teaspoon cumin.

1. Drain the chick-peas, saving 1/4 cup of the liquid.
2. In a blender or food processor, mix the chick-peas, 1/4 cup liquid, lemon juice, garlic, tahini, and seasonings.
3. Blend until smooth. If you don't have a blender, mash the chick-peas with the back of a fork.
4. Serve with pita or as dip for vegetables.

Nutrition Information: Total calories: 625
Calories per serving (1/4 cup): 80

Nutrients	%	Grams
Carbohydrate	55	11
Protein	15	3
Fat	30	3

Beverages

Water always has been and always will be an appropriate fluid replacement for thirsty athletes. When you tire of plain old water, try some of these liquid refreshers. They not only quench your thirst, but they also refuel your muscles with carbohydrates and replace other nutrients that you might lose through sweating.

BEVERAGE RECIPES

HOMEMADE SPORTS DRINK
SUNSHINE REFRESHER
FRUIT SMOOTHIE
BANANA FROSTIE
ORANGE-PINEAPPLE DELIGHT
STRAWBERRY FIZZ
MAPLE GRAHAM SHAKE
PROTEIN SHAKE
HOMEMADE GINGERALE
HOT SPICED TEA MIX
LOW-CAL CAPPUCCINO
WARM MILK IDEAS

HOMEMADE SPORTS DRINK

For a low-cost fluid replacer that has a nutritional profile similar to the more expensive commercial sports drinks, try this simple recipe.

Yield: 1 quart

4 tablespoons sugar

1/4 teaspoon salt

1/4 cup boiling water

1/4 cup orange juice (*not* concentrate) or 2 tablespoons lemon juice

3-3/4 cups cold water

1. In the bottom of a pitcher, dissolve the sugar and salt in the hot water.
2. Add the juice and the remaining water; chill.
3. Quench that thirst!

Nutrition Information: Total calories: 200
Calories per 8 ounces: 50

Nutrients	%	Grams
Carbohydrate	100	12
Sodium		110 mg
Potassium		30 mg

SUNSHINE REFRESHER

Light and tasty, this is a refreshing recovery drink after a hot workout.

Yield: 2 servings (about 12 ounces each)

1 cup (8 ounces) plain or vanilla yogurt

1/2 cup milk, skim or low-fat

1/2 cup orange juice

8 ice cubes

1 tablespoon honey, sugar, or sweetener as desired

1. Combine all ingredients in a blender.
2. Whip until smooth and frothy.

Nutrition Information: Total calories (made with skim milk and yogurt): 250
Calories per serving: 125

Nutrients	%	Grams
Carbohydrate	80	25
Protein	20	6
Fat	—	—

FRUIT SMOOTHIE

Fruit smoothies are popular for breakfasts and snacks. The ingredients can vary according to individual tastes. Some tried-and-true combinations include banana and strawberries in orange juice and melon and pineapple in pineapple juice. Almost any combination works! For a thick, frosty shake, use fruit that has been frozen. When you have a surplus of ripe fresh fruit, prevent spoilage by slicing the fruit into chunks and freezing them; then the fruit is ready for blending into a smoothie.

Yield: 1 serving

1/2 cup yogurt (plain or flavored) or milk
1 cup fruit juice
1/2 to 1 cup fruit, fresh, frozen, or canned

Optional: 1/4 cup milk powder, Grape-Nuts, wheat germ, oat bran, or graham crackers.

1. Place all ingredients in a blender and whip until smooth.

Nutrition Information: Calories per serving: 250

Nutrients	%	Grams
Carbohydrate	80	50-60
Protein	10	5
Fat	10	3

BANANA FROSTIE

This wonderful shake tastes sinfully good, and it's also excellent poured over your morning bowl of cereal! If you use less milk, you'll end up with banana "ice cream" thick enough to be eaten with a spoon.

Whenever you have a surplus of bananas, peel them, cut them into chunks, and freeze them so they'll be ready and waiting to be whipped into this frosty treat.

Yield: 1 serving

1 banana, in frozen chunks
1 cup milk, preferably low-fat

Optional: honey, brown sugar, or a sugar substitute; dash of cinnamon; 1/4 teaspoon vanilla.

1. Put frozen banana chunks into a blender with milk.
2. Blend on medium speed until smooth.
3. If desired, add sweetener and flavorings.

Nutrition Information: Calories per serving: 220 (made with 1% milk)

Nutrients	%	Grams
Carbohydrate	75	40
Protein	15	8
Fat	10	3

ORANGE-PINEAPPLE DELIGHT

A thirst-quenching way to boost potassium intake.

Yield: 1 serving

1/2 cup orange juice
1/2 cup pineapple juice
1 medium banana, cut into chunks

Optional: 4 ice cubes or 1/2 cup seltzer.

1. Combine the juices and banana in a blender.
2. Cover and blend at high speed until smooth and thick, about 1 minute.
3. Serve over ice or blend the ice cubes in the juice for a frosty drink. Add seltzer for a sparkling treat.

Nutrition Information: Calories per serving: 240

Nutrients	%	Grams
Carbohydrate	99	59
Protein	1	1
Fat	—	0

STRAWBERRY FIZZ

Seltzer makes a wonderfully fun and foamy treat when added to blender drinks. Try lots of combinations: peaches, pineapple chunks, whatever!

Yield: 1 serving

1 cup vanilla yogurt or low-fat milk
1/2 cup strawberries, fresh or frozen
1/2 cup seltzer

1. Combine yogurt and strawberries in a blender.
2. Cover and mix well.
3. Add seltzer; blend 2 to 3 seconds to mix.
4. Pour into a tall glass. Be prepared for it to foam up.

Nutrition Information: Calories per serving: 210

Nutrients	%	Grams
Carbohydrate	70	37
Protein	20	10
Fat	10	2

Maple Graham Shake

This is popular for a quick breakfast or snack. To make it into a higher calorie weight-gain supplement, add 1/4 cup milk powder and 2 or 3 more graham crackers. For variety, replace the graham crackers with breakfast cereals.

Yield: 1 serving

1 cup milk, preferably low-fat
1 to 2 tablespoons maple syrup
4 graham cracker sheets (8 squares), crumbled

Optional: dash cinnamon or nutmeg; a banana.

1. Combine ingredients in a blender.
2. Cover and blend 1 minute on medium speed, or until smooth.

Nutrition Information: Calories per serving: 400 (made with 1% milk)

Nutrients	%	Grams
Carbohydrate	70	70
Protein	10	12
Fat	20	8

Protein Shake

This shake is a simple way to not only boost protein and calcium but also your intake of health-protective tofu (see chapter 2). This recipe uses silken tofu, which has about 5 grams of protein per quarter-cake. Extra-firm tofu has more protein (10 grams per quarter-cake), but it blends poorly. Dry milk powder, with 11 grams of protein per quarter-cup, boosts protein as well.

Yield: 1 serving

1/4 cake silken tofu   1/4 cup dried milk powder
1 cup low-fat milk   2 tablespoons chocolate milk mix

1. Combine ingredients in a blender.
2. Cover and blend for 1 minute, or until smooth.

Nutrition Information: Total calories: 350

Nutrients	%	Grams
Carbohydrate	60	52
Protein	30	26
Fat	10	4

HOMEMADE GINGERALE

This has a delightfully refreshing taste—worth the preparation. Ginger is known to calm upset stomachs and reduce morning sickness.

Yield: 4 servings

2 tablespoons fresh ginger root, chopped
2 lemon rinds
3 to 4 tablespoons honey or other sweetener to taste
1 cup boiling water
1 quart seltzer

1. Put the chopped ginger and lemon rinds in a small bowl with the honey.
2. Pour in 1 cup of boiling water (or just enough to cover). Let steep for 5 minutes.
3. Strain and chill.
4. When ready to serve, add the seltzer water.

Nutrition Information: Total calories: 260
Calories per serving (10 ounces): 65

Nutrients	%	Grams
Carbohydrate	100	16
Protein	—	—
Fat	—	—

HOT SPICED TEA MIX

This recipe, submitted by a member of the National Ski Patrol, is a welcome energizer on winter days. Its high sugar content quickly replaces the glycogen depleted by cold-weather exercise.

Yield: 20 to 30 servings (about 2 tablespoons of mix per 6 ounces of liquid)

1 cup instant tea (unsweetened)
2 cups sugar
2 cups Tang
1 cup lemonade powder mix
1 teaspoon cinnamon
1 teaspoon cloves

1. Combine all ingredients, mix well, and store in a sealed container.
2. To prepare hot tea, add 2 level tablespoons of the mix per 6 ounces of hot water. *Note:* Many mugs hold 10 to 12 ounces.

Nutrition Information: Total calories: 3,700
Calories per serving (2 level tablespoons): 90

Nutrients	%	Grams
Carbohydrate	100	22
Protein	—	—
Fat	—	—

LOW-CAL CAPPUCCINO

If you are a coffee lover, you can enjoy this frothy treat at home, with no special equipment other than a blender.

Yield: 1 8-ounce serving

4 ounces (1/2 cup) low-fat milk
4 ounces (1/2 cup) hot brewed double-strength coffee (regular
   or decaffeinated)
Dash of ground cinnamon
Sweetener, as desired

1. In a small saucepan over low heat, heat the milk until tiny bubbles form around the edge of the pan. Do not let the milk boil!
2. Carefully pour the hot milk into a blender or food processor, cover with a vented lid, and blend at high speed until frothy.
3. To serve, pour the hot coffee into a mug. Pour the frothy milk over the coffee; sprinkle with cinnamon and add sweetener, as desired.

Nutrition Information: Calories per serving (unsweetened): 40

Nutrients	%	Grams
Carbohydrate	60	6
Protein	40	4
Fat	—	—

WARM MILK IDEAS

Calcium-rich milk is an important sports drink for athletes of all ages. It's nutrient-dense, and a great way to boost your intake of protein, calcium, riboflavin, and vitamin D. To add excitement to the recommended 3 to 4 daily servings, try adding any of these ingredients to a mug of warm milk.

- Honey
- Dash of cinnamon or nutmeg
- A few drops of vanilla, rum, almond, or peppermint extract
- Chocolate syrup (most brands are very low in fat)
- 2 crushed butterscotch candies
- 2 crushed peppermint candies
- Instant coffee (decaffeinated or regular) and chocolate milk powder and dash of cinnamon

Snacks and Desserts

Snacks and desserts are major parts of Americans' meal style. Fresh fruits are ideal choices for either, yet there is a time and a place for other sweets. The trick is to choose the ones low in fat and high in carbohydrates. These recipes provide healthy alternatives to empty-calorie temptations. To transform many of your own baked goods into low-fat versions, try substituting applesauce or prune puree for most or all of the fat. The prune puree works best in recipes featuring chocolate, while applesauce is fine in most other recipes. Experiment to see how much you find acceptable!

SNACKS

NO-BAKE PEANUT BUTTER BALLS
PEANUT BUTTER IDEAS
POTATO SNACKS
SEASONED POPCORN
LOW-FAT CHEESECAKE SQUARES
FROZEN FRUIT NUGGETS

DESSERTS

APPLE BROWN BETTY
LOW-FAT OATMEAL COOKIES
CHOCOLATE LUSH
ZUCCHINI CAKE
A TO Z CAKE
BLUEBERRY BUCKLE

See also: Applesauce Raisin Bread, Banana Bread, Honey Bran Muffins, and the other bread recipes, Granola, Banana Frostie.

NO-BAKE PEANUT BUTTER BALLS

These are great for hiking, biking, and cross-country skiing. They travel best in cool weather. At home, store them in the refrigerator. They are a high-calorie, nutrient-dense snack that is a good addition to a weight-gain diet.

Yield: 16 balls

1/2 cup peanut butter
1/2 cup honey
3/4 cup nonfat dry milk
3/4 cup wheat germ

Optional: 1/2 cup raisins.

1. Blend the peanut butter and honey. Add the milk and wheat germ. Mix well.
2. Shape into balls the size of a walnut. If desired, roll the balls in additional wheat germ.

Nutrition Information: Total calories: 2,000
Calories per serving (1 ball): 125

Nutrients	%	Grams
Carbohydrate	50	14
Protein	20	6
Fat	35	5

PEANUT BUTTER IDEAS

Peanut butter is a staple for hungry athletes who want a satisfying, wholesome snack. Although peanut butter is fat-ladened, it can fit into the fat budget for most sports diets (see table 2.3). If you are a peanut butter lover, the following ideas might add some variety to plain old peanut butter!

Bread or tortillas with peanut butter and

- Jelly (of course!)
- Honey
- Banana slices
- Apple slices
- Raisins
- Cinnamon or cinnamon sugar
- Applesauce, raisins, and cinnamon
- Sprouts
- Cottage cheese
- Granola or sunflower seeds
- Dill pickle slices (no kidding!)

Milk shake: 1 cup milk, 1 banana, 1 tablespoon peanut butter, sweetener as desired.

POTATO SNACKS

This is a tasty way to use leftover (or planned-over) baked potatoes.
Yield: 1 serving

1 large (8-ounce) potato, baked
1 ounce shredded cheese, preferably low-fat
Seasonings as desired, such as garlic powder, chili powder, Italian seasonings, salt, and pepper

1. Slice the baked potato into 1/3" thick coins.
2. Sprinkle with cheese and seasonings as desired.
3. Heat in the toaster oven or microwave until cheese is melted.

Nutrition Information: Calories per serving: 200

Nutrients	%	Grams
Carbohydrate	70	35
Protein	20	10
Fat	10	2

SEASONED POPCORN

Popcorn makes a fun, wholesome snack as long as it's prepared without lots of butter or oil. Note that even lite popcorn has a significant amount of calories that quickly add up when eaten in quantity.

Cooking method	Calories per cup
Air popped	25 to 40
Microwave bags	70 to 90
Oil popped	40 to 80
Oil popped plus butter	75 to 100
Smartfood	80
Lite brands	60 to 80

Popcorn pops because each kernel contains a small amount of moisture surrounded by a hard covering, the hull. When heated to 350°, the water within the kernel turns to steam, which expands and bursts the kernel open, resulting in popped corn. One-quarter cup of kernels yields about 7 or 8 cups popped corn.

If you don't have an air popper or a no-fat microwave popper, try this low-fat method for stovetop popcorn.

Yield: 1 serving (4 cups)

> 1 tablespoon oil, preferably canola
> 2 tablespoons popcorn kernels

1. Heat the oil in the bottom of a saucepan. Add the corn kernels.
2. When the popcorn is just about to start popping, carefully drain off half the oil but leave the kernels behind.
3. Resume cooking, allowing the corn to pop without the oil.

Season with any of these ingredients.

Garlic powder or garlic salt
Onion powder or onion salt
Curry powder
Oregano, basil, or other Italian seasonings
Powdered salad dressing mixes
Combination of red pepper and paprika
Soy sauce
Parmesan cheese or grated mozzarella
Taco seasoning mix
Cinnamon

To get the seasonings to stick without butter, take these tips from some of my ingenious clients:

- Spray the popcorn with cooking spray, such as Pam, then sprinkle on the seasonings. (Or you can buy seasoned popcorn sprays.)
- Mix salt and water or soy sauce in a spray bottle and mist the popcorn with the salt solution. People with high blood pressure should limit their intake of salted popcorn (see chapter 2).

Nutrition Information: Calories per serving (with half of the oil drained): 150

Nutrients	%	Grams
Carbohydrate	55	20
Protein	5	3
Fat	40	7

LOW-FAT CHEESECAKE SQUARES

In place of the graham crackers, try stone ground wheat crackers, flour tortillas, or English muffins. For variety, use cottage cheese instead of the cream cheese or mix honey with the cream cheese and freeze the dessert before serving. You'll end up with a healthy snack that most kids love. It tastes remarkably like an ice cream sandwich!

Yield: 1 serving

2 graham cracker squares
1 teaspoon cream cheese, low-fat or fat-free
1 teaspoon jam or fruit spread

Optional: sprinkling of cinnamon.

1. Spread one graham cracker with low-fat cream cheese.
2. Add the jam; sprinkle with cinnamon, if desired.
3. Top with the second graham cracker, making it into a sandwich.

Nutrition Information: Calories per serving: 90

Nutrients	%	Grams
Carbohydrate	70	16
Protein	10	2
Fat	20	2

FROZEN FRUIT NUGGETS

Popping a few of these frozen fruit chunks into your mouth is a refreshing treat after a hot summer workout. Frozen bananas are particularly good—similar to banana ice cream! These frozen chunks also whip up into delightful frosty shakes when mixed in the blender with milk, yogurt, or juice.

Grapes	Watermelon
Bananas	Cantaloupe
Strawberries	Other fruits of your choice

1. Cut the fruit into bite-sized pieces.
2. Spread the fruit pieces on a flat pan and put in the freezer for 1 hour. When frozen, put the pieces into baggies and return to the freezer. They'll be ready for you to eat when the munchies strike!

Nutrition Information: Approximate calories per cup of
nuggets: 50

Nutrients	%	Grams
Carbohydrate	95	12
Protein	5	trace
Fat	—	—

APPLE BROWN BETTY

This has always been a family favorite.

Yield: 8 servings

> 1/3 box (11 sheets) graham crackers
> 1/4 cup margarine, melted
> 6 large apples, unpeeled
> 3/4 cup brown sugar
> 1 teaspoon cinnamon
> 1/2 cup water

Optional: 1/4 teaspoon nutmeg, 1/4 teaspoon cloves; 2 tablespoons lemon juice; 1/2 cup raisins or chopped nuts.

1. Crush the graham crackers into crumbs by placing them in a plastic bag and rolling them with a rolling pin or a bottle.
2. In a bowl, combine the crumbs with melted margarine.
3. Put 1/3 of the mixture in the bottom of a 2-quart casserole dish.
4. Core and slice the apples into thin wedges and put them into a
   bowl. Sprinkle the apple wedges with sugar, cinnamon, and other
   spices as desired.
5. Put the apple slices into the baking dish; add 1/2 cup water then
   the rest of the graham cracker crumbs.
6. Cover and bake at 350° for 25 minutes; uncover, then bake another
   15 minutes to crispen.

Nutrition Information: Total calories: 2,500
Calories per serving: 310

Nutrients	%	Grams
Carbohydrate	75	58
Protein	2	1
Fat	23	8

LOW-FAT OATMEAL COOKIES

This recipe offers a low-fat alternative to most cookies, which get 40 to 60 percent of their calories from fat. These have a soft, chewy texture. Yum!

Yield: 22 cookies

2 tablespoons oil, preferably canola
1/4 cup applesauce
1/2 cup brown sugar
1/2 cup white sugar
1 egg or 2 egg whites
1 teaspoon vanilla
1/2 teaspoon cinnamon
1/2 teaspoon salt
1/2 teaspoon baking soda
1 teaspoon baking powder
1-1/2 cups uncooked oats
1 cup flour, preferably half white and half whole wheat

Optional: 1/2 cup raisins, 1/2 cup chopped nuts.

1. Preheat the oven to 375°.
2. Mix together the oil, applesauce, sugar, egg, vanilla, cinnamon, and salt. Beat well.
3. Add the soda, powder, oats, (and raisins); mix well, then gently stir in the flour.
4. Drop by rounded tablespoons onto a baking sheet treated with cooking spray.
5. Bake for 10 to 12 minutes or until firm when lightly tapped with a finger.

Nutrition Information: Total calories: 2,000
Calories per cookie: 90

Nutrients	%	Grams
Carbohydrate	75	17
Protein	5	0.5
Fat	20	2

CHOCOLATE LUSH

This brownie pudding is a tasty treat for those who want a high-carbohydrate dessert after a wholesome meal. It forms its own sauce during baking.

Yield: 9 servings

1 cup flour
3/4 cup sugar
2 tablespoons unsweetened dry cocoa
2 teaspoons baking powder
1 teaspoon salt
1/2 cup milk
2 tablespoons oil, preferably canola
2 teaspoons vanilla
3/4 cup brown sugar
1/4 cup unsweetened dry cocoa
1-3/4 cups hot water

Optional: 1/2 cup chopped nuts.

1. Preheat the oven to 350°.
2. In a medium bowl, stir together the flour, white sugar, 2 tablespoons cocoa, baking powder, and salt; add the milk, oil, and vanilla. Mix until smooth. (Add nuts.)
3. Pour into an 8" × 8" square pan that is nonstick, lightly oiled, or treated with cooking spray.
4. Combine the brown sugar, 1/4 cup cocoa, and hot water. Pour this mixture on top of the batter in the pan.
5. Bake at 350° for 40 minutes, or until lightly browned and bubbly.

Nutrition Information: Total calories: 2,100
Calories per serving: 230

Nutrients	%	Grams
Carbohydrate	80	46
Protein	5	3
Fat	15	4

ZUCCHINI CAKE

This popular version of the A to Z Cake (see the next recipe) is a tried-and-true favorite.

Yield: 12 servings

1 cup brown sugar
2 eggs or 4 egg whites
1/2 cup oil, preferably canola
2 teaspoons vanilla
2 teaspoons cinnamon
1 teaspoon salt
2 cups grated zucchini
2 teaspoons baking soda
1 teaspoon baking powder
2 cups flour, preferably half whole wheat and half white

Optional: 1 cup raisins.

1. Preheat the oven to 350°.
2. Combine the sugar, eggs, oil, vanilla, cinnamon, and salt. Mix well.
3. Stir in the grated zucchini, then the baking powder, baking soda, and flour (and raisins). Blend gently.
4. Pour into a 9" × 9" baking pan that is nonstick, treated with cooking spray, or lined with wax paper. Bake for 40 to 45 minutes, or until a toothpick inserted near the center comes out clean.

Nutrition Information: Total calories: 3,000
Calories per serving: 250

Nutrients	%	Grams
Carbohydrate	55	35
Protein	5	3
Fat	40	11

A TO Z CAKE

The zucchini in the preceding recipe for Zucchini Cake is the Z in the A to Z Cake. To customize your cake, follow the steps in the preceding recipe, but replace the zucchini with your choice of 2 cups of any of these foods:

Apples, grated

Applesauce

Apricots, chopped

Bananas, mashed

Carrots, grated

Cherries, pitted and chopped

Coconut, fresh ground

Dates, finely chopped

Eggplant, ground

Figs, finely chopped

Grapes, seedless

Honey (omit sugar)

Lemons (use only
    1/2 cup juice)

Marmalade (omit sugar)

Mincemeat

Oranges, chopped

Peaches, fresh or canned,
    chopped

Pears, chopped

Peppermint (use only 1/2 cup)

Pineapple, crushed and drained

Prunes, chopped (1 cup)

Pumpkin, canned

Raisins

Raspberries

Rhubarb, finely chopped

Strawberries, fresh or
    frozen, drained

Sweet potato, coarsely grated

Tapioca, cooked

Tomatoes (use only
    1/2 cup sugar)

Yams, cooked and mashed

Yogurt, plain or flavored

Zucchini, grated

BLUEBERRY BUCKLE

There are few things that smell nicer than homebaked desserts. This cake is a favorite, not only for dessert but also as a coffee cake for Sunday brunch.

Yield: 12 servings

1/2 cup sugar
1/4 cup oil, preferably canola
1 egg or 2 egg whites
1/2 cup milk
1/2 teaspoon salt
2 teaspoons baking powder
2 cups flour, preferably half whole wheat and half white
2 cups blueberries, fresh or frozen
Topping:
1/3 cup sugar
1/3 cup flour, preferably whole wheat
1 teaspoon cinnamon
2 tablespoons margarine

1. Preheat the oven to 375°.
2. Mix together the sugar, oil, and egg; add the milk, salt, and baking powder, and then the flour.
3. Fold in the blueberries.
4. Pour into a nonstick or lightly oiled 8" x 8" baking pan.
5. Make topping by combining the sugar, flour, and cinnamon and mashing in the margarine using the back of a spoon. Crumble the topping over the batter.
6. Bake for 40 to 50 minutes, or until toothpick inserted near center comes out clean.

Nutrition Information: Total calories: 2,600
Calories per serving: 215

Nutrients	%	Grams
Carbohydrate	65	35
Protein	5	3
Fat	30	7

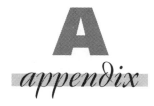

A
appendix

Recommended Reading

This list provides additional reading for many of the topics discussed in this book. A few titles are primarily for professionals, but most are appropriate for the general public. Many are available through the following sources of reliable nutrition materials:

- Nutrition Counseling and Education Services (NCES)
  1904 East 123rd Street, Olathe, KS 66061   800-445-5653
- Gurze Eating Disorders Bookshelf Catalogue
  PO Box 2238, Carlsbad, CA 92018   800-756-7533

You can also look for the books in your local library or bookstore, or order them directly through the publishers.

Adult Children of Alcoholics

Black, C. 1987. *It will never happen to me*. New York: Ballantine.

Bradshaw, J. 1990. *Homecoming: Reclaiming and championing your inner child*. New York: Bantam.

Woititz, J. 1993. *The intimacy struggle*. Deerfield Beach, FL: Health Communications.

Woititz, J. 1990. *Adult children of alcoholics*. Deerfield Beach, FL: Health Communications.

Body Image

Hirschmann, J. and C. Munter. 1995. *When women stop hating their bodies*. New York: Ballantine.

Hutchinson, M. 1985. *Transforming body image: Learning to love the body you have*. Freedom, CA: Crossing Press.

Metcalfe, L. 1994. *Reshaping your body, rethinking your mind: A practical guide to enhancing body image & improving self esteem*. 450 W. Valle del Oro, Tucson, AZ 85737.

Newman, L. 1991. *SomeBody to love: A guide to loving the body you have.* Chicago: Third Side Press.

Thomas Cash Body Image Therapy. 1993. *A program for self-directed change.* Sound cassette series. New York: Guilford Publications.

Calories

Netzer, C. 1994. *The complete book of food counts.* New York: Dell.

Pennington, J. 1992. *Bowes & Church's food values of portions commonly used.* 16th ed. Philadelphia: Lippincott.

Cancer

Nixon, D. 1994. *The cancer recovery eating plan: The right foods to help fuel your recovery.* New York: Random House.

Children

Hess, M.A., A. Hunt, and B. Motenko. 1991. *A healthy head start: A worry-free way to feeding young children.* New York: Holt.

Hirschmann, J. and L. Zaphiropoulos. 1993. *Preventing childhood eating problems: A practical approach to raising children free of food and weight conflicts.* New York: Ballantine.

Ikeda, J. and P. Naworski. 1992. *Am I fat? Helping young children understand differences in body size.* Santa Cruz, CA: ETR.

Jennings, D. and S.N. Steen. 1995. *Play hard, eat right: A parent's guide to sports nutrition.* Minneapolis, MN: Chronimed.

Satter, E. 1991. *Child of mine: Feeding with love and good sense.* Palo Alto, CA: Bull.

Cookbooks (See also Vegetarian and Vegetarian Cookbooks)

Baird, P. 1993. *The pyramid cookbook: Pleasures of the food guide pyramid.* New York: Holt.

Clark, N. 1994. *The New York City Marathon cookbook: Nutrition tips and recipes for high-energy eating and life-long health.* 830 Boylston St., Brookline, MA 02167.

Ponichtera, B. 1991 and 1995. *Quick & healthy recipes and ideas.* 2 vols. The Dalles, OR: ScaleDown.

Diabetes

Berg, K. 1986. *Diabetic's guide to health and fitness: An authoritative approach to leading an active lifestyle.* Champaign, IL: Human Kinetics.

Gordon, N. 1993. *Diabetes: Your complete exercise guide.* Champaign, IL: Human Kinetics.

Diet Analysis Software

DINE Healthy. Dine Systems Inc., 586 N. French Road, Amherst, NY 14228. 800-688-1848.

Nutri-Calc. Cande Corp., 449 East Saratoga St., Gilbert, AZ 85296. 602-926-2632.

Diet Balancer. PO Box 769, Wappinger Falls, NY 12590. 800-927-2988.

Eating Disorders

Goodman, L. 1992. *Is your child dying to be thin? A workbook for parents and family members on eating disorders.* Pittsburgh: Dorrance.

Hall, L. 1993. *Full lives: Women who have freed themselves from food and weight obsessions.* Carlsbad, CA: Gurze.

Hirschmann, J. and C. Munter. 1989. *Overcoming overeating: Living free in a world of food.* New York: Fawcett/Columbine.

Hirschmann, J. and C. Munter. 1995. *When women stop hating their bodies: Freeing yourself from food & weight problems.* New York: Ballantine.

Kano, S. 1989. *Making peace with food.* New York: Harper-Row.

Patterson, C., et al. 1992. *Nutrition & eating disorders: Guidelines for the patient with anorexia nervosa and bulimia nervosa.* Van Nuys, CA: PM, Inc.

Rodin, J. 1992. *Body traps: Breaking the binds that keep you from feeling good about yourself.* New York: Morrow.

Roth, G. 1986. *Breaking free from compulsive eating.* New York: Signet.

Roth, G. 1992. *When food is love.* New York: Penguin.

Yates, A. 1991. *Compulsive exercise and the eating disorders.* New York: Bruner/Mazel.

Eating Disorders (primarily for professionals)

Black, D.R., ed. 1991. *Eating disorders among athletes: Theories, issues and research.* Reston, VA: American Alliance for Health, Physical Education, Recreation and Dance.

Brownell, K. and J. Foreyt. 1986. *Handbook of eating disorders: Physiology, psychology and treatment of obesity, anorexia and bulimia.* New York: Basic.

Brownell, K., J. Rodin, and J. Wilmore. 1992. *Eating, body weight and performance in athletes: Disorders of modern society.* Philadelphia: Lea & Febiger.

Eating Disorders Review, a bimonthly newsletter available through Raven Press, Ltd., 1185 Avenue of the Americas, New York, NY 10036.

NCAA videotapes available through Karol Media, 350 N. Pennsylvania Ave., Wilkes-Barre, PA 18773.

   Afraid to eat: Eating disorders and the student athlete (17 minutes).

   Out of balance: Nutrition and weight (16 minutes).

   Eating disorders: What can you do? (15 minutes).

Thompson, R. and R. Trattner Sherman. 1993. *Helping athletes with eating disorders.* Champaign, IL: Human Kinetics.

Ergogenic Aids

Barrett, S. and V. Herbert. 1993. *The vitamin pushers.* New York: Prometheus.

Bucci, L. 1994. *Nutrients and ergogenic aids for sports and exercise.* Boca Raton, FL: CRC Press.

Williams, M. 1989. *Beyond training: How athletes enhance performance, legally and illegally.* Champaign, IL: Human Kinetics.

Exercise Physiology

McArdle, W., F. Katch, and V. Katch. 1994. *Essentials of exercise physiology.* Philadelphia: Lea & Febiger.

Noakes, T. 1991. *The lore of running.* Champaign, IL: Human Kinetics.

Wilmore, J. and D. Costill. 1994. *Physiology of sport and exercise.* Champaign, IL: Human Kinetics.

Fast Foods

Franz, M. 1994. *Fast food facts.* 4th ed. Minneapolis: Chronimed.

Tribole, E. 1992. *Eating on the run.* Champaign, IL: Human Kinetics.

Warshaw, H. 1993. *The healthy eater's guide to family and chain restaurants: What to eat in over 100 chain restaurants across America.* Minneapolis: Chronimed.

General Nutrition

Brody, J. 1985. *Jane Brody's good food book: Living the high carbohydrate way.* New York: Bantam.

Brody, J. 1987. *Jane Brody's nutrition book.* New York: Bantam.

Herbert, V. and G. Subak-Sharpe. 1995. *Total nutrition: The only guide you'll ever need. From the Mt. Sinai School of Medicine.* New York: St. Martens.

Somers, E. 1993. *Nutrition for women: The complete guide.* New York: Holt.

Stein, P. and N. Winn. 1992. *The CAN HAVE diet and more!: The easy guide to informed exercise and food choices.* Olathe, KS: NCES, Inc.

Heart Disease

Goor, R. and N. Goor. 1992. *Eater's choice. A food lover's guide to lower cholesterol.* 3rd ed. New York: Houghton Mifflin.

Ornish, D. 1990. *Dr. Dean Ornish's program for reversing heart disease.* New York: Random House.

Winston, M. 1991. *American Heart Association cookbook.* New York: Random House.

Lactose Intolerance

Kidder, B. 1991. *The milk-free kitchen: Living well without dairy products.* New York: Holt.

Pregnancy

Erick, M. 1990. *D.I.E.T. during pregnancy.* Brookline, MA: Grinnen-Barret.

Erick, M. 1993. *No more morning sickness: A survival guide for pregnant women.* New York: Penguin.

Melpomene Institute. 1990. *The bodywise woman.* Champaign, IL: Human Kinetics.

Swinney, B. 1993. *Eating expectantly: The essential eating guide and cookbook for pregnancy.* Colorado Springs, CO: Fall River.

Sports Nutrition

Applegate, L. 1991. *Power foods: High performance nutrition for high performance people.* Emmaus, PA: Rodale.

Berning, J. and S. Nelson Steen. 1991. *Sports nutrition for the 90s: The health professional's guidebook.* Gaithersburg, MD: Aspen.

Brouns, F. 1993. *Nutritional needs of athletes.* Chichester, England: Wiley.

Coleman, E. and S. Nelson Steen. 1996. *The ultimate sports nutrition handbook.* Palo Alto, CA: Bull.

Clark, N. 1994. *The New York City Marathon cookbook: Nutrition tips and recipes for high-energy eating and life-long health.* 830 Boylston St., Brookline, MA 02167.

Kleiner, S.M. and M. Greenwood-Robinson. 1996. *High performance nutrition.* New York: Wiley.

Williams, M. 1995. *Nutrition and fitness for sport.* Dubuque, IA: William C. Brown.

Vegetarian Cookbooks

Baird, P. 1991. *Quick harvest: A vegetarian's guide to microwave cooking.* Englewood Cliffs, NJ: Prentice Hall.

Havala, S. and M. Clifford. 1993. *Simple, lowfat and vegetarian: Unbelievably easy ways to reduce the fat in your meals.* Baltimore: Vegetarian Resource Group.

Hinman, B. 1995. *The meatless gourmet: Favorite recipes from around the world.* Rocklin, CA: Prima.

Oster, M. 1996. *The soy of cooking.* Minnetonka, MN: Chronimed.

Robertson, L., C. Flinders, and B. Rupenthal. 1986. *The new Laurel's kitchen.* Berkeley, CA: Ten Speed.

Wasserman, D. and R. Mangels. 1991. *Simply vegan: Quick vegetarian meals.* Baltimore: The Vegetarian Resource Group.

Vitamins, Supplements, and Herbs

Hands, E. 1995. *Food finder: Food sources of vitamins and minerals.* Salem, OR: ESHA Research.

Somer, E. 1992. *The essential guide to vitamins and minerals.* New York: Holt.

Tyler, V. 1994. *Herbs of choice: The therapeutic use of phytomedicinals.* Binghamton, NY: Hawthorn.

Weight Control

Erdman, S. 1995. *Nothing to lose: A guide to sane living in a large body.* San Francisco, CA: Harper.

Foreyt, J. 1992. *Living without dieting.* Houston: Harrison.

Kostas, G. 1994. *The balancing act: Nutrition and weight guide.* Dallas: Balancing Act Nutrition Books.

Lohman, T. 1992. *Advances in body composition assessment: Current issues in exercise science. Monograph 3.* Champaign, IL: Human Kinetics.

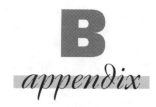

Where to Go for More Information

The following associations are reliable sources of additional nutrition, sports nutrition, or exercise information. Many have publications to which you can subscribe. You will find additional newsletters listed in this appendix. And because I am frequently asked how to become a sports nutritionist, I have included at the end of this appendix some information on getting started down that road.

Aerobics and Fitness Association of America (AFAA)
15250 Ventura Blvd., Suite 200, Sherman Oaks, CA 91403   800-233-4886
Magazine: *American Fitness*

American Anorexia/Bulimia Association
c/o Regents Hospital, 425 East 61st St., 6th floor
New York, NY 10021   212-981-8686

American Cancer Association
1599 Clifton Road NE, Atlanta, GA 30329   800-227-2345

American College of Sports Medicine
PO Box 1440, Indianapolis, IN 46206-1440   317-637-9200
Journal: *Medicine and Science in Sports and Exercise*

American Diabetes Association, Communications Department
1660 Duke St., Alexandria, VA 22314   800-232-3472, ext. 290
Journals: *Diabetes, Diabetes Care, Diabetes Review,* and *Diabetes Forecast*

American Dietetic Association, National Center for Nutrition and Dietetics
216 West Jackson Blvd., Chicago, IL 60606-6995   800-366-1655
Journal: *Journal of the American Dietetic Association*

American Heart Association, National Center
7272 Greenville Ave., Dallas, TX 75231   800-242-8721

American Running and Fitness Association
4405 East West Highway, Suite 405, Bethesda, MD 20814   301-913-9517
Newsletter: *Running & FitNews*

Center for Science in the Public Interest
1875 Connecticut Ave. NW, Suite 300, Washington, DC 20009-5728   202-332-9110
Newsletter: *Nutrition Action Health Letter*

Food and Nutrition Information Center, National Agricultural Library
USDA Room 304, 10301 Baltimore Blvd., Beltsville, MD 20705-2351 301-504-5719

Gatorade Sports Science Institute
PO Box 9005, Chicago, IL 60604   312-222-7704
Newsletter: *Sports Science Exchange*

IDEA, The International Association for Fitness Professionals
6190 Cornerstone Court East, Suite 204, San Diego, CA 92121   619-535-8979
Publication: *IDEA Today*

National Center Against Health Fraud (NCAHF)
PO Box 1276, Loma Linda, CA 92354   909-824-4690
Newsletter: *NCAHF Newsletter*

National Dairy Council, O'Hare International Center
10255 West Higgins Rd., Suite 900, Rosemont, IL 60018   708-803-2000
Newsletter: *Dairy Council Digest*

National Strength and Conditioning Association
PO Box 38909, Colorado Springs, CO 80934   719-632-6722
Journals: *Journal of Strength and Conditioning Research* and *Strength and Conditioning*

Women's Sports Foundation
Eisenhower Park, East Meadow, NY 11554   800-227-3988
Newsletter: *Women's Sports Experience*

ADDITIONAL NEWSLETTERS

Eating Disorders Review, Raven Press
1185 Avenue of the Americas, New York, NY 10036   800-853-2478

Environmental Nutrition
PO Box 420451, Palm Coast, FL 32142-0451   800-829-5384

Harvard Medical School Health Letter
PO Box 420300, Palm Coast, FL 32142-0300   800-829-9045

Nutrition & the MD, Raven Press
1185 Avenue of the Americas, New York, NY 10036   800-853-2478

Penn State Sports Medicine Newsletter
PO Box 6568, Syracuse, NY 13217-9976   800-825-0061

Sports Medicine Digest, Raven Press
1185 Avenue of the Americas, New York, NY 10036   800-853-2478

Tufts University Diet and Nutrition Letter
PO Box 57857, Boulder, CO 80322-7857   800-274-7581

How to Become a Sports Nutritionist

Every week I get letters from people who have read my books or articles, they ask me where they can go to school to learn more about nutrition and exercise. Some even want to become a sports nutritionist. Here's what I tell them.

• To date, relatively few institutions have a sports nutrition major, but many of the larger state universities do have departments in both Nutrition and Exercise Science. You can often combine the two programs to create a major that suits your needs. For a list of academic programs in nutrition that are accredited and approved by the American Dietetic Association, call or write

> The American Dietetic Association
> 216 West Jackson Boulevard
> Chicago, IL 60606-6995
> 312-899-0040

For a list of academic programs in exercise science, write to

> The American College of Sports Medicine
> PO Box 1440
> Indianapolis, IN 46206-1440
> 317-637-9200

If you just want to further your personal knowledge, you can take one or two classes in nutrition or exercise science without committing to four years of advanced education. However, the full program is recommended for people who want to develop a career in sports nutrition.

If you want to become a sports nutritionist, you need not have a double major in nutrition and exercise science. Rather, you can major in nutrition and take two or three elective courses in exercise science. For example, my master's degree at Boston University is in nutrition, but I took several courses in exercise physiology.

• If you want to do nutrition counseling, you should become a registered dietitian (RD). This means you will be recognized by the American Dietetic Association, the nation's largest organization of nutrition professionals, career doors will open up to you. Some people take short, certificate courses, but these cannot match the education you receive in four years of undergraduate schooling, plus an internship, plus perhaps even a master's degree in nutrition. Getting proper education and credentials is a very important professional responsibility.

By becoming a registered dietitian, you will also be eligible to join SCAN, the special interest group of the American Dietetic Association that handles the nutritional aspects of sports, cardiovascular disease, wellness, and eating disorders. SCAN members are the leading sports nutritionists.

• Although your career goals may be to work with athletes and other active, healthy people, I strongly recommend that students and new graduates work first in a clinical setting, such as a hospital, to learn more about how to handle heart disease, diabetes, cancer, and many of the ailments of aging. This knowledge will help you to keep people well and will also enhance your work experience. I strongly believe that one or two years of clinical work is a good investment in your career. I have no regrets about the time I spent working in hospitals!

• Most sports nutritionists practice what they preach and are familiar with the nutritional needs of a variety of sports. I've found that my personal interests in hiking, camping, bike touring, running, and marathoning have enriched the knowledge I can offer my clients. Being involved in your sport adds to your credibility.

• Get involved—either as a volunteer for Little League, youth soccer, the YMCA, or any sport that interests you. Work on nutrition and fitness programs sponsored by your state's dietetic association or council on physical fitness. Write articles for your local bike or running club's newsletter or the local newspaper. By developing networks that will help you meet other local sports nutritionists and sports medicine professionals, you might open doors that eventually lead to paid work.

• Although sports nutrition should be an integral part of most training programs, when it comes to finding a job, you are still unlikely to see numerous "Sports Nutritionist Wanted" notices. Some places for you to try to create a job include health clubs, YMCAs, corporate wellness programs, sports medicine practices, high schools, and college and university athletic departments. Be creative!

Most people knock on several doors before finding a welcoming venue. Or, they make their own jobs using their personal contacts. For example, some registered dietitians who are mothers of teenage athletes have started sports nutrition classes targeted for other parents, coaches, and students. Some RDs who love tennis, ballet, or gymnastics have become known as the sports nutritionist for their sport. Many who work out at a health club have started to work with the members of the club. You can create your dream job, and with lots of hard work and time, you'll achieve your goals. Be patient, no one becomes a sports nutritionist overnight.

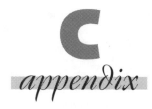

appendix

Selected References

Acheson, K., Y. Schutz, T. Bessard, et al. 1984. Nutritional influences on lipogenesis and thermogenesis after a carbohydrate meal. *Am J Physiol* 246: E62-E70.

Alford, B.A., A. Blankenship, and D.R. Hagen. 1990. The effects of variations in carbohydrates, protein, and fat content of the diet upon weight loss, blood values, and nutrient intakes of adult obese women. *J Amer Diet Assoc* 90: 534-540.

American College of Sports Medicine. 1994. Eating disorders and athletes: A guide for coaches, parents and friends. Indianapolis, IN: American College of Sports Medicine.

American College of Sports Medicine. 1996. Position stand: Exercise and fluid replacement. *Med Sci Sports Exerc* 28 (1): i-vii.

American Dietetic Association. 1993. Position of The American Dietetic Association: Use of nutritive and nonnutritive sweeteners. *J Am Diet Assoc* 93 (7): 816-821.

American Dietetic Association. 1996. Position of The American Dietetic Association: Vitamin and mineral supplementation. *J Am Diet Assoc* 96 (1): 73-77.

American Psychiatric Association. 1994. *Diagnostic and statistical manual of mental disorders.* 4th ed. Washington, DC: American Psychiatric Association.

Anderson, J., B. Johnstone, and M. Cook-Newell. 1995. Meta-analysis of the effects of soy protein intake on serum lipids. *N Engl J Med* 333: 276-282.

Andon, M., K. Smith, M. Bracker, D. Sartoris, P. Saltman, and L. Strause. 1991. Spinal bone density and calcium intake in healthy postmenopausal women. *Am J Clin Nutr* 54: 927-929.

Applegate, L. 1991. Nutritional considerations of ultradistance performance. *Intl J Sports Nutrition* 1 (1): 3-27.

Ardell, D. 1986. *High level wellness: An alternative to doctors, drugs and disease.* Berkeley, CA: Ten Speed Press.

Ascherio, A., E. Rimm, M. Stampfer, E. Giovannucci, and W. Willett. 1995. Dietary intake of marine n-3 fatty acids, fish intake, and the risk of coronary heart disease among men. *N Engl J Med* 332 (15): 977-982.

Barr, S., K.C. Janelle, and J.C. Prior. 1995. Energy intakes are higher during the luteal phase of ovulatory menstrual cycles. *Am J Clin Nutr* 61: 39-43.

Belko, A. 1987. Vitamins and exercise—an update. *Med Sci Sports Exerc* 19 (Suppl): S191-S196.

Bergstrom J., L. Hermansen, E. Hultman, et al. 1967. Diet, muscle glycogen, and physical performance. *Acta Physiol Scand* 71: 140-150.

Bernadot, D., (ed.) and Sports and Cardiovascular Nutritionists. 1992. *Sports nutrition: A guide for the professional working with active people.* 2d ed. Chicago: American Dietetic Association.

Bouchard, C. 1991. Heredity and the path to overweight and obesity. *Med Sci Sports Exerc* 23 (3): 285-291.

Brisman, J. and M. Siegal. 1984. Bulimia and alcoholism: Two sides of the same coin? *J Substance Abuse Treatment* 1: 113-118.

Brodie, D. and R Eston. 1992. Body fat estimations by electrical impedance and infrared interactance. *Intl J Sports Med* 13 (4): 319-325.

Brouns, F. 1993. *Nutritional needs of athletes.* West Sussex, England: Wiley & Sons.

Brouns, F., W. Saris, and N. Rehrer. 1987. Abdominal complaints and gastro-intestinal function during long lasting exercise. *Intl J Sports Med* 8: 175-189.

Burke, L. and V. Deakin. 1994. *Clinical sports nutrition.* Sydney: McGraw-Hill.

Burkes-Miller, M. and D. Black. 1988. Male and female college athletes: Prevalence of anorexia nervosa and bulimia nervosa. *Athletic Training* 23: 137-140.

Cassidy, A., S. Bingham, and K. Setchell. 1994. Biological effects of a diet of soy protein rich in isoflavones on the menstrual cycle of premenopausal women. *Am J Clin Nutr* 60: 333-340.

Clancy, S.P., P.M. Clarkson, M.E. DeCheke, K. Nosaka, et al. 1994. Effects of chromium picolinate supplementation on body composition, strength, and urinary chromium loss in football players. *Intl J Sports Nutr* 4: 142-153.

Clark, N., M. Nelson, and W. Evans. 1988. Nutrition education for elite women runners. *Phys Sportsmed* 16: 124-135.

Clarkson, P. 1993. Nutritional ergogenic aids: Caffeine. *Intl J Sport Nutr* 3: 103-111.

Coggan, A. and E. Coyle. 1987. Reversal of fatigue during prolonged exercise by carbohydrate infusion or ingestion. *J Appl Physiol* 63: 2388-2395.

Cohen, G. 1991. *Exercise in pregnancy.* Vol 3 (13) of *Sports Science Exchange,* Gatorade Sports Science Institute, Chicago, IL.

Colins, G., M. Kotz, J. Janesz, et al. 1985. Alcoholism in the families of bulimic anorexics. *Cleve Clin Q* 52: 65-67.

Costill, D.L. 1988. Carbohydrates for exercise: Dietary demands for optimal performance. *Intl J Sports Med* 9: 1-18.

Costill, D., R. Bowers, G. Branam, et al. 1971. Muscle glycogen utilization during prolonged exercise on successive days. *J Appl Physiol* 31: 834-838.

Costill, D., E. Coyle, G. Dalsky, et al. 1977. Effect of plasma FFA and insulin on muscle glycogen usage during exercise. *J Appl Physiol* 43: 695-699.

Costill, D., G. Dalsky, and W. Fink. 1978. Effects of caffeine ingestion on metabolism and exercise performance. *Med Sci Sports Exerc* 10: 155-158.

Costill D.L., D.S. King, R. Thomas, and M. Hargreaves. 1985. Effects of reduced training on muscular power in swimmers. *Phys Sportsmed* 13 (2): 94-101.

Costill, D. L., W. Sherman, W. Fink, C. Maresh, M. Witten, and J. Miller. 1981. The role of dietary carbohydrate in muscle glycogen resynthesis after strenuous exercise. *Am J Clin Nutr* 34: 1831-1836.

Costill, D.L., R. Thomas, R.A. Robergs, D. Pascoe, C. Lambert, S. Barr, and W. Fink. 1991. Adaptations to swimming training: Influence of training volume. *Med Sci Sports Exerc* 23 (3): 371-377.

Coyle E.F., M. Hagberg, B. Hurley, W. Martin, A. Ehsani, and J. Holloszy. 1983. Carbohydrate feeding during prolonged strenuous exercise can delay fatigue. *J Appl Physiol* 55 (1): 230-235.

Coyle, E.F. and S.J. Montain. 1992. Benefits of fluid replacement with carbohydrates during exercise. *Med Sci Sports Exerc* 24 (Suppl): 324-330.

Davis, J. M. 1995. Carbohydrates, branched-chain amino acids, and endurance: The central fatigue hypothesis. *Intl J Sport Nutr* 5 (Suppl): S29-S38.

DeSouza, M.J. and D. Metzger. 1991. Reproductive dysfunction in amenorrheic athletes and anorexic patients: A review. *Med Sci Sports Exerc* 23 (9) : 995-1007.

Devine, A., R.A. Criddle, I. Dick, D. Kerr, and R. Prince. 1995. A longitudinal study of the effect of sodium and calcium intakes on regional bone density in post-menopausal women. *Am J Clin Nutr* 62 (4): 740-745.

Evans, William. 1994. Is exercise really damaging your body? *Penn State Sports Medicine Newsletter* 3 (2).

Foster-Powell, K. and J. Brand Miller. 1995. International tables of glycemic index. *Am J Clin Nutr* 62: 871S-983S.

Ginsberg, H.N., et al. 1995. Increases in dietary cholesterol are associated with modest increases in both LDL and HDL cholesterol in healthy young women. *Arteriosclerosis, Thromb, and Vasc Biol* 15: 169-178.

Gisolfi, C. and J. Copping. 1993. Thermal effects of prolonged treadmill exercise in the heat. *Med Sci Sports Exerc* 25 (3): 310-315.

Goldberg, G.R., A.M. Prentice, W. Coward, H. Davies, P. Murgatroyd, C. Wensing, A. Black, M. Harding, and M. Sawyer. 1993. Longitudinal assessment of energy expenditure in pregnancy by the doubly labeled water method. *Am J Clin Nutr* 57: 494-505.

Gomez, T., P. Mole, C. Meredith, and R. Gregorek. 1994. Body composition changes with moderate dietary restrictions in strength-trained men. *Med Sci Sports Exerc* 26 (5 Suppl): Abstract 988.

Greenhaff, P. 1995. Creatine and its application as an ergogenic aid. *Intl J Sport Nutr* 5 (Suppl): S100-S110.

Halberg, F. 1983. Chronobiology and nutrition. *Contemporary Nutrition* 8, no.9, Minneapolis, MN: General Mills.

Hall D.C., D.A. Kaufman. 1987. Effects of aerobic and strength conditioning on pregnancy outcomes. *Am J Obstet Gynecol* 157: 1199-1203.

Hallmark, M., J. Reynolds, C. DeSouza, C. Dotson, R. Anderson, and M. Rogers. 1996. Effects of chromium and resistive training on muscle strength and body composition. *Med Sci Sports Exerc* 28 (1): 139-144.

Hargreaves, M., D. Costill, W. Fink, et al. 1987. Effect of pre-exercise carbohydrate feedings on endurance cycling performance. *Med Sci Sports Exerc* 19: 33-36.

Hennekens, C., J. Burns, J. Mansen, M. Stampfer, B. Rosner, et al. 1996. Lack of effect of long-term supplementation with beta carotene on the incidence of malignant neoplasms and cardiovascular disease. *N Engl J Med* 334 (18): 1145-1149.

Hickner R., C. Horswill, J. Welker, J. Scott, J. Roemmich, and D. Costill. 1991. Test development for the study of physical performance in wrestlers following weight loss. *Intl J Sports Med* 12 (6): 557-562.

Hill, J.O., W. McArdle, J. Snook, and J. Wilmore. 1992. *Commonly asked questions regarding nutrition and exercise: What does the scientific literature suggest?* Vol. 9 of *Sports science exchange.* Chicago: Gatorade Sports Science Institute.

Hooper, S.L., L.T. Mackinnon, A. Howard, R. Gordon, and A. Bachmann. 1995. Markers for monitoring overtraining and recovery. *Med Sci Sports Exerc* 27 (1): 106-112.

Horowitz, J.F. and E.F. Coyle. 1993. Metabolic responses to preexercise meals containing various carbohydrates and fat. *Am J Clin Nutr* 58: 235-241.

Horswill, C. 1995. Effects of bicarbonate, citrate, and phosphate loading on performance. *Intl J Sport Nutr* 5 (Suppl): S111-S119.

Houmard, J.A., D.L. Costill, J.B. Mitchell, S.H. Park, R.C. Hickner, and J.N. Roemmich. 1990. Reduced training maintains performance in distance runners. *Intl J Sports Med* 11 (1): 46-52.

International Food Information Council. 1993. *Caffeine and health: Clarifying the controversies.* Washington, DC: IFIC.

Ivy, J., D. Costill, W. Fink, et al. 1979. Influence of caffeine and carbohydrate feedings on endurance performance. *Med Sci Sports Exerc* 11: 6-11.

Ivy, J., A. Katz, C. Cutler, W. Sherman, and E. Coyle. 1988. Muscle glycogen synthesis after exercise: Effect of time on carbohydrate ingestion. *J Appl Physiol* 64 (4): 1480-1485.

Jandrain, B., G. Krentowski, F. Pirnay, et al. 1984. Metabolic availability of glucose ingested three hours before prolonged exercise in humans. *J Appl Physiol* 56: 1314-1319.

Jenkins, D.J., T.M. Wolever, R.H. Taylor, et al. 1981. Glycemic index of foods: A physiological basis for carbohydrate exchange. *Am J Clin Nutr* 34: 362-366.

Jenkins, D.J., T.M. Wolever, A. Venketeshwer Rao, et al. 1993. Effect on blood lipids of very high intakes of fiber in diets low in saturated fat and cholesterol. *N Engl J Med* 329: 21-26.

Kaiserauer, S., A. Snyder, M. Sleeper, and J. Zierath. 1989. Nutritional, physiolgical, and menstrual status of distance runners. *Med Sci Sports Exerc* 21 (2): 120-125.

Kant, A., R. Ballard-Barbash, and A. Schatzkin. 1995. Evening eating and its relation to self-reported weight and nutrient intake in women, CSFII 1985-1986. *J Am College Nutr* 14 (8): 358-363.

Katch, F., P. Clarkson, W. Knoll, et al. 1984. Preferential effects of abdominal exercise training on regional adipose cell size. *Research Quart Exerc Sport* 55: 249.

Kavouras, S., J. Berning, K. Ratcliff, P. Hackbarth, and J. Troup. 1994. Effect of a high-carbohydrate and high-fat diet prior to 45 minutes of intense exercise cycling. *Med Sci Sports Exerc* 26 (5 Suppl): Abstract 49.

Kulpa, P.J., B.M. White, and R. Visscher. 1987. Aerobic exercise in pregnancy. *Am J Obstet Gynecol* 156: 1395-1403.

Leibel, R.L., M. Rosenbaum, and J. Hirsch. 1995. Changes in energy expenditure resulting from altered body weight. *N Engl J Med* 332: 621-628.

Lemon, P. 1991. Protein and amino acid needs of the strength athlete. *Intl J Sports Nutr* 1 (2): 127-145.

Lemon, P. 1995. Do athletes need more protein and amino acids? *Intl J Sport Nutr* 5 (Supplement): S39-S61.

Lemon, P., M. Tarnopolsky, J. MacDougall, and S. Atkinson. 1992. Protein requirements and muscle mass/strength changes during intensive training in novice bodybuilders. *J Appl Physiol* 73: 767-775.

Lloyd, T., J. Buchanan, S. Bitzer, C. Waldman, C. Myers, and B. Ford. 1987. Interrelationships of diet, athletic activity, menstrual status and bone density in collegiate women. *Am J Clin Nutr* 46: 681-684.

Lloyd, T., S. Triantaflyllou, E. Baker, P. Houts, J. Whiteside, A. Kalenak, and P. Stumpf. 1986. Women athletes with menstrual irregularity have increased musculoskeletal injuries. *Med Sci Sports Exerc* 18 (4): 374-379.

Loucks, A. and S. Horvath. 1985. Athletic amenorrhea: A review. *Med Sci Sports Exerc* 17 (1): 56-72.

Lukaski, H.C. 1987. Methods for the assessment of human body composition. *Am J Clin Nutr* 46: 537.

Lutter, J. and S. Cushman. 1982. Running while pregnant. *J Melpomene Institute* 1 (1): 2-4.

Mason, W.L., G. McConell, and M. Hargreaves. 1993. Carbohydrate ingestion during exercise: Liquid vs. solid feedings. *Med Sci Sports Exerc* 25 (8): 966-969.

Matkovic, V., J. Ilich, M. Andon, L. Hsieh, et al. 1995. Urinary calcium, sodium, and bone mass of young females. *Am J Clin Nutr* 62: 417-425.

Metcalfe, L. 1994. Reshaping your body, rethinking your mind: A practical guide to enhancing body image and improving self-esteem. 450 West Valle del Oro, Tucson, AZ 85737.

Murray B., G. Paul, J. Seifert, and D. Eddy. 1991. Responses to varying rates of carbohydrate ingestion during exercise. *Med Sci Sports Exerc* 23 (6): 713-718.

National Research Council. 1989. *Recommended dietary allowances,* 10th ed. Washington, DC: National Academy Press.

Nelson, M., M. Fiatarone, C. Morganti, I. Trice, R. Greenberg, and W. Evans. 1994. Effects of high-intensity strength training on multiple risk factors for osteoporosis fractures. *JAMA* 272 (24): 1909-1914.

Nelson, M., E. Fisher, P. Catsos, et al. 1986. Diet and bone status in amenorrheic runners. *Am J Clin Nutr* 43: 910-916.

Neufer, P.D., D. Costill, M. Flynn, J. Kirwan, J. Mitchell, and J. Houmard. 1987. Improvements in exercise performance: Effects of carbohydrate feedings and diet. *J Appl Physiol* 62 (3): 983-988.

Nishimune, T., T. Yakushiji, T. Sumimoto, et al. 1991. Glycemic response and fiber content of some foods. *Am J Clin Nutr* 54: 414-419.

Otis, C. 1990. Amenorrhea and bone density. *Sports Medicine Digest,* November.

Pasman, W., M. van Baak, A. Jeukendrup, and A. de Haan. 1995. The effects of different dosages of caffeine on endurance performance time. *Intl J Sports Med* 16: 225-230.

Pedersen, A., M. Bartholomew, L. Dolence, L. Aljadir, K. Netteburg, and T. Lloyd. 1991. Menstrual differences due to vegetarian and non-vegetarian diets. *Am J Clin Nutr* 53: 879-885.

Phillips, P., B. Rolls, J. Ledingham, et al. 1984. Reduced thirst after water deprivation in healthy elderly men. *N Engl J Med* 311: 753-759.

Pollitt, E. 1995. Does breakfast make a difference in school? *J Am Diet Assoc* 95 (10): 1134-1139.

Rauch L.H.G., I. Rodger, G. Wilson, J. Belonje, S. Dennis, T. Noakes, and J. Hawley. 1995. The effects of carbohydrate loading on muscle glycogen content and cycling performance. *Intl J Sports Nutr* 5 (1): 25-35.

Rehrer, N., E.J. Beckers, F. Brouns, F.T. Hoor, and W. Saris. 1990. Effects of dehydration on gastric emptying and gastrointestinal distress while running. *Med Sci Sports Exerc* 22 (6): 790-795.

Rimm, E.B., M.J. Stampfer, A. Ascherio, et al. 1993. Vitamin E consumption and the risk of coronary disease in men. *N Engl J Med* 328 (20): 1450-1466.

Rokitzki, L., E. Logemann, G. Huber, E. Keck, and J. Keul. 1994. Alpha-tocopherol supplementation in racing cyclists during extreme endurance training. *Intl J Sport Nutr* 4: 253-264.

Rosen, L., D. McKeag, D. Hough, and V. Curley. 1986. Pathogenic weight-control behavior in female athletes. *Phys Sportsmed* 14: 79-86.

Sanborn, C., B. Albrecht, and W. Wagner. 1987. Athletic amenorrhea: Lack of association with body fat. *Med Sci Sports Exerc* 19 (3): 207-212.

Sherman, W. 1989a. Muscle glycogen supercompensation during the week before athletic competition. *Sports Science Exchange* Vol 2 (6). Chicago, IL: Gatorade Sports Science Institute.

Sherman, W. 1989b. Pre-event nutrition. *Sports Science Exchange*. Vol 2 (2). Chicago, IL: Gatorade Sports Science Institute.

Sherman, W., G. Brodowicz, D. Wright, W. Allen, J. Simonsen, and A. Dernbach. 1989. Effects of 4 h preexercise carbohydrate feedings on cycling performance. *Med Sci Sports Exerc* 21 (5): 598-604.

Sherman, W., D. Costill, W. Fink, and J. Miller. 1981. Effect of exercise-diet manipulation on muscle glycogen and its subsequent utilization during performance. *Intl J Sports Med* 2: 114-118.

Sherman, W. and N. Leenders. 1995. Fat loading: The next magic bullet? *Intl J Sports Nutr* 5 (Suppl): S1-S12.

Sherman, W. and E. Maglischo. 1991. Maximizing chronic fatigue among swimmers: Special emphasis on nutrition. *Sports Science Exchange* 4 (35). Chicago, IL: Gatorade Sports Science Institute.

Sherman, W., M. Peden, and D. Wright. 1991. Carbohydrate feedings 1 hour before exercise improves cycling performance. *Am J Clin Nutr* 54: 866-870.

Sims, E. 1976. Experimental obesity, dietary induced thermogenesis, and their clinical implications. *Clin Endo Metab* 5: 377-395.

Sims, E. and E. Danforth. 1987. Expenditure and storage of energy in man. *J Clin Invest* 79: 1-7.

Stampfer, M.J., C.H. Hennekens, J.L. Manson, et al. 1993. Vitamin E consumption and the risk of coronary disease in women. *N Engl J Med* 328 (20): 1444-1449.

Sternfeld, B., C. Quesenberry, B. Eskenazi, and L. Newman. 1995. Exercise during pregnancy and pregnancy outcome. *Med Sci Sports Exerc* 27 (5): 634-640.

Stewart, M., J. McDonald, A. Levy, et al. 1985. Vitamin/mineral supplement use: A telephone survey of adults in the United States. *J Amer Diet Assoc* 85: 1585-1590.

Stout, J., J. Eckerson, T. Housh, G. Johnson, and N. Betts. 1994. Validity of body fat estimations in males. *Med Sci Sports Exerc* 26 (5): 262.

Suitor, C.W. 1991. Perspectives on nutrition during pregnancy: Part I, weight gain; part II, nutrient supplements. *J Amer Diet Assoc* 91 (1): 96-98.

Thomas, D.E., J.R. Brotherhood, and C. Brand. 1991. Carbohydrate feeding before exercise: Effect of glycemic index. *Intl J Sports Med* 12 (2): 180-186.

Thompson, J., M. Manore, J. Skinner, E. Ravussin, and M. Spraul. 1995. Daily energy expenditure in male athletes with differing energy intakes. *Med Sci Sports Exerc* 27 (3): 347-354.

Trice, I. and E. Haymes. 1995. Effects of caffeine ingestion on exercise-induced changes during high-intensity, intermittent exercise. *Intl J Sports Nutr* 5 (1): 37-44.

Van Horn, L., K. Liu, D. Parker, et al. 1986. Serum lipid response to oat product intake with a fat modified diet. *J Amer Diet Assoc* 86: 759-764.

Varner, L. 1995. Dual diagnosis: Patients with eating and substance-related disorders. *J Am Diet Assoc* 95 (2): 224-225.

Ventura, J.L., A. Estruch, G. Rodas, and R. Segura. 1994. Effect of prior ingestion of glucose or fructose on the performance of exercise of intermediate duration. *Eur J Appl Physiol* 68: 345-349

Walberg, J.L., M.K. Leidy, D.J. Sturgill, et al. 1988. Macronutrient content of a hypoenergy diet affects nitrogen retention and muscle function in weight lifters. *Intl J Sports Med* 94 (4): 261-266.

Watson, R. and T. Leonard. 1986. Selenium and vitamins A, E, and C: Nutrients with cancer preventive properties. *J Amer Diet Assoc* 86: 505-510.

Webb, P. and J. Annis. 1983. Adaptation to overeating in lean and overweight men and women. *Human Nutr: Clin Nutr* 37C: 117-131.

Weir, J., T. Noakes, K. Myburgh, et al. 1987. A high-carbohydrate diet negates the metabolic effects of caffeine during exercise. *Med Sci Sports Exerc* 19: 100-105.

Wemple, R.D., D. Lamb, and A. Blostein. 1994. Caffeine ingested in a fluid replacement beverage during prolonged exercise does not cause diuresis. *Med Sci Sports Exerc* 26 (5 Suppl): Abstract 1146.

Wilmore, J. and D. Costill. 1994. *Physiology of sport and exercise.* Champaign, IL: Human Kinetics.

Wilmore, J., K. Wambsgans, M. Brenner, C. Broeder, I. Paijmans, J. Volpe, and K. Wilmore. 1992. Is there energy conservation in amenorrheic compared with eumenorrheic distance runners? *J Appl Physiol* 72 (1): 15-22.

Woititz, J. 1990. *Adult children of alcoholics.* Deerfield Beach, FL: Health Communications.

Yates, A. 1991. *Compulsive exercise and the eating disorders: Toward an integrated theory of activity.* New York: Brunner/Mazel.

Zachwieja, J., D. Costill, G. Beard, R. Robergs, D. Pascoe, and D. Anderson. 1992. The effects of carbonated carbohydrate drink on gastric emptying, gastrointestinal distress, and exercise performance. *Intl J Sports Nutr* 2: 239-250.

Zarkadas, P., J. Carter, and E. Banister. 1994. Taper increases performance and aerobic power in triathletes. *Med Sci Sports Exerc* 26 (Suppl): Abstract 194.

Zawadzki, K.M., B.B. Yaspelkis, and J. Ivy. 1992. Carbohydrate-protein complex increases the rate of muscle glycogen storage after exercise. *J Appl Physiol* 72 (5): 1854-1859.

Zelasko, C. 1995. Exercise for weight loss: What are the facts? *J Am Diet Assoc* 95 (12): 1414-1417.

Index

About the Author

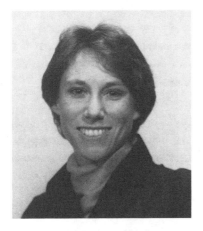

Nancy Clark, MS, RD, is the director of nutrition services at SportsMedicine Brookline, one of the largest athletic injury clinics in New England. A registered dietitian specializing in sports nutrition, wellness, and the nutritional management of eating disorders, Nancy counsels both casual exercisers and competitive athletes. Her more famous clients include members of the Boston Red Sox and Boston Celtics, as well as many elite and Olympic athletes.

Nancy is a nutrition columnist for the *Physician and SportsMedicine*, *New England Runner*, *Adventure Cycling*, and *Rugby*. She is a regular contributor to *SHAPE* and *Runner's World*, and she writes a monthly nutrition column called "The Athlete's Kitchen" which appears in over 100 sports and health publications. In addition, Nancy is the author of two other books: *The New York City Marathon Cookbook* and *The Athlete's Kitchen*.

A well-known lecturer, Nancy has given presentations to such groups as the American Dietetic Association (ADA), the American College of Sports Medicine (ACSM), and the International Food Information Council. She has also led workshops for athletes at the Olympic Training Centers in Colorado Springs and Lake Placid. Nancy received her undergraduate degree in nutrition from Simmons College in Boston and her master's degree in nutrition from Boston University. She is a Fellow of the ADA, recipient of their 1995 Media Excellence Award, and an active member of ADA's practice group of sports nutritionists (SCAN) and a recipient of its 1992 Honor Award. In addition, Nancy is a Fellow of the ACSM and recipient of the 1994 Honor Award from ACSM's New England Chapter.

An athlete herself, Nancy has hiked across America, run marathons, and trekked in the Himalayas. A bike commuter and member of the Greater Boston Track Club, Nancy lives in Waltham, Massachusetts, with her husband, John McGrath; son, John Michael; and daughter, Mary.

Additional Resources from HK

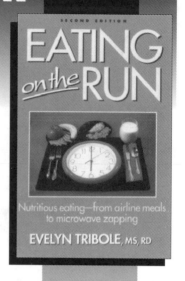